Healing
Basics

Prevent Cancer or its Recurrence

Achieve Ideal Weight Without Hunger

Build the Foundation of True Health

Nicolette M. Dumke

**HEALING BASICS
PREVENT CANCER OR ITS RECURRENCE
ACHIEVE IDEAL WEIGHT WITHOUT HUNGER
BUILD THE FOUNDATION OF TRUE HEALTH**

All quotations from the Bible in this book are taken from the New King James Version © 1982 by Thomas Nelson, Inc. Used by permission. All rights reserved.

Published by
Allergy Adapt, Inc.
1877 Polk Avenue
Louisville, Colorado 80027
303-666-8253

©2018 by Nicolette M. Dumke
Printed in the United States of America

Publisher's Cataloging-in-Publication

Names: Dumke, Nicolette M., author.
Title: Healing basics : prevent cancer or its recurrence , achieve ideal weight without hunger , build the foundation of true health / Nicolette M. Dumke.
Description: Includes bibliographical references and index. | Louisville, CO: Allergy Adapt, Inc., 2018
Identifiers: ISBN 978-1-887624-22-0 | LCCN 2017951262
Subjects: LCSH Glycemic index--Popular works. | Reducing diets. | Cancer--Diet therapy. | Integrative medicine. | Cooking. | Low-carbohydrate diet--Recipes. | BISAC HEALTH & FITNESS / Diet & Nutrition / General | HEALTH & FITNESS / Diseases / Cancer
Classification: LCC RM237.73 .D86 2018 | DDC 613.2/833--dc23

Dedication

To my husband, Mark, who meant it
when he said, "for better or for worse."
During cancer and difficult breathing,
he has been my motivation to persist, fight, learn,
and do everything I could to regain my health.

And to our sons, Joel and John,
who add so much joy to our lives.
They are the best of the "better."

Disclaimer

The information contained in this book is merely intended to communicate food preparation material and information about possible treatment options which are helpful and educational to the reader. It is not intended to replace medical diagnosis or treatment, but rather to provide information and recipes which may be helpful in implementing a diet prescribed by your doctor. Please consult your physician for medical advice before embarking on any treatment or changing your diet.

The author and publisher declare that to the best of their knowledge all material in this book is accurate; however, although unknown to the author and publisher, some recipes may contain ingredients which may be harmful to some people and some treatments and natural remedies may be harmful to some people.

There are no warranties which extend beyond the educational nature of this book, either expressed or implied, including, but not limited to, the implied warranties of merchantability, fitness for a particular purpose, or non-infringement. Therefore, the author and publisher shall have neither liability nor responsibility to any person with respect to any loss or damage alleged to be caused, directly or indirectly, by the information contained in this book. Your use of the information is at your sole risk.

If you do not wish to be bound by the above, you may return this book to the publisher for a full refund.

Website

www.healingbasics.life

Table of Contents

A Learning Experience 8

In a Nutshell. 10

How Did We Get Here? 11

Back to Basics 18

Nutrition for True Health 24

Why You Must Help Yourself 40

The Foundation of True Health 58
  Satisfaction With Food 59
  The Breath of Life 70
  Peace 75
  Ultimate Peace. 77

Putting Good Nutrition into Practice 81
When Cooking is Difficult 82
  About the Recipes and Ingredients 84
  Easy Dinners 94
  Cultured Vegetables 108
  Cultured Dairy Products 120
  Bone Broth 128
  Grains 141
  Legumes 174
  Nuts 181
  Beverages 185
  Treats 193

Appendices
  Appendix A – Using the Glycemic Index for Weight Loss Without Hunger . . 208
  Appendix B – Glycemic Index Values for Foods 211
  Appendix C – Allergies, Inflammation and Weight Loss 224
  Appendix D – Anti-inflammatory Foods 227
  Appendix E – Additional Advice for Cancer Patients 230
  Appendix F – Mold Remediation 232
  Appendix G – How To Read Food Labels 236

Appendix H – Bread Machine Information 242
Appendix I – Buteyko Breathing Experiences 246
Appendix J – Table of Measurements 249

References 250

Sources of Special Foods, Products, and Information 251
Prepared Foods 251
Supplies and Ingredients for Cooking 258
Other Products and Services 268
Information 272

A Personal Postscript: Details of My Learning Experience. 275

Index 285

Acknowledgements

I would like to acknowledge my husband Mark. I thank him for his love, encouragement and support that have made my books, our family, and everything else possible.

I acknowledge my son John. He told me that he and the other software engineers at his workplace performed quality control by trying to "break" each other's programs. John suggested that I try to make the recipes in this book fail and I followed his suggestion. Most important for health reasons, I attempted to get the cultured vegetable recipes fail to produce the correct lactic acid bacteria fermentation. In some cases, such as using pre-peeled mini-carrots, failure occurred. In others, such as less diligence in removing asparagus stalk leaves, the change did not create a problem with the fermentation. I thank John for all the help he gave me with this book.

I acknowledge my son Joel for being the inspiration to include acknowledgments in this book. The acknowledgments for his dissertation were the best part of the paper, as well as being almost the only part a non-electrical engineer could understand. What he did[1] at age 27, I am just getting around to doing at age 64.

I must thank God for every breath I have taken, labored or free, for every lucid thought I have, and for the ability to do everything I do, from brushing my teeth to writing this book to loving my family. I thank Him for the love He has given me and all of humankind (who are willing to accept His love) and for all the people named above. I thank Him for the gift of life, which I no longer take for granted, and most importantly for the assurance of eternal life.

If my books have helped you and you feel inclined to thank me, don't. Thank God who has ordered all the circumstances of my life to produce the books. In His grace and providence, He is turning what seemed to be trials for me into blessings for some of you, hopefully both health blessings now and eternal blessings in the future.

---

1 Dumke, Joel M. *EM/MPM-Based Segmentation Techniques with Improved Boundary Accuracy*, Purdue University, March, 2010. A paragraph from his acknowledgments follows:

Although there are those who may find this distasteful in an academic setting, I must acknowledge that every accomplishment and achievement of my life has come from God. I did not create myself. I did not choose or define my own abilities. I am inadequate to sustain myself. I have listed many people who were always willing to help me, but there were many times when they were simply not able. I have entirely depended on God in those times, and though I have had a few disappointments, I have never been forsaken. What He has given me is far better than anything I could have earned, controlled, or devised myself.

A Learning Experience

This book was born out of a learning experience I have been having for about three and a half years at the time of this writing. I was not seeking to learn new ways to improve my health. I was comfortable with the "status quo" of living in a body which requires a food allergy rotation diet containing uncommon foods, LDA treatment twice a year (see pages 48 to 50 for more about LDA and EPD) and supplements. I had not had a flare-up of Crohn's disease in about 20 years since shortly after I started EPD shots. I was grateful for being in better condition that anyone else I know with inflammatory bowel disease.

However, during the last few years, I have been repeatedly led to information that, when applied, has helped me make progress on the road to better health. I feel compelled to tell you what I have learned so you don't have to learn it in a similar way. The process of applying the information in this book is a journey, but given time, I hope you too will have the opportunity to achieve better health than would have been possible without this book.

The details of the learning experience are recorded at the end of the book beginning on page 275. A short summary is that I got viral pneumonia three and a half years ago which went into asthma that was continual and uncontrolled. Inhalers did not help. Nine months into the journey, my doctor discovered a bacterial sinus infection. He started treatment with antibiotic nasal rinses which were ineffective. The oral antibiotics that did rid me of the infection led to a sinus infection with *Candida albicans*. A post-treatment comprehensive stool test revealed opportunistic resistant yeast and bacteria, no *Lactobacillus*, chemical markers that were way off, and impaired digestion. Drug-based medicine had been ineffective in restoring my health. However, if the bacterial sinus infection had been left untreated, I would have been stuck where I was. Because of the severe state my asthma was in, antifungal drugs were used to treat the *Candida* sinus infection and intestinal yeast, but herbal products and probiotics were also used. They were effective in restoring some beneficial intestinal flora to acceptable levels although I still have opportunistic bacteria and have yet to reach "normal."

The next step my allergy doctor took was based on his intuition about why I had infection after infection. Thyroid test lab results were within the normal range but my TSH (thyroid stimulating hormone) and T3 (triiodothyronine) were at the lower limits of normal. My TSH had been at the high end of the normal range a few years before, which he thought might indicate a common pattern of post-menopausal thyroid decline. Addressing my thyroid problem was pivotal. He also decided to order a dust test on our house. To read everything I learned about mold remediation in the wake of this, see pages 232 to 235.

Because I always try to treat any problem with food, early on I made changes in my diet. At my first office visit when asthma symptoms returned after a 40 year hiatus, my allergy doctor's physician's assistant told me I should eat cultured vegetables to improve my intestinal flora which would help the asthma. She rightly realized that asthma, like many chronic health problems, has roots in intestinal health.

As I was learning about cultured vegetables, I came across information about bone broth, soaking and dehydrating nuts to make them more digestible, and other traditional ways of making foods more digestible and making it easier to absorb their nutrients. Traditional food preparation methods are steps back to a nutritionally better time.

That diet was crucial to good health was nothing new to me. A surprising discovery came when a friend of mine told me about the Buteyko breathing method for asthma. It is important that we take our breathing back to the way it used to be before modern occupations, lifestyles, and diets.

Then a crisis led me through a detour of willingness to use standard medical practices. Although I eschewed drug-and-surgery medicine for most of my life, the diagnosis of breast cancer made me agree to surgery without a pause. Initially, I said there was no way I would take chemotherapy, being an allergy-sensitive person. However, due to my husband's distress over the diagnosis, I told him I would take chemotherapy if needed. Thankfully, it was not needed. Now that I know more about chemotherapy for breast cancer, I have returned to my original no-chemotherapy position.

There are times when invasive or toxic conventional treatments are warranted for life-threatening diseases. Some forms of cancer are highly responsive to chemotherapy, such as lymphocytic leukemia in children. However, even in these situations, natural strategies can also be used to help people tolerate and recover from the treatment better and even make the treatment more effective.

Although there are times when we must use conventional medicine, there are often less invasive or toxic alternatives which this book presents. Some conventional treatments do not actually help and may even do more harm than good. We need to know all of our options and make the best decisions *for ourselves*. This book strives to give you information you need to make decisions based on what is best for you rather than what standard (sometimes meaning most profitable) practice is.

After the crisis had passed, I returned to my usual approach to health problems and made changes in my diet and lifestyle to give me the best chance of preventing a cancer recurrence. I learned that what is good for the allergy patient is good for the cancer patient is good for the heart patient or diabetic who needs to lose weight, and so on. My habits due to allergies put me on my holistic oncologist's "You're doing everything right" list, and the changes I made due to cancer were good for allergies. A wide range of health conditions can be helped by many of the same nutritional and lifestyle principles.

The discovery of this broader perspective is the impetus behind this book. Almost everyone can improve their health using the principles in this book. If your health is good, read and apply these principles to help prevent future problems. Then I hope we all will enjoy the sunrise of good health.

In a Nutshell

There are times when conventional medical treatment is the wisest choice, such as after a major accident or for life-saving surgery. However, for most chronic illness the medical system manages rather than even attempts to cure disease. We keep paying exorbitant sums to refill prescriptions month after month for the rest of our lives but never really feel good, healthy or even normal.

This book offers an alternative: It provides well-documented information demonstrating that a better way to improve health often is naturally by improving lifestyle and diet. Helpful lifestyle changes include avoiding exposure to toxic substances, moderate exercise, correct breathing, and pursuing peace.

The best help for health problems is often found in the kitchen. I discovered much useful advice in the Weston Price Foundation book *Nourishing Traditions*. Their principles for returning to dietary basics are very wise; unfortunately many of us with food allergies or gluten intolerance cannot eat the ever-present favored foods that are included in many of their recipes. Therefore, I have adapted their principles to be friendly for people following food allergy or gluten-free diets and have done the same with advice from other sources. The recipes in this book focus on easy digestibility and maximum nutrition, as well as fitting requirements of the special diets discussed in this book.

The incidence of cancer in the United States is over forty percent and is rising. Therefore, in my opinion, everyone should consume a diet that will help prevent cancer and promote good health. The basic principles of this basic diet are (1) to eat whole natural foods, not processed foods, including many fruits and vegetables and (2) to keep blood sugar and insulin levels low and stable. For individuals with food allergies or gluten intolerance, an additional principle is avoiding foods which cause reactions. For individuals whose health may be improved by weight loss, such as those with heart disease and diabetes, strict glycemic control also is a principle that is added to the anti-cancer diet. Low energy can be improved by the circadian rhythm diet which advises eating high-carbohydrate and high-protein foods at the time of day when needed metabolically. Individuals with candidiasis, autism, irritable bowel syndrome, inflammatory bowel disease and other conditions may consider adding the dietary principles specific for their condition to the anti-cancer diet. See pages 25 to 39 for more information about how to eat to treat specific health problems.

Although this book does not contain as many recipes as I often include, the recipes here offer a good start. These recipes are mostly special-diet-friendly recipes not available elsewhere. For more options, recipes from other sources are referenced at the end of each recipe chapter.

My hope is that by implementing the nutritional and lifestyle advice in this book, you will be able to optimize your health and prevent future health problems.

How Did We Get Here?

Americans' health has changed dramatically in the last several decades, with major diseases striking people at ever younger ages. Type 2 diabetes used to be a disease of people middle aged and older. Now it is not unusual to find it in people as young as their late teens. A Centers for Disease Control (CDC) report on diabetes from 1980 through 2014 showed that it rose from two to two and a half times its 1980 incidence for all age groups (18 to 79 years old) by 2014.[1] Over one quarter of people over 65 currently have diabetes, and the CDC projects that one in three adults could have diabetes by 2050.[2] In 1940, women under age 50 almost never got breast cancer. The breast cancer rate in younger women has tripled since World War II.[3] Very few people had allergies then. Those who did usually had simple problems like hayfever from pollen or an allergy to cats. Now one billion people world-wide suffer from allergies, many of them life-threatening.[4] Weight problems have skyrocketed since the 1980s when a third of Americans were overweight and only 15% obese. Now two thirds of people are overweight and over one third are obese.[5] What happened? Why did our health deteriorate so terribly in the span of these decades?

Many things changed when we entered World War II. Food rationing was necessary to supply the military with food, which created changes both good and bad. A positive change was the advent of Victory Gardens that encouraged many people to grow their own vegetables. However, I remember my parents describing a change that, in retrospect, we know was terrible for health. With most of the butter going to the military, the substitute was a stick of rubbery white oleomargarine which came with a little packet of yellow coloring that could be kneaded into the substance if you wanted it to look more like butter. The slogan, "Better living through chemistry," also was coined about that time. In the 1950s, TV made us more sedentary than in previous years. That was coupled with the birth of fast food when McDonald's Hamburgers franchises opened in the mid-1950s. Less cooking was done at home, so processed foods became a major part of most people's diets. Finally, as small family farms were replaced by agribusiness, changes occurred in farming methods and animal husbandry.

1 Incidence of Diagnosed Diabetes per 1,000 Population Aged 18-79 Years, by Age, United States, 1980-2014. https://www.cdc.gov/diabetes/statistics/incidence/fig3.htm

2 Diabetes in the United States. http://stateofobesity.org/diabetes/

3 Servan-Schreiber, David, MD, PhD. *AntiCancer: A New Way of Life.* (New York: Penguin Group, Inc., 2009), 62.

4 Galland, Leo, MD. *The Allergy Solution.* (Carlsbad, CA, Hay House, Inc., 2016), 19.

5 Kash, Peter Morgan, and Jay Lombard, DO. *Freedom from Disease.* (New York, NY, St. Martin's Press, 2008), xiv.

Changes in Our Diet

How did the standard American diet (SAD, and it certainly is sad) become so unhealthy? Profit motives were part of the change. Today, corn and soy are in almost all commercially-made foods because they are inexpensive. Trans fats do not go rancid, so it is economically advantageous to use them for whatever fat is in a processed food to extend the shelf life of the food almost indefinitely. Profit is a large part of why cattle and chickens are raised by current methods. Genetically modified foods (GMOs) with their patented seeds bring in untold profit for Monsanto in sales of both seeds and pesticides without, in my opinion, any regard for the health of our planet or the people living on it.

Tastes have also changed. Sugar consumption began rising in the early 1800s and was 11 pounds per person per year in 1830. By the year 2000, it had risen to 150 pounds per person per year. Corn syrup consumption has also skyrocketed and is in many processed foods. One of the largest dietary sources of sugar or corn syrup is soft drinks, and their manufacturers are determined to keep Americans drinking sodas. They pay for research to be done on how "energy balance," not sugar, is the cause of obesity, and have connections with the CDC to support them.[6] It is indeed true that eating significantly more than you are burning in exercise will cause weight gain, but sugar causes high insulin which leads to depositing fat even if you are not eating too much. High insulin also causes hunger, which drives you to eat more. High fructose corn syrup, with its higher glycemic index, is even worse for us than sugar. See pages 28 to 29 for the details of why high insulin levels caused by sugary foods are the most important cause of obesity, not calories.

Sugar, which the body makes into glucose, should be avoided by cancer patients. It is the preferred food of cancer cells where it is used rapidly and instead of other foods. The way positron emission tomography (PET) scans detect cancer is, after infusing the patient with radioactively labeled glucose, by scanning for areas where it is taken up in large amounts. Cancer patients should also avoid sugar and the ever-present white flour in baked goods because they stimulate a large release of insulin and insulin-like growth factor (IGF). Both hormones promote inflammation which stimulates the growth of cancer cells. IGF also increases the capacity of cancer cells to invade other tissues.[7]

The second change in our diets was in the types of fat we eat. We now eat too much inflammation-promoting omega-6 fat and very little omega-3 fat. This is due to the preponderance of corn, soy and sunflower oils in processed foods as well as to the way animals are now raised. Beginning in the 1950s, cattle were no longer raised on pasturelands, but instead were fed corn, wheat and soy in feedlots. Chickens no longer

---

6 Gillam,Carey. More Coca-Cola Ties Seen Inside U.S. Centers For Disease Control. August 1, 2016.
https://usrtk.org/food-related-diseases/more-coca-cola-ties-seen-inside-u-s-centers-for-disease-control/
7 Apple, Sam. May 26, 2016. An Old Idea Revived: Starve Cancer to Death.
https://www.nytimes.com/2016/05/15/magazine/warburg-effect-an-old-idea-revived-starve-cancer-to-death.html?_r=0

pecked at bugs and seeds but were fed an unnatural diet of corn. As a result, the ratio of omega-3 to omega 6 fatty acids in the body fat of these animals has changed from a healthy 1 to 1 ratio to between 1 to 15 and 1 to 40. Feeding animals linseed as 5% of their diet improves the ratio of fatty acids but is rarely done.[8]

An additional change in the fat we eat was hydrogenation, which makes the omega-6 oils usually used even more pro-inflammatory. Also, hydrogenated fats contain trans- rather than cis- bonds and thus are stiff when incorporated in cell membranes. This does not allow the cell membranes to function normally.

The International Study of Asthma and Allergies in Childhood showed that eating fast food three or more times a week resulted in more asthma, eczema, and rhinitis. Trans fats also have been connected to an increase in asthma in other research.[9]

Another change in our food is the widespread use of inorganic phosphate compounds which are used in sodas and to improve the texture of processed foods. These compounds promote the growth of non-small-cell lung cancer. They are found in a wide variety of foods such as processed cheese, lunch meats, pastries, fruit syrups, ice cream, frozen pizza and fish sticks. The amount of inorganic phosphates Americans consume has more than doubled since the 1990s.[10]

Cattle are now given estrogenic hormones and rBGH (recombinant bovine growth hormone) to increase milk production. Treatment with rBGH causes the cows to produce IGF which is excreted in their milk and not destroyed by pasteurization. As discussed above, our endogenous IGF released after eating sugar stimulates cancer cells.[11] Monsanto's rBGH drug, Posilac™, poses even more of a problem. The FDA approved this drug in 1993.[12] A 1996 International Journal of Health Services report said that milk from cows treated with rBGH contained ten times the level of IGF-1 (insulin-like growth factor-1) as milk from untreated cows, and more recent reports say it is as much as twenty times higher.[13] In 1998, the British medical journal *The Lancet* reported that women with small increases in levels of IGF-1 were up to seven times more likely to get breast cancer at a pre-menopausal age.[14] This timeline of events since the introduction of rBGH suggests a reason for the increased incidence of breast cancer in young women.

An even more frightening change in our food supply is the introduction of genetically modified organisms (GMOs) which are made in a laboratory by inserting genes from a totally unrelated organism. GMO plants are usually engineered to be resistant to

---

8 Servan-Schreiber, 72-73.

9 Galland, Leo, MD. *The Allergy Solution*. (Carlsbad, CA, Hay House, Inc., 2016), 21.

10 Servan-Schreiber, 86.

11 Servan-Schreiber, 75.

12 O'Brien, Robyn. *The Unhealthy Truth: How Our Food Is Making Us Sick and What We Can Do About It*. (New York, Broadway Books, Random House, 2009), 98.

13 O'Brien, 102.

14 O'Brien, 102.

the herbicide Roundup™ which is used to kill weeds. Thus high amounts of Roundup™ can be used on crops without killing the crop. In addition to the pesticides that remain on these foods, GMOs are recognized by the body as foreign. The timeline of events of the last 20 years suggests consuming GMOs results in more food allergies. (See pages 31 to 32 for details about the timeline). Several states have tried to pass or have passed initiatives to require labeling of GMO foods, but they have been struck down by the expenditure of millions of dollars from Monsanto to thwart allowing shoppers knowledge of whether a food contains GMOs.[15] Yet, although there has been no testing done, the FDA insists that GMO foods are safe. The "safety" of Roundup™ is also being protected as the Environmental Protection Agency (EPA) has acted to stall a toxicology review of the herbicide by the Centers for Disease Control (CDC).[16] However, the World Health Organization's International Agency for Research on Cancer declared glyphosate (the chemical name of the active ingredient in Roundup™) a probable human carcinogen.[17]

Over ten years ago I received a phone call from a mother about her recently diagnosed allergic daughter. She was most concerned with why her daughter was severely allergic. She spent much time and effort discovering the reason. Her research led her disagree with the FDA about the safety of GMOs and she has had the opportunity to discuss this on television programs such Oprah and CBN TV.

Until 2006, Robyn O'Brien was an ordinary mother of four children. Then her one-year old daughter had her first small taste of eggs for breakfast and had an immediate severe allergic reaction. How could she be so allergic? Her pediatrician told Robyn that this was not her daughter's first exposure to eggs because she had been immunized against flu a few months previously. A pediatric allergist said she was at risk for more food allergies and more severe reactions. In response to her questions, he told Robyn not to worry about the "whys" but to concentrate on her job of keeping her daughter safe.[18] Desperate to protect her daughter and other allergic children, Robyn thoroughly researched the "whys" and started a crusade to help "allergy kids" by providing much needed information for parents of allergic children. (See her website at AllergyKids. com). The most important health-changing information she learned was that consuming a diet of processed foods can dysregulate the immune system, leading to allergies.[19] Changing her family's diet to all organic non-GMO foods has kept her daughter safe.

15 Chow, Lorraine. 8 Battleground States in the GMO Food Labeling Fight. http://www.ecowatch. com/8-battleground-states-in-the-gmo-food-labeling-fight-1882162099.html .

16 Gilliam, Carey. Collusion or Coincidence? Records Show EPA Efforts to Slow Herbicide Review Came in Coordination With Monsanto. *Huffington Post*, August 17, 2017, http://www.huffingtonpost. com/entry/5994dad4e4b056a2b0ef02f1

17 International Agency for Research on Cancer, World Health Organizaion. *Evaluation of Five Organophosphates Insecticides and Herbicides.* IARC Monographs Volume 112, March 20, 2015. http://www.iarc. fr/en/media-centre/iarcnews/pdf/MonographVolume112.pdf

18 O'Brien, 9-11,

19 O'Brien, 45-47.

Environmental Problems:
Exposure to a Myriad of Chemicals

Changes in our environment have also affected our health negatively. In the 1960s, millions of barrels of oil were being pumped from the ground, making gas and petroleum products cheap and available for use in new profitable ventures.[20] Everyone owned or wanted to own an automobile. The emissions from vehicles and factories caused air pollution, which not only increases inflammation in general, but it increases airway response to allergens and worsens asthma.[21]

The abundance of petroleum also led to the development of many new chemical products such as plastics, pesticides, herbicides, cleaning products, building products, synthetic perfumes, etc. Since 1940, more than 100,000 new chemicals have been used in consumer products.[22] Unfortunately, many of these are unregulated and untested.

The World Health Organization's International Agency for Research on Cancer tracks potentially carcinogenic substances in the environment. Of the nine hundred substances they have tested, only one was recognized as non-carcinogenic. Four hundred two are known or probable carcinogens, many of which are still widely used. Four hundred ninety seven have not been classified yet. In 1995 the National Toxicology Program carried out animal trials. Their conclusion was that we are regularly exposed to over 3,750 carcinogens. Although we may be getting a dose of each that is considered non-problematic, their combined toxicity is thirty seven to seventy five times the dose considered toxic to animals.[23]

A most worrisome group of environmental toxins is those that disrupt hormones. They trigger inflammation and amplify allergic responses.[24] They are found in herbicides, pesticides, plastics, household products and beauty products. The most commonly known of these is bisphenol A (BPA) which promotes the progression of several cancers. It also blocks the effects of some chemotherapeutic drugs.[25]

Another group of endocrine disruptors, the phthalates, has been linked to allergies. Diethyl hexyl phthalates (DHEPs) cause wheezing in children. They are in adhesives, coatings, toys, childcare products, and cosmetics. Butyl benzyl phthalates, associated with asthma, rhinitis and eczema, are found in plastics, floor tile, and carpet backings.[26]

Formaldehyde is emitted from wood products such as plywood and particle board, floor finishes, paint, wallpaper, new fabrics, laser printers, copiers and personal comput-

20 Galland, 25.
21 Galland, 33.
22 Galland, 26.
23 Servan-Schreiber, 83.
24 Galland, 33-34.
25 Servan-Schreiber, 83.
26 Galland, 84.

ers.[27] Exposure to it is associated with increased sensitization to common airborne allergens. A 1999 study published in the journal *Allergy* found that the increase in allergies and asthma over the last few decades has paralleled the use of formaldehyde containing products in homes.[28]

The slogan I heard as a child, "Better living through chemistry," was untrue. We should support environmental activism and do whatever we can to encourage change, but it is not likely to happen quickly because of the economic forces at work. The one thing we can do about chemicals is wisely select what we allow in our homes. Use unscented natural cleaning products, wash all new clothing and fabric items thoroughly and with a pre-soak before you wear them, and buy solid wood furniture rather than particle board furniture. If that is too pricey, explore your options in antique stores, flea markets, etc. Also consider purchasing unfinished solid wood furniture and finishing it yourself with non-toxic coating or paint from a source such as American Formulating and Manufacturing. (For more about AFM cleaners and their Safecoat™ paint, sealants and stains, see page 20 and "Sources," page 269).

Lifestyle Changes

Our lifestyles have also changed since the 1940s. The rise in automobiles contributed to a more sedentary lifestyle. Instead of walking, or at least walking to a bus stop, everyone began driving. Our occupations now are also sedentary; many involve sitting in front of a computer all day. Television became a major consumer of time in some families. Therefore, sedentary habits and lack of exercise have contributed to obesity, diabetes, and other health problems.

Lack of exercise contributes to the development of cancer. Only 14% of active Americans will get cancer, much lower than the 42% national average.[29] My oncologist was pleased at my first office visit to hear that I take at least one, sometimes two, walks every day. You don't have to do a lot of intense exercise to reap major benefits.

Growing up as part of a large Italian extended family in an Italian neighborhood, I thought every home had a garden and every family's dinners contained a bountiful supply of home grown vegetables dressed with olive oil. We canned and froze much of the harvest from my father's garden and our fruit trees so we had nutritious home-grown food year round. In the 1970s, when economic changes caused most families to need two incomes to survive, there was not enough time for gardening nor the amount of home cooking I had grown up with. Today's apartment and condominium living also prevents gardening most of the time.

---

27 Servan-Schreiber, 86.

28 Galland, 36-37.

29 Quillin, Patrick, PhD, RD, CNS. *Beating Cancer with Nutrition,* (Carlsbad, CA,, Nutrition Times Press, 2005), 49.

The decline of gardening, rise of automobiles and thus less walking have affected our health in an additional way. Because we spend less time in the sun than our great-grandparents did, vitamin D deficiency is common and rising.

Over ten years ago my allergy doctor learned that low vitamin D levels are associated with leaking of the tight junctions between intestinal cells,[30] thus allowing food fragments to escape into the bloodstream. Because this contributes to food allergies, he suggested I have a blood test for vitamin D. My blood level was 7 ng/ml, far below the 50 ng/ml that he considered optimal.

In addition to food allergies, low vitamin D levels are associated with bone health issues (see pages 50 to 51), high blood pressure, cardiovascular disease, cancer, inflammatory diseases, infections,[31] and increased all-cause mortality.[32] Low vitamin D increases the risk of developing cancer as well as decreasing survival rates, so cancer patients should have blood levels checked and supplement if needed.

The articles cited below recommend the blood level of vitamin D be 30 ng/ml or above. For cancer prevention and general good heath, supplementing with vitamin D3, the active form, is recommended if blood testing shows a level below 30ng/ml. Then the blood level should be monitored at least until the dosage required for maintaining an optimal level has been determined. Vitamin D supplementation is a wise step for preventing and addressing many health problems.

There is no way to turn the clock back, but we can personally enjoy regular exercise, carefully read labels on the commercially made foods we buy, and do as much cooking from scratch as we can. Knowing how we as a nation reached our current state of health helps us understand what we can do to regain our health. Now, and for the future, we need to get back to basics and take charge of our diets and health.

30 Sun, Jun. "Vitamin D and mucosal immune function." *Curr Opin Gastroenterol.* 2010 Nov; 26(6): 591-595. https://www.ncbi.nlm.nih.gov/pmc/articles/PMC2955835/

31 Pilz S, Kienreich K, Tomaschitz A, Ritz E, et al. "Vitamin D and cancer mortality: systematic review of prospective epidemiological studies." *Anticancer Agents Med Chem.* 2013 Jan;13(1):107-17. https://www.ncbi.nlm.nih.gov/pubmed/2309492

Pilz S, Tomaschitz A, Obermayer-Pietsch B, et al. "Epidemiology of vitamin D insufficiency and cancer mortality." *Anticancer Res.* 2009 Sep;29(9):3699-704. https://www.ncbi.nlm.nih.gov/pubmed/19667167

32 Whiteman, Honor. Study links vitamin D deficiency to 'all-cause mortality and cancer prognosis.'" Medical News Today, June 18, 2014. https://www.medicalnewstoday.com/articles/278323.php

Back to Basics

We must make changes if we want to be exceptions to the current American state of health. If you are a parent, take this opportunity to prevent your children from being part of the trend toward progressively worse health. If you currently have a health condition, possibly one that is part of a national epidemic, work on improving the outcome by changing your diet and lifestyle now. In my opinion, treatments offered by conventional medicine will usually not significantly improve your lot. You must help yourself.

Since our health started spiraling downward after 1940, we might think we should take our diets and lifestyles back to the way they were in the 1930s. However, this is not back far enough; you may remember that sugar consumption was already on the rise in the 1800s. It's also difficult to re-create diets and lifestyles from history books or memory, and we can't ask great-grandma about her personal health in detail. A good way to determine what an ideally healthy diet is would be to find and study ideally healthy people. This is what Dr. Weston Price did in the 1930s when he visited and studied fourteen isolated societies around the world. They were like small pockets of traveling back in time.

Although the diets of these traditional groups differed in what they specifically ate, there were dietary principles they all held in common. They ate fruits, vegetables, legumes, whole grains, fats, nuts, seeds, and meat or fish in their whole, natural state. No part of an animal was left unused. When fish were eaten, the heads and skeletons were made into soup. Their diets contained both cooked and raw foods.[33] Organ meats were prized because they seemed important for fertility and children.[34] The groups that consumed milk drank it "as is" or ate it as yogurt or cheese.[35]

Although isolated from each other, the groups had food preservation and preparation techniques in common, such as using lactofermentation to preserve vegetables, fruits and meats, allowing milk to ferment to produce yogurt and cheese and the making of bone broths. Highly nourishing broth served as an extender of the animal by providing a nutrient-dense easily digested base for meals. These isolated groups also shared the practice of soaking cereals, grains and legumes before cooking them.[36]

The animal fats and tropical oils they ate had antimicrobial properties.[37] Animal fats also supplied vitamins A and D, the meat supplied protein, B vitamins, and minerals. Because people ate everything in its entirely, they undoubtedly obtained nutrients that

---

33 Fallon, Sally with Mary Enig, PhD. *Nourishing Traditions.*, (Brandywine, MD, NewTrends Publishing, 2001), xi.
34 Fallon with Enig, 16.
35 Fallon with Enig, 25.
36 Fallon with Enig, xii.
37 Fallon with Enig, 13.

have yet to be discovered. Rather than dissecting and analyzing foods as we do, they simply enjoyed their traditional diets.

When I was a child, we were closer food-wise to the cultures that Dr. Price studied than most of us are now. Americans of some ethnic extractions still cooked almost everything "from scratch." I remember helping my mother make chicken soup from a chicken, learning to make bread with my grandmother, and lessons on crimping the edge of a pie crust from my aunt. My mother and I made pasta together with a crank-type pasta maker, and my grandmother made pasta with a chitarra (wooden frame with metal wires strung across it) that came from Italy.

We had dessert only on special occasions such as birthdays and holidays. Candy was strictly rationed. When we received Halloween or Easter candy, we ate a few pieces, and the rest was put in a high cupboard. Every Saturday night we could choose one piece of candy to eat, and then we brushed our teeth.

I have fond memories of closeness enjoyed while doing food-related tasks with friends and family. When the cherries on our neighbor's tree had been picked and were ready to can or make into pies, the women and girls on our block sat under the tree and pitted cherries for hours, and then each took some cherries home. When my dad picked Italian beans from his garden, I always helped him snap them. I remember sitting on the patio in the cool of the evening talking while we snapped beans. My mother and I talked for hours while peeling apples from our trees to make into applesauce or freeze for pies.

When I was first married, my husband taught me some new habits, like eating sugar more freely and picking up "broasted chicken" for dinner. We ate out once a week. I did not go so far as making the open-and-pour casseroles[38] my mother-in-law told me about, hoping to make my kitchen time easier. There were, and still are, some things no self-respecting Italian will do! I taught my husband to eat many vegetables instead of just peas and corn. He quickly became accustomed to foods made from scratch and has never returned to eating meals made of highly processed foods. He even eventually gave up sugar, after a childhood of having dessert every night and a candy drawer in the kitchen that he could snack from whenever he wished.

When I developed food allergies after a few years of marriage, I didn't experience the panic that many people do because I knew it was possible to make everything from scratch and thus eliminate the problem ingredients.

When you begin to take your diet and cooking back to basics, start with small changes, such as reading labels and purchasing bread, crackers, etc. that are made from whole grains and healthy fats with no added sugar. Then prepare meals at home from whole foods. If there are nights when you need a shortcut to dinner, avoid highly pro-

---

38 Open-and-pour casseroles were made from cans of cream of mushroom soup, spam, and other unthinkable things, opened and poured into a casserole dish, mixed, sometimes sprinkled with crushed potato chips and then baked until warm.

cessed foods and substitute pre-made foods from a health food store. Use frozen rather than fresh vegetables to save washing and chopping time. Take your diet back to basics by doing the type of cooking done by the traditional cultures Dr. Price studied. With the information and recipes on beginning on page 94, you will be able to make your food easier to digest and extremely nutritious.

Taking your home environment back to healthy basics is easier than the transition to mostly home cooking. Though the world around you is swimming in chemicals, you can improve what you are exposed to in your home. Start with cleaning out the cupboards where you store cleaning and laundry products and the cabinet under the kitchen sink. Throw away everything that is fragranced or carries a long list of chemicals or warnings on the label. That will probably be almost everything you purchased at a grocery or discount store.

What is wrong with fragrance if you are not sensitive to it? It is there to cover the smell of toxic cleaning ingredients. Also, chemical fragrances are themselves toxic. A study was done in on what was in the air clothes dryers vented to the outside. Laundry done with fragranced detergents produced twenty one harmful volatile organic compounds (VOCs). If both fragranced detergents and dryer sheets were used, the list was much longer. There were no VOCs emitted from the laundry washed with unscented detergent.[39]

Air fresheners don't actually freshen the air, they just cover unpleasant odors with chemical perfumes that are as toxic as those in laundry products. The use of air fresheners is linked to allergies and worsening asthma.[40] Remove whatever is causing offensive odors, like garbage in your kitchen wastebasket. Then open the windows to really freshen the air.

Alternatives to chemical cleaning products can be found at health food stores, but read the labels even there. I am unable to give recommendations for products you can find at the health food store because, like the packaged foods there, the ingredients change often. Old standbys for non-toxic cleaning include vinegar, baking soda, borax and BonAmi™ scouring powder. When you need serious cleaning power, try some AFM SuperClean™. A bottle of this concentrate will last you a long time. The label directs how to dilute if from between 1:15 to 1:2 to clean everything from kitchen counters to walls to diifficult-to-remove soap scum deposits. For soap scum, you may want to moisten the surface with 1:2 SuperClean™, let it stand a while, and then scrub with BonAmi™. For information on where to get SuperClean™, see "Sources," page 269.

Microfiber cloths and dusters can eliminate the need to use many cleaning products. My old favorite cloths contained 80% polyester and 20% polyamide fibers and were reasonably priced but, unfortunately, came from a company that recently closed. Since then I have tried several brands of microfiber cloths in all price ranges. Cloths sold by multi-level marketing are not more effective than my favorites but are much more expensive. (The marketing method adds to the price). The cloths sold at grocery stores

---

39 Galland, Leo, MD. The Allergy Solution. (Carlsbad, CA, Hay House, Inc., 2016), 88.
40 Galland, 93.

and discount stores seemed much less effective to me. When I inspected the labels on the few cloths that came with fiber content information, I discovered that they contained no polyamide. Before purchasing such cloths, feel them. Microfiber that works well contains polyamide and feels sticky. The surface of most microfiber cloths is covered with loops. If washing windows, use looped cloths for washing and a smooth window cloth for drying the windows. Unfortunately, I have been unable to find a smooth cloth that works as well as the multi-level marketing window cloth and is reasonably priced. My new favorite looped cloths contain 20% polyamide like my old favorites and are made by VibraWipe™. See "Sources," page 269, for more information.

Use water with microfiber cloths when cleaning, either by wetting the cloths or with a spray bottle. Although microfiber can be used dry for dusting, I slightly dampen cloths before dusting to minimize the amount of dust that escapes the cloth and is inhaled. I also change cloths frequently while cleaning and deposit the soiled cloths in the washer to wash when I finish cleaning. Do not wash microfiber cleaning cloths with cotton fabrics or they will pick up lint that destroys their effectiveness. Wash the cloths in cool water with laundry detergent only and hang them to dry.

Although I usually use non-toxic cleaning agents, there are times when what you are trying to get rid of is worse than a "big gun" cleaner. See pages 232 to 235 for more about getting rid of mold. If you must use something like Clorox™, open the windows so the fumes will be diluted with fresh air rather than building up. If you are sensitive to the smell of Clorox™, have someone else treat a moldy area with Clorox™, let it dry and sit for an hour or for as long as overnight, and then rinse the area thoroughly and air out thoroughly before you use the room. Be sure to buy unscented Clorox™.

When you buy an item of new clothing, remove the chemicals it is laden with before wearing. I have always washed new clothing before wearing, but recently read about a new twist on this. In *The Allergy Solution*, Dr. Galland recommends soaking new clothing overnight in the washer with warm water first, and then washing it repeatedly until it smells all right.[41] I was surprised when I soaked a rust-colored turtleneck top overnight and the water was deep orange the next morning.

Personal care products should be natural, unscented products, not petroleum-based and without parabens or phthalates.[42] Shop for them at health food stores and read the labels. Interestingly, recent studies have linked the rapidly rising incidence of peanut anaphylaxis in children to early exposure to peanut oil in skin care products.[43] Thus, be careful of what you put on your skin because it will be absorbed. The practice of slathering children with toxic DEET to prevent mosquito bites is ludicrous considering that vitamin B1 works better and is non-toxic. For more about this, see pages 42 to 43.

---

41 Galland, 91-92.

42 Servan-Schreiber, David, MD, PhD. *AntiCancer: A New Way of Life*. (New York: Penguin Group, Inc., 2009), 6 of "AntiCancer Action" section in the center of the book.

43 Galland, 49.

We also must get back to exercise basics. A few generations ago, many Americans got plenty of exercise in their daily lives. Farmers, manual laborers, and hard-working housewives did not have modern appliances or equipment to help with the heavy work. When I was a child, we had a washtub and scrub board that were saved as a memento of my Grandma Jiannetti who had used it for family laundry. I remember watching my aunt wash clothes with the time-saving device that came next, a wringer washing machine. The clothes agitated in a tub of soapy water, and then she lifted heavy, wet clothes to the wringer. Here she fed them through the rollers to remove most of the soapy water. The process was then repeated a time or two with pure water before she carried a heavy laundry basket outside to hang clothing on the clothes line. After clothes were dry, we had to do the ironing. (I did plenty of ironing as a teenager). A lot of exercise was certainly involved in doing laundry years ago.

Now we have appliances to help us at home. At our workplaces, we are much more likely to sit at a computer all day than to lift a shovel or do any kind of physical exertion. Thankfully, many Americans exercise regularly. If you don't, start now on exercise that is simple to do and that you enjoy. You might try taking a brisk thirty-minute walk most days. Some people do this on their lunch hour. With a healthy lunch brought from home, you can eat at your desk while working and then use your lunch time to walk.

Exercise is important for everyone. Moderate exercise, used with a glycemic control diet, is a vital tool for weight loss. Asthmatics especially benefit from exercise, although some avoid it for fear of provoking an asthma attack. (Consult your doctor before you begin an exercise program if you are asthmatic). A gradually built up walking program is an ideal place to start. Walk with your mouth closed and breathe through your nose. Start each walk at a slow pace and gradually increase the speed. If you feel you must breathe through your mouth, slow down. Opening your mouth during exercise thwarts the purpose of exercise for asthmatics and may lead to an asthma attack.[44] For more about Buteyko breathing see pages 70 to 73 and 273. The advice Patrick McKeown, a major force in promoting the Buteyko breathing method, gives to all asthmatics is, "Spend as much time as possible outdoors and take some form of exercise."[45]

While exercise is important for everyone, it is essential for people with cancer. Our defenses against cancer can be directly stimulated by exercise. It helps rid the body of excess fat, which is where carcinogenic toxins are stored. Exercise improves our hormonal balance, decreasing excess estrogen and testosterone that stimulate reproductive system cancers. For all cancers, exercise is beneficial because of its effect on natural killer (NK) cells. If people who regularly exercise hear bad news (as in a threatening medical report), their level of natural killer (NK) cells remains relatively stable. In non-exercisers,

44 McKeown, Patrick, MA, H Dip. *Asthma-Free Naturally*. (San Francisco, CA, Conari Press 2008),102-104.
45 McKeown, 97.

the number of NK cells may drop rapidly.[46] Cancer cells metabolize best in anaerobic environments (with little or no oxygen), so exercise, which sends more oxygen to tissues, slows their metabolism.[47] An editorial in the *Journal of Clinical Oncology* reported that exercise decreases the chance of relapse 50 to 60 percent for breast cancer, including cases that are not sensitive to estrogen.[48]

In *AntiCancer*, Dr. Servan-Schreiber gives cancer patients advice on how to succeed in an exercise program. His advice, useful for anyone, is to begin slowly and gently with exercise like walking, possibly progressing to running. Walking to get wherever you can get easily on foot is very beneficial. He emphasizes exercising anywhere and everywhere, just get into the habit. By exercising in small doses, a person gets a lot of exercise without becoming exhausted. Exercises such as yoga or tai chi stimulate the body gently and can be done by almost anyone, regardless of their physical condition. As you are able to take on more, if you're ready for a change, choose the exercise you most enjoy. Join an exercise group if that suits you. Exercise on an exercise bicycle, treadmill or elliptical trainer while you watch a movie DVD.[49]

A friend who had a mastectomy about three months after mine and learned about what she should do to help prevent a recurrence told me that she could not believe how good she felt after starting to eat better and walk every day. You too can make changes that will help you improve your health. How to eat in the way that is *best for you* is discussed in the next chapter.

---

46 Servan-Schreiber, David, MD, PhD. *AntiCancer: A New Way of Life.* (New York: Penguin Group, Inc., 2009), 197-198.

47 Quillin, Patrick, PhD, RD, CNS. *Beating Cancer with Nutrition*, (Carlsbad, CA,, Nutrition Times Press, 2005), 45.

48   Servan-Schreiber, 201.

49 Servan-Schreiber, 202-203.

Nutrition for True Health

Good nutrition is a cornerstone of optimal health. As a person with food allergies, I focused on foods that were different from what "normal" folks eat. However, in the last few years I've learned that there are over-arching dietary principles that we all can benefit from following. Dr. David Servan-Schreiber's anti-cancer diet[50] is good for all of us to follow because 42% of Americans will get cancer. This diet's principles will not only lessen cancer risk, but maintenance of stable blood sugar and insulin levels is also helpful for weight issues and inflammation which can promote allergies, arthritis, etc. The types of fat eaten on the anti-cancer diet, in addition to less concentrated carbohydrates eaten for blood sugar control, will be helpful for heart patients, diabetics, and anyone who does not want to be pressured to take statins as discussed on page 57.

Because so much chronic disease is connected to overweight, if you need more weight loss help than the anti-cancer diet provides, try the glycemic control diet (pages 27 to 30) which will allow you to lose weight without experiencing hunger. Hunger is absent because the diet keeps your insulin level low and stable and blood sugar stable. Feeling hungry occurs when blood sugar is falling or low or insulin is high. On this diet, at the first feeling of hunger, you should eat a small protein-containing snack. Many of us know we need to lose weight. However, those who are slim may also need to control their blood sugar and insulin levels for optimal health even though their appearance does not suggest health problems.

The most basic advice for a healthy diet is to eat food in the most natural state you can find. If it won't rot or sprout, don't eat it. Avoid highly processed foods. Cook most of what you eat from basic whole-food ingredients. For foods like bread that can take more time to make than you have, read ingredient labels carefully and choose the item with the "cleanest" ingredients. Look for bread which contains no high-fructose corn syrup or sugar, no hydrogenated fats, little or no refined white flour, little or no sweeteners in general, and no long list of chemicals on the ingredient list. Be aware that if the item contains any white flour, vitamins that it was enriched with will be at the end of the ingredient list. These vitamins are acceptable ingredients unless you are allergic to yeast. The B vitamins required for enrichment of foods made with white flour usually are made from yeast because this is the least expensive source. To avoid yeast-derived vitamins, you must avoid all products made with white flour as well as white rice.

This chapter contains information about a variety of diets in addition to the anti-cancer and glycemic control diets. They include diets for food allergies, for a number of intestinal conditions, and the circadian rhythm diet for energy when you need it. You may need to combine the principles of a few of these diets for your own best diet.

---

50 Servan-Schreiber, David, MD, PhD. *AntiCancer: A New Way of Life.* (New York: Penguin Group, Inc., 2009), 104-145.

Forsake unhealthy eating habits and old ideas about foods (as in what foods can be eaten for breakfast) and follow the diet that is best for *your* health. Nothing tastes as good as healthy feels.

The Anti-Cancer Diet

The anti-cancer diet Dr. David Servan-Schreiber presents in his book *Anti-Cancer: A New Way of Life* resembles the Mediterranean diet[51] with one important difference: it puts great emphasis on blood sugar control. This is because sugar feeds and stimulates the growth of cancer cells. In 1923, Otto Warburg studied cancer cells and discovered "the Warburg Effect," which is that cancer cells consume sugar voraciously and metabolize it without oxygen. The idea then was to treat cancer by starving the cancer cells. With the discovery of DNA in 1953, all attention was turned to mutations and other genetic aspects of cancer cells. We are now taking a step in the right direction by returning to a natural dietary way to control cancer.[52]

The most important principle of the anti-cancer diet is control of your blood sugar and insulin levels. This means eating little or no sugar or other refined sweeteners and few or no baked goods made of mostly white flour. For those on allergy or gluten-free diets, baked goods made with brown rice flour are as bad as those made with white flour for raising your blood sugar and insulin levels. Traditional long-fermemted sourdough breads and breads made with whole grain flour plus nuts, seeds and whole grains[53] are advised because they have a lower glycemic index.[54] For an explanation of and more information about the glycemic index, see pages 208 to 210.

Eliminating sugar and corn syrup is the most important change a cancer patient can make because sugar is the preferred food of cancer cells. High fructose corn syrup is even worse than sugar, and it is found in most processed foods, which should be avoided. Stevia is the best substitute for sugar. Dr. Servan-Schreiber also allows lower glycemic index nutritive sweeteners such as agave, coconut sugar, and acacia or orange blossom honey to be used occasionally in moderation.[55]

---

51 A traditional Mediterranean diet contains fruits and vegetables (veggies were the stars of meals in my childhood), proteins from legumes, cheese, and nuts, grain products such as pasta (not overcooked, so it has a low glycemic index), good crusty bread, olive oil, and fish and meat in moderation.

52 Apple, Sam. "An Old Idea Revisited: Starve the Cancer to Death". *New York Times*, 5-16-2016. https://www.nytimes.com/2016/05/15/magazine/warburg-effect-an-old-idea-revived-starve-cancer-to-death.html?_r=0

53 To make bread more easily using much less of your time, see *Easy Breadmaking for Special Diets,* 3rd Edition as described on the last pages of this book. The third edition contains recipes to make fermented sourdough with a variety of grains, including gluten-free grains. Theses recipes use a freeze-dried gluten-free starter so you do not have to maintain a sourdough culture.

54 Servan-Schreiber, 68-69.

55 Servan-Schreiber, 71.

Anything you eat that causes the release of a large amount of insulin also provokes the release of insulin-like growth factor (IGF) which stimulates the growth of cancer cells.[56] Before I learned this, I'd eat a large bunch of grapes for a snack without eating protein at the same time to balance the carbohydrate. After the cancer diagnosis, I realized how I had been raising my insulin level, so I switched to fruits that provoke very little release of insulin, such as cherries, blueberries, raspberries, peaches, plums, and apples. I eat them in moderate quantities, usually with nuts, or eat only nuts for a snack.

The second principle of the anti-cancer diet is to eat only healthy fats. Hydrogenated fats should be completely avoided. Olive, canola and nut oils are good oils that do not promote inflammation. Butter and cheese from free-range animals are also good choices.[57]

Eat meat that has a healthy ratio of omega-3 to omega-6 fatty acids. Corn and soy-fed meat and poultry are very high in omega-6 fatty acids, which promote inflammation and stimulate the growth of cancer cells. Meat from free-range raised animals is your meat of choice. Be aware that not all organic meat is free-range. Game meat is an excellent choice[58] as is wild-caught fish.

The third principle of the anti-cancer diet is to eat a wide range of fruits and vegetables including highly-colored produce. My oncologist, who is far above her peers on prevention, tells me at every visit that the more fruits and vegetables I eat, the less chance I have of a recurrence. A six-year study published in the *British Journal of Cancer* showed that breast cancer patients who consumed many fruits and vegetables rich in carotenoids lived longer than those who consumed few.[59]

Most fruits and vegetables can be eaten cooked or raw. However, cooking with oil is essential for making the anti-cancer lycopenes in tomatoes available for our use. Cabbage family vegetables are most helpful eaten raw. Freezing preserves the anti-cancer substances in foods, so enjoy frozen berries when fresh berries are not in season or are more expensive. Although organic is ideal, the positive effects of the anti-cancer agents in the foods overrides the negative impact of contaminants, so if you can't find or afford organic, eat as wide a variety of thoroughly washed conventional produce as you can find. Eat locally grown produce whenever you can; it spends less time in transit and may retain more nutrients.[60]

A number of foods have anti-cancer properties. They include green tea at three or more cups per day, olive oil, berries, cherries, peaches, plums, nectarines, cruciferous and onion family vegetables, tomatoes, turmeric, ginger, and terpene-rich herbs such as

---

56 Servan-Schreiber, 80.

57 Servan-Schreiber, 75-58, 143.

58 Servan-Schreiber, 80.

59 Ingram, D. "Diet and Subsequent Survival in Women with Breast Cancer." *British Journal of Cancer* 69:3. 1994, 592-595.

60Servan-Schreiber, 123-125.

mint, thyme, marjoram, oregano, basil, and rosemary. See *AntiCancer* for more about which foods are best for you and your type of cancer if you are a cancer patient.[61]

The type of water you drink is also critical for cancer patients.[62] I switched from bottled water to water from a purifier when I found out that the bottles water comes in, even the "safest," leach a variety of phthalates, inorganic phosphate, and other chemicals used to produce the plastic. Avoiding BPA (Bisphenol A) is not enough! Do not use canned goods because the plastic can linings leach the same cancer-stimulating chemicals into the food. Get rid of your Tupperware™ and purchase some Glasslock™ food storage containers, or use glass and ceramic jars and bowls to store your food. Substitute cellophane bags and wrap for plastic. For sources of these products, see pages 270 to 271. For more about how to store food without plastic visit the "Treading My Own Path" website here: http://treadingmyownpath.com/2016/08/04/the-definitive-guide-to-storing-food-without-plastic/

Cancer patients with allergies must "deal with your allergies," says Patrick Quillin, PhD, in *Beating Cancer With Nutrition.* He says that the immunoglobulins responsible for allergies depress the production of cancer-fighting immune factors such as natural killer cells and tumor necrosis factor. Eating foods you are allergic to distracts your immune system from its most important job of fighting cancer cells to attack food allergens. He recommends a rotation diet for those who have multiple food allergies.[63]

Cancer patients who are recovering from surgery or taking chemotherapy may be too exhausted to shop or cook for the anti-cancer diet. My hope is that you have a friend or family member or can hire someone to do some cooking and shop for nourishing food, avoiding processed foods, sugar and unhealthy fats. Good nutrition will help you endure and recover from treatments and give you the best outcome. For more ideas about how to eat well at this stage of your treatment, see "When Cooking is Difficult' on pages 82 to 83.

The Glycemic Control Diet for Weight Loss
Achieve Your Ideal Weight Without Suffering Hunger

The focus of a glycemic control diet is to keep your blood sugar and insulin levels low and stable. Anyone beginning the diet will have unstable levels at first, causing hunger, which is a sign of high insulin and/or falling blood sugar. When hunger strikes, you should immediately eat a snack that contains protein to return your blood sugar and insulin to healthy levels. Starvation and deprivation are the hallmark of high-car-

---

61 Servan-Schreiber, 110-120.

62 Servan-Schreiber, 86.

63 Quillin, Patrick, PhD, RD, CNS. *Beating Cancer with Nutrition*, (Carlsbad, CA,, Nutrition Times Press, 2005), 102-110.

bohydrate low-fat and calorie counting diets. You will have a whole new mindset with glycemic control eating, which is to correct your blood sugar and insulin levels quickly and banish hunger. This means you can forget about willpower. You won't need it.

The glycemic control diet is useful for many conditions in addition to overweight including diabetes and heart disease. Glycemic control can be simple if your blood sugar doesn't take wild swings, as in my description of giving up grapes and instead eating low glycemic index fruits and/or nuts in the anti-cancer diet section above. Simple control is good for slim people on the anti-cancer diet. However, if you want to make consistent progress on weight loss, you may be better off with a formal balancing of carbohydrates and proteins. You should eat protein-containing snacks two to three times per day and follow other guidelines as presented on the next few pages. With either approach, simple or formal, most of the carbohydrates you eat should be low on the glycemic index (GI), with some moderate GI foods in small quantities. For more about the glycemic index and tables of these values for foods, see pages 208 to 223.

Glycemic control is the best way to lose weight because (1) you do not have to experience hunger and (2) it enables you to work with your body rather than struggling against your body in the weight loss process, as in calorie counting diets, which often end up making us fatter in the long term. To lose weight, we need to control the hormones that determine whether the body stores or burns fat. These hormones include insulin, cortisol, and leptin, among others. In optimally healthy people of normal weight, the leptin system raises metabolic rate and reduces appetite if we overeat, thus restoring us to a normal weight. Decreasing your level of inflammation helps leptin to function normally. Inflammation can be reduced by eating anti-inflammatory fats and anti-inflammatory foods. See page 227 to 229 for a list of anti-inflammatory foods.

Insulin is the most important hormone for controlling weight. To burn fat rather than store it, you must also keep your insulin level low and stable. The way to accomplish this is to always balance carbohydrates with protein and to eat protein or balanced protein plus carbohydrate snacks between meals, eating something every two to three hours. **If you feel hungry, it means your insulin level is high. You need to eat a protein snack immediately.** A more detailed discussion of how to balance proteins and carbohydrates is below

The reason insulin levels are critical for weight control is because a high level of insulin activates an enzyme called lipoprotein lipase. This enzyme catalyzes the production of triglycerides from any fatty acids (digested fat units in the form that is absorbed by the intestine) eaten in a meal. Thus, excess insulin promotes storage of fat by our fat cells rather than using it for fuel after a meal.[64] In a person with normal insulin levels, any recently eaten fats could have been used for energy during the two hours after a meal. **If insulin levels are high, dietary fat is more likely to be stored in the fat cells.**

---

64 Montignac, Michel. Scientific Principles: Basic Principle Behind the Montignac Method. http://www.montignac.com/en/scientific-principles/

In addition, high insulin levels in the blood inhibit the activity of the enzyme trig-lyceride lipase which breaks down stored fat for use as energy. Thus, **if you have chronically high insulin, you cannot burn your own body fat!**[65] For more about how hormones control weight loss, see *Food Allergy and Gluten-Free Weight Loss* as described on the last pages of this book or visit www.foodallergyandglutenfreeweightloss.com.

Here is a list of the most important things to do to lose weight with this no-hunger plan. Following these principles here will stabilize your blood sugar, insulin, and other hormone levels and enable you to burn fat. Do not allow the numbers below to make you legalistic about counting as if you were on a calorie counting diet. Weigh a portion of the food once when starting this eating plan, and then eat about that amount the next time. See the glycemic index tables on pages 211 to 223 to determine what amount of a specific food is one unit, meaning that it contains 15 grams of carbohydrate (for carbohydrate foods) or 7 grams of protein (for protein foods).

1. **All of your meals should contain the correct balance of protein to carbohydrate.** Consume carbohydrates low on the glycemic index as much as possible. Keep your carbohydrate intake at or below two units (30 grams at 15 grams per carbohydrate unit) per meal and balance it with the same or a greater number of units of protein (7 grams per protein unit). Add a little fat (especially if the protein food doesn't provide some) and enough additional protein and non-starchy vegetables to satisfy your hunger.

2. **Every morning eat a breakfast which contains enough protein to satisfy you plus carbohydrates in the correct amount to balance the protein or less.** Eat breakfast early, ideally within the first hour after arising.

3. **Eat protein-containing snacks three times a day**, mid-morning, mid-afternoon, and at bedtime. They don't have to be large; a handful of nuts will do. If you desire, sometimes you can add carbohydrates to your snack in the correct balance with the protein you are eating. Eat enough at each snack to quell any hunger.

4. **Think nutrients.** Eat plenty of the anti-inflammatory foods listed on pages 227 to 229 and consider taking a supplement that provides general nutritional support as well as the nutrients most important for control of insulin levels and inflammation such as chromium and omega-3 fatty acids. Eat lots of low-carb fruits and vegetables, and make sure you're eating healthy fats as described in the anti-cancer diet section on page 26. Fat is a friend with this type of weight loss, so do eat healthy fats.

5. **Do some moderate exercise** or brisk walking. Intense or prolonged exercise, especially without food, can cause your body to hold onto fat and burn muscle, which will decrease your metabolism and make weight loss more difficult. Never exercise when you are hungry; have a protein-containing snack first. See the "Exercise Right" page here http://www.foodallergyandglutenfreeweightloss.com/exercise_right.html for what type and how much exercise is right for you.

---

65 Hart, Cheryle R., MD and Mary Kay Grossman, RD, *The Insulin Resistance Diet*, (New York: McGraw-Hill, 2001, 2007), 5; and www.montignac.com/en/la_methode_scientifique.php

See *Food Allergy and Gluten-Free Weight Loss* for more information about weight loss, exercise that is right for you, and recipes. See Appendix C on pages 224 to 226 if you have food allergies and want to lose weight.

The Circadian Rhythm Diet
for Energy When You Need It

In *The Circadian Prescription*, Dr. Sidney Baker presents a diet that he developed after learning about the research of Dr. Charles Ehret on human circadian rhythms. The principle behind this diet is to give our bodies the foods they need when they need them for optimal energy, cognitive function, mood, detoxification and healing. This diet helps stabilize blood sugar, so it is useful for weight loss. The diet's rhythmic shake (recipe on page 190) which is consumed every morning also contains phytonutrients that decrease the risk of reproductive cancers.

If you are eating a healthy diet without processed foods, adopting this system of eating probably will not change what you eat in the course of a day, just when you eat it. All or almost all carbohydrates should be eaten at dinner time or in the evening. Breakfast consists of the rhythmic shake either alone or with other high protein foods. Lunch is also mostly protein foods.

A breakfast heavily reliant on protein is the opposite of what most people eat. We think the carbohydrates in cereal, toast, orange juice, etc. are what we need for energy. Actually, protein is what we need for morning energy. Our bodies need to make adrenal hormones to get us going in the morning, and protein is required for that. The window for making these hormones is brief, and if the required substances are not available then, the hormones will not be made in sufficient quantities. Protein eaten in the morning can be saved by the body for use later in the day. Tryptophan, the amino required to make serotonin for sleep, can be absorbed most easily in the morning and, with sufficient carbohydrates consumed in the evening, will be used to make the serotonin we need to sleep well.[66]

While we are asleep at night, detoxification, biochemical replenishment, and synthesis of new substances needed for repairs are all occurring. Carbohydrates provide the fuel for all of this activity. In order to get rid of worn-our molecules or toxic substances, the liver must add something (usually a methyl group) on to them before they can be excreted. Carbohydrates are also needed to transport tryptophan into the brain where it is converted into serotonin, which is needed for sleep.[67]

Dr. Baker writes that he has always felt the amount of carbohydrate allowed on some anti-*Candida* diets was too low for good health. He finds that those with *Candida* can

---

66 Baker, Sidney M., MD. *The Circadian Prescription.* (New York: Berkley Publishing Group- Penguin Putnam Inc., 2000), 64-65.
67 Baker, 45-47.

eat more healthy carbohydrates without problems as long as they eat them late in the day. However, sugars and sweeteners, refined flour, and yeast-containing foods must still be avoided at all times of the day if you have *Candida*.[68]

Dr. Baker's rhythmic shake contains dairy products or rice dairy products, soy, flaxseed, and blueberries. Except for the blueberries, these foods are not tolerated by many people with food allergies. Therefore, in addition to including his shake recipe in this book, there are recipes for four shakes without these ingredients that can be used for each day of a rotation diet. See pages 187 to 189 for these recipes. I try to have one of these shakes every morning, and they improve my energy as well as giving me enough omega-3 fatty acids to keep the skin on my fingertips crack-free and in good condition.

The Food Allergy Elimination Diet

Individualized elimination diets are commonly used to treat food allergies. If the patient is allergic to only one or two foods, eliminating the offending foods in all of their forms may be the only treatment necessary. This is the course usually taken in the case of children with peanut anaphylaxis. My father was able to treat the milk allergy he developed from drinking large quantities of milk for an ulcer by simply eliminating dairy products. He was allergic to no other foods.

The problem with elimination diets is that if you replace wheat in your diet with rice, for example, in a few years you may find yourself allergic to rice. Rice allergy used to be uncommon, but now that so many people are on gluten-free diets and daily eat rice at every meal, rice allergy is no longer rare. If you can eliminate the offending few foods without relying on the same replacements often, and if there is not a continuing problem like a leaky gut that led to your food allergies, an elimination diet can be very effective and less work than a rotation diet. See the next page for more about rotation diets.

All of us with food allergies should avoid genetically modified foods to avoid developing more food allergies. Although the FDA did no testing before approving GMOs and insists that they are safe, the timeline associated with the epidemic of peanut anaphylaxis in children casts grave doubt on the safety of GMOs. In 1996, GMO soy, the first GMO food the FDA approved, came into widespread use. Soy and peanuts are both in the legume family, and it is not unusual for a person allergic to one member of a food family to react to other members as well. In 1997, the incidence of peanut anaphylaxis rose by 20%.[69] This trend in the United State has continued every year so at the time of this writing one in thirteen children have peanut anaphylaxis. Their lives are at risk if they are exposed to peanuts.

---

68 Baker, 106-107.

69 O'Brien, Robyn. *The Unhealthy Truth: How Our Food Is Making Us Sick and What We Can Do About It.* (New York, Broadway Books, Random House, 2009), 65.

In 1998, GMO soy was introduced in the United Kingdom, and the rate of soy allergies rose 50% in 1999.[70] These examples may not constitute proof that consuming GMOs is unsafe, but since I personally do not want to develop more food allergies, I avoid GMO foods.

At this time, the list of GMO foods in the United States includes soy, corn, sugar beets (beet sugar), canola (oil), cottonseed (oil), papaya, zucchini, yellow summer squash, some tomatoes, some apples (including non-browning apples), some potatoes (but not sweet potatoes or yams), and alfalfa. When you shop for these foods, if you want to avoid GMOs, you must buy organic produce. For packaged foods, look for a logo that says the food is certified GMO free. So far the government has not prohibited producers of healthy foods from putting this non-GMO logo on their products.

The World Health Organization (WHO) has developed a protocol for determining whether GMOs might cause the development of allergies to those foods, but unfortunately none of the GMO foods developed in the United States has been tested using the protocol.[71] Some European countries take the "better safe rather than sorry" approach and do not allow GMOs to be used in their food. The powers that be in the United States have not followed the example of the Europeans. However, nothing keeps us from personally avoiding GMO foods and instead supporting organic food production with our dollars.

The Food Allergy Rotation Diet

The purpose of a rotation diet is to prevent the development of new food allergies. For additional allergy prevention, readers of this section will want to follow the advice in the previous section and also strictly avoid GMO foods. In my opinion, everyone with food allergies in their family should avoid GMOs in order to prevent the development of allergies.

If you have multiple food allergies, you may have some degree of allergy to many foods that you do not suspect. A way to help yourself is to "rotate" your foods, or eat a rotation diet. A rotation diet is a system of controlling food allergies by eating biologically related foods on the same day and then waiting at least four days before eating them again. Such a diet will help those with food allergies in several ways. It may help prevent the development of allergies to new foods. Any food, if eaten repetitively, can cause food allergies in allergy-prone individuals. A rotation diet also helps you detect allergies to foods for which you were not tested and may not have suspected were problems. A rotation diet may enable you to eat foods to which you have a mild or borderline allergy and which you might not tolerate if you ate them often.

---

70 O'Brien., 66, 89-90.

71 O'Brien., 138.

You may need to expand the number of foods you include in your diet to include foods you may have never heard of or eaten so you have a wide variety of foods to rotate. This will give you the best nutrient intake and also prevent you from having a rotation day with, for example, only two or three foods. In that case, you would be eating those few foods in large quantities and may sensitize to them in spite of rotating. To discover less common foods and learn how to prepare them, see *The Ultimate Food Allergy Cookbook and Survival Guide*. This book contains food family tables to explore for new foods, everything you need to know to follow a rotation diet, a diet that can be personalized to fit your allergies, and recipes that fit the diet. For more information about *The Ultimate Food Allergy Cookbook and Survival Guide* see the last pages of this book.

Another option if you are allergic to many foods is to undergo treatment with LDA (low dose allergens) or EPD (enzyme potentiated desensitization). These two treatments are very much alike, with LDA containing allergens that Americans are exposed to and EPD having been developed for the British. (EPD is not available in the United States). The treatments involve taking injections every two months initially and at longer intervals as time progresses. Dietary and environmental controls must be adhered to around the time of your shots. For more about this type of treatment, see pages 48 to 50.

The Gluten-Free Diet

The gluten-free diet is a diet that eliminates one protein, gluten. It was originally developed for people with celiac disease. Although the immunological mechanisms behind celiac disease and food allergies are different, how to implement an elimination diet is the same. The principle behind both diets is to eliminate all sources of foods that cause you problems. See pages 238 to 239 for hidden sources of gluten.

Gluten damages the intestinal lining in people with celiac disease. They must strictly avoid all gluten to allow their intestinal lining to heal and sometimes must also avoid other foods such as dairy products during the initial healing time. After the lining is healed, they must avoid gluten for life to maintain a healthy intestinal lining.

The gluten-free diet eliminates wheat (by all of its names[72]), rye, kamut, spelt, triticale and barley. Until recently, oats were also avoided on the gluten-free diet. Now the "rules" have been liberalized to allow some patients to have ½ cup per day of oats processed under gluten-free conditions after a year of avoidance of gluten. All oats, includ-

---

72 Wheat of various strains or processed in various ways goes by these names: bulgur, couscous, durum, farina, semolina and graham flour. When reading labels, watch for and avoid starch, modified starch, or modified food starch from an unspecified source, dextrin, hydrolyzed vegetable protein, textured vegetable protein, seitan, germ, bran, and grain vinegar. This list is not exhaustive, and wheat derivatives can be hiding in places like the solutions injected into frozen poultry, etc. For information on how to recognize wheat and other common allergens when reading food labels, see pages 238 to 241 of this book.

ing gluten-free oats, contain a protein called avenin which is very similar to gluten and may be a problem for some celiacs. [73]

However, there are many grains and grain alternatives left to eat on a gluten-free diet in addition to ubiquitous rice. They include amaranth, buckwheat, corn, Job's tears, millet, montina, quinoa, sorghum, teff, and wild rice. These can be ground into flour or you can use flours and starches from other plants such as arrowroot, beans, cassava, flax, nuts, peas, potatoes, tapioca, and yucca. This is not an exhaustive list. If you find another flour or grain you would like to try, consult this Celiac Support Association list to see if it is allowed: https://www.csaceliacs.org/grains_and_flours_glossary.jsp .[74] The Celiac Support Association (formerly called the Celiac Sprue Association) is the definitive source for information on the gluten-free diet. To learn more, visit www.csaceliacs.org .

The incidence of celiac disease in the United States has increased four-fold in the last few decades.[75] As with the recent spike in the incidence of food allergies discussed earlier in this chapter, we might wonder why this rapid change occurred. Dr. William Davis, MD thinks it is because wheat ceased being the tall, flexible "amber waves of grain" we sing about and was replaced with high-yielding dwarf wheat during those decades.[76] This is not a GMO strain: it was developed between 1948 and 1980 by intensive hybridization. The yield from this wheat may be ten-fold that of what was common in the mid-20th century, but it cannot survive and thrive without chemical pest control and high-nitrogen chemical fertilization. It has enormous seed heads and stiff short stalks and is easier than the older strains of wheat to harvest and thresh.[77]

Dr. Davis, who is wheat sensitive, did an experiment using himself as the test subject. He obtained some einkorn (see "Sources," page 263), the wild 14-chromosome grain that is the original parent of all wheat, and made bread from it. He also made bread from organic modern 42-chromosome whole wheat. He ground each grain into flour and added only water and yeast to make each grain into a loaf of bread. He ate four ounces of the einkorn bread with no reaction. On another day he ate four ounces of the modern wheat bread and had a reaction that lasted for one and a half days.[78] Dr. Davis wondered what difference between einkorn and modern wheat could have caused the reaction. Therefore, he searched scientific journals for an answer to this question and learned that the types gluten in modern wheat are about 95% from their parent strains of wheat, but 5% of the gluten is different, unique to modern wheat, and not found in the older plants. In one hybridization experiment, fourteen unique new gluten proteins

73 Celiac Support Association. "The Scoop on Oats." https://www.csaceliacs.org/guide_to_oats.jsp
74 Celiac Support Association. "Grains and Flours Glossary: Grains and Flours for Those With Gluten-related Conditions." https://www.csaceliacs.org/grains_and_flours_glossary.jsp
75 Davis, William, MD. *Wheat Belly*. (New York, NY, Rodale, Inc., 2011), 78-79.
76 Davis, 17-18.
77 Davis, 22-24; also Shewry, PR. "Wheat." *Journal Exp Botany* 2009;60(6):1537-53 .
78 Davis, 26-27.

were produced.[79] Additionally, he learned that the quantity of genes in modern wheat that code for gluten types associated with celiac disease is higher than in the wheat we ate fifty years ago.[80]

In recent years, many individuals who test negative for celiac disease have discovered that removing gluten from their diets provides relief from a variety of chronic conditions and symptoms. This has lead to an abundance of gluten-free commercially prepared foods which are usually made with rice. Because of their convenience, these foods are often eaten at every meal. Eating any food every day, including rice, can lead to an allergy to that food. If you have developed intolerance to rice, see *Gluten-Free Without Rice* as described on the last pages of this book.

The Anti-*Candida* Diet

Candida albicans is a yeast that is normally present in our intestines in small numbers. The presence of large amounts can cause a wide range of symptoms. There are drugs than help eradicate *Candida*, but no drug will solve the problem unless you also follow an anti-*Candida* diet. About 25 years ago, I heard Dr. William Crook speak in Boulder, Colorado, and he said, "No amount of Diflucan™ will get rid of yeast if you keep eating sugar."

Diets for *Candida* control vary in their strictness. Initially, you may be required to follow a low-carbohydrate diet that permits unprocessed meat, fish, non-starchy vegetables, nuts and oils in quantities sufficient to satisfy hunger. Some fruits, some starchy vegetables, milk, and non-yeast baked goods may be allowed in very small quantities. As your health improves, you may be able to add more fruit, starchy vegetables and grains. Foods that are strictly prohibited on *Candida* control diets include all sugar and sweeteners (except stevia), processed foods, yeast-containing baked goods, long-aged cheese (farmer's or pot cheese is allowed), vinegar, dried fruit, fruit juices, melons, mushrooms, malted products, coffee, tea, and alcoholic beverages.[81]

The reason for avoiding foods like mushrooms, tea, and coffee is not because these foods will stimulate the growth of *Candida* in your body, but that you may have an allergic cross-reaction to them if you have a *Candida* problem. As your health improves, you may be able to enjoy them occasionally. Sugar does stimulate yeast growth and must be avoided entirely.[82]

---

79 Davis, 25-26; also Song, X; Ni, Z; Yao, Y et al. "Identification of differentially expressed proteins between hybrid and parents in wheat seedling leaves." *Theory Applied Genetics* 2009 Jan;118(2):213-25.

80 Davis, 25-26; also Gao, X; Liu, SW, et al. "High frequency of HMW-GS sequence variation through somatic hybridization between *Agropyron elongatum* and common wheat." *Planta* 2010 Jan;23(2)245-50.

81 Crook, William G., MD. *The Yeast Connection,* 2nd Edition. (Jackson, TN, Professional Books, 1984), 75-78, 95-100.

82 Crook, 94.

A final suggestion for overcoming *Candida* permanently is to have your thyroid function checked and treated correctly. (See pages 54 to 55 for more about correct treatment). Although conventional medicine does not concur, it has long been suspected that there is a connection between thyroid problems and *Candida* overgrowth.[83] I struggled with yeast related intestinal problems for decades and was treated with drugs off-and-on and herbs and diet continuously. I never really felt the problem was solved until I had been on thyroid replacement medication for about a year.

The Specific Carbohydrate Diet

The specific carbohydrate diet (SCD) is the first of three diets presented here whose purpose is controlling the bacterial flora in the intestine. Which of these diets suits a person depends on the type of problem individuals have with their intestinal flora. The SCD was developed to treat inflammatory bowel diseases (IBD) such as ulcerative colitis and Crohn's disease. The GAPS diet below was developed from the SCD to treat autism.

The SCD began its journey from obscurity when Elaine Gottschall's eight year old daughter was on the brink of needing surgery for ulcerative colitis after every kind of medical treatment had failed. Elaine took her to Drs. Sidney and Merrill Haas, who put the girl on a diet that eliminated starch and sugars composed of two single sugar molecules (disaccharides) such as table sugar and lactose in milk. After being on the diet less than two years, she was symptom-free. A few years later she returned to eating starches and sugars in moderation and has been healthy ever since.[84]

The principle behind the SCD is that some people can not digest disaccharides and some starches. These remain in the intestine and fuel the growth of bacteria rather than being absorbed and nourishing the person. Then intestinal bacteria ferment the sugars and starches, and byproducts of bacterial metabolism injure the surface of the small intestine, which increases the inability to digest sugars and starches. It is a vicious cycle. Some of the products of the bacterial fermentation may be absorbed and produce symptoms outside the intestine such as behavioral problems.[85]

There are two kinds of starch in plant foods, amylose and amylopectin. Amylose is chains of single sugars that are broken down into single sugars fairly easily. Amylopectin is a complex branched molecule that is much harder to digest. The SCD permits vegetables that contain mostly amylose and it forbids foods containing amylopectin, including all grains and starchy vegetables.[86]

---

83 Shomon, Mary. "Yeast Overgrowth, Candidiasis, and Thyroid Disease: Is There a Relationship Between Yeast and Your Thyroid?" July 17, 2017.
https://www.verywell.com/candidiasis-yeast-overgrowth-and-thyroid-disease-3231788
84 Gottschall, Elaine, BA, MSc. *Breaking the Vicious Cycle: Intestinal Health Through Diet.* (Baltimore, Ontario, The Kirkton Press, 2000), 1.
85 Gottschall, 17-18.
86 Gottschall, 29-30.

Foods that are absolutely prohibited on the SCD include sugar (sucrose), milk (which contains lactose) and all dairy products except homemade yogurt that has been fermented at least 24 hours to remove the lactose, maltose and isomaltose (in malt and candies), all grains, including non-grain family members like amaranth, buckwheat and quinoa, all types of starch such as tapioca or corn starch, and starchy vegetables. Baked goods, pasta, and products made from grains or starches are not allowed. Some legumes are high in amylopectin and must be avoided. These include garbanzo beans, bean sprouts, soybeans, mungbeans, and fava beans.

The foods permitted on the SCD include unprocessed meats, non-starchy vegetables, some legumes (see exceptions above), fruits that are fresh, frozen, canned or dried without sugar or starch, natural nuts (no starch coating used for roasting), homemade yogurt that has been fermented for at least 24 hours, honey, very dry wine, and weak coffee or tea. For more details about allowed and restricted foods, see *Breaking the Vicious Cycle* or the legal/illegal food list on the SCD website here: http://www.breakingtheviciouscycle.info/legal/listing/ . The SCD is also good for other intestinal diseases. In addition to ulcerative colitis and Crohn's disease, celiac disease that does not respond to a gluten-free diet and irritable bowel syndrome may respond well to the SCD.

The Gut and Psychology Syndrome (GAPS) Diet

The GAPS diet was developed for autistic children by Dr. Natasha Campbell-McBride. She is the mother of an autistic son who recovered from autism after being on the GAPS diet. Her book contains numerous examples of other recovered autistic children.

Autistic children almost always have some kind of digestive problem. When Dr. Campbell-McBride asks parents about their child's stools, it is very rare for them to respond that they are normal.[87]

The GAPS diet was developed from the SCD but has an introductory phase designed to heal the intestine and put the patient on the road to recovery quickly. I tried the GAPS diet when I was making no progress on reducing diarrhea seven weeks after having finished a course of antibiotics. It got me back to normal stools within a week.

The introductory phase of the GAPS diet begins with a diet of bone broth, thoroughly cooked meat used in making the broth, all of the gelatinous tissues and fat from the bones and broth, and the marrow from the bones. She has her patients eat all of the fat because it is highly saturated fat and its short chain fatty acids can be absorbed directly into intestinal cells without needing any digestion first, so it nourishes the intestinal cells quickly and easily to speed their healing. Thoroughly cooked non-starchy vegetables can

---

87 Campbell-McBride, Natasha, MMedSci. *Gut and Psychology Syndrome: Natural Treatment for Autism, Dyspraxia, ADD, Dyslexia, ADHD, Depression, Schizophrenia*, Revised and Expanded Edition. (Cambridge, Medinform Publishing, 2010), 9.

be added to make the broth a soup. Probiotic foods are also in the introductory phase, starting with cultured vegetables. Cultured dairy products are introduced as soon as possible. After the first several days, avocados, ghee and egg yolks are introduced, and then eggs and cooked peeled apples.[88] Finally, the patient moves to the full GAPS diet which includes all of the foods permitted by the SCD.

Dr. Campbell-McBride says that healing the intestine and establishing healthy flora will clear up food allergies. As you can see from the foods on the introductory diet, she is generous with dairy products and eggs. She says that homemade ghee is so pure that her patients, even those with severe dairy allergy, tolerate it.[89] (I made ghee from goat butter and did not tolerate it. I also ate avocado every day for three weeks and began reacting to it). This diet is a good natural treatment for autistic children and is excellent for quick intestinal healing, but if you have food allergies and try this diet, you should be careful and take your allergies more seriously than the GAPS diet does.

The Low FODMAP Diet

The low FODMAP diet is a third diet that aims to control the bacterial flora of the intestine. It was developed to help irritable bowel syndrome. It eliminates several kinds of short-chain carbohydrates and sugar alcohols, and gets its name from the substances it eliminates which are Fermentable Oligosaccharides, Disaccharides, Monosaccharides And Polyols. These substances are poorly absorbed in the small intestine and are fermented by bacteria to produce gas. They can also cause diarrhea by drawing water into the intestine.

Foods may contain one or more of the eliminated carbohydrates, and how much is present of all of them combined in a food determines if that food is acceptable on this diet. Furthermore, there is individual variation in how much of each kind of carbohydrate can be tolerated. Although some foods are to be strictly avoided and there is a list of foods that possibly may be used, there is no list of foods that will be tolerated by everyone on the low FOODMAP diet. Each individual must test foods to determine what he or she can tolerate.

Your Personalized Combination of Diets

In my opinion, all of us should follow the principles of the anti-cancer diet. Some of you may have more than one of the health problems discussed in this chapter, and will also need to follow principles from other diet(s). You may feel that if you combine

88 Campbell-McBride, 142-152.
89 Campbell-McBride, 121.

the "rules" of more than one diet, you will starve, but this is not true. Because food is your best medicine and other treatment may have side effects, may fail, or may not work as well alone as if with good dietary support, you should use a combination diet. Your body will thank you, and you will be happy you made all needed dietary changes as you begin to feel better.

Combining diets is not as hard as it may seem. I will use myself as an example so you can see that it is do-able. I started with an allergy elimination diet. When I developed many more food allergies, I went to a rotation diet. Adding the anti-*Candida* diet to that meant that I used no nutritive sweeteners and no longer ate bread made with yeast. Since I was not eating wheat already, this was not much of a loss.

When I added the rules of the specific carbohydrate diet (SCD), it did seem like a loss. There were no more homemade crackers or starchy foods of any kind. So I made stevia-sweetened cookies out of nut butters (four varieties) and had a baked good to eat every rotation day. My Crohn's disease improved to the point that I have almost forgotten I have it. Using the SCD was well worth doing. After two years on the SCD, starchy foods are allowed occasionally. I do occasionally eat sweet potatoes and eat white potatoes rarely. I no longer miss baked goods at all and don't bother to make the nut butter cookies any more.

The anti-cancer diet was very easy to add. The only dietary change I made was to control my blood sugar better. I no longer eat high-glycemic fruits and instead eat nuts for most snacks. I got a water filter and stopped drinking bottled water unless it is in glass bottles. I now use glass and cellophane for food storage instead of plastic.

When I have an office visit with the oncologist, I usually have to wait a while. Seeing the other patients in the multi-doctor waiting room is disturbing. Often I am the only patient with abundant hair, good facial color, always-open eyes, and normal weight. The anti-cancer diet is very much worth following because it may give me a better chance of never being in the same condition as the other patients in the waiting room. In addition, the better blood sugar control has eliminated ever feeling ravenous hunger.

Adding the circadian rhythm diet meant eating fruit later in the day and adding the allergy versions of the rhythmic shakes to my breakfasts of game meat and vegetables. The shakes are delicious and give me more energy. The only "problem" is that I sometimes neglect to keep up with making a supply of frozen seed milk (the base ingredient of the shakes). Then I either skip my shake for the day or get cooking right away. Cooking right away is well worth it, but I really should keep a good supply of seed milk at all times. However, perfect discipline is unrealistic, so cut yourself some slack.

Once you reach the point of feeling healthy, dietary changes are worth the time and effort you've put into them. Go for it! You'll be glad you did.

Why You Must Help Yourself

Up to this point, the focus of this book has been on nutrition and lifestyle practices that will enable us optimize our health. "What to do" has been the subject, and now we move to considering what not to do.

The medical system is an influence on our health that we should use carefully and with caution. It is essential that we be fully informed when making medical decisions, including knowing the potential benefits, possible side effects, and other options we may have for treatment. This chapter is a primer in learning how to weigh all factors when making decisions about using common medical treatments. It is not exhaustive coverage of the subject, does not include the vast majority of treatments, and will not be current for very long. If you are faced with a medical decision, *you must help yourself* by thoroughly researching your options. You need to protect yourself.

Reasons why *you* must help yourself:

1. Others may not protect you as well you can. The medical system as a whole does not exist to help you with your health[1], although some individual medical professionals are devoted to helping others. Many of them honestly believe that drugs and surgery are the best treatments and nearly all of them know little or nothing about nutritional and natural options. Medical professionals may help you medically, family members and friends can help you with researching medical decisions, cooking, etc., but *you* must take charge.

2. No one else can carry out certain advice, such as using breathing techniques and managing your peace of mind.

3. The feeling of helplessness has a detrimental effect on health. You escape helplessness when you realize that *you* are in charge and can be doing any number of things to help yourself.

Following the nutritional and lifestyle advice in this book which applies to you will give you the best chance of optimizing your health. Do read the references to studies, etc. so you know this advice has as much or more scientific relevance as drugs and conventional treatments. However, taking charge and realizing *you are not helpless* or at the mercy of the system is the most basic of the options for improving your health. If you take charge and do anything to help yourself, you will banish the feeling of helplessness and increase your chances of a good outcome. The study discussed in the next paragraph demonstrates how amazingly beneficial non-medical help can be.

---

1 Rosenthal, Elizabeth, MD. *An American Sickness: How Healthcare Became Big Business and How You Can Take It Back.* (New York, NY, Penguin Press, 2017),1. In the first paragraph of the book Rosenthal writes, "In the past quarter century, the American medical system has stopped focusing on health or even science. Instead it attends more or less single-mindedly to its own profits."

Psychiatrist David Spiegel, MD, was upset with those who attributed cancer to psychological problems, feeling that this placed a burden of guilt on patients for possibly causing their own cancer. He devised a study to prove that this was not true. For the study, groups of eight to ten women with metastatic breast cancer met weekly in support groups. They were compared with women who had the same diagnoses and treatments but did not attend support groups. The women who attended the groups confronted their fear, expressed their feelings, and developed close relationships. They also experienced significantly less anxiety, depression, and pain than the women in the control group.[2]

Dr. Spiegel experienced a surprise when he followed up with these women about ten years after they'd been diagnosed with cancer and participated in the support groups. Three of the fifty women who attended the groups answered the phone themselves when he called. No women in the control group had survived that long. The support group women who did not survive lived twice as long as the control group women. There was even a difference between those who went to the support group regularly versus sporadically. The more often a woman attended, the longer she lived. Dr. Spiegel's study proved that doing something to help yourself, such as attending a support group, increased survival time.[3] (Concerning the question this study was designed to answer, Dr. Servan-Schreiber reports that no psychological factor starts the cancer process, but such factors can influence its progression.[4])

After the publication of this study, a prospective study was done on the impact of the feeling of helplessness on mortality of young men in an area of Finland where young men had an excessively high rate of mortality, especially from cardiac disease. Men who answered both study questions to indicate that they felt helpless had three times the mortality rate six years later and also developed 160% more fatal cancers than those who did not feel helpless.[5] Furthermore, a number of studies have shown that women with breast cancer who were in good psychological condition had NK (natural killer) cells that were much more active than the NK cells of women who felt persistent discouragement or helplessness.[6]

Although I have not seen information on feelings of helplessness with other medical conditions, I remember a time when I was facing seemingly unsolvable intestinal dysbiosis. I decided to research every possible natural treatment and follow as many

---

2 Servan-Schreiber, David, MD, PhD. *AntiCancer: A New Way of Life*. (New York: Penguin Group, Inc., 2009), 155. Also Spiegel, D., J.R. Bloom, and I. Yalom. "Group Support for Patients with Metastatic Cancer, a Randomized Outcome Study." *Archives of General Psychiatry* 38:5. 1981:527-533.

3 Servan-Schreiber, 156. Also Spiegel, D, et al., "Effect of Psychosocial Treatment of Survival of Patients with Metastatic Breast Cancer." *Lancet*. 2:8673. Nov. 18, 1989: 1209-1210.

4 Servan-Schreiber, 147.

5 Servan-Schreiber, 156-157.

6 Servan-Schreiber, 159.

treatments as I could. This activity immediately improved my attitude, and progress on eradicating the dysbiosis[7] also improved. I also learned not to be too upset about things like stool test results and accept the fact that mine would probably never be perfect.

Long before this, I had worked as a medical technologist with a woman whose husband was a medical student. One day she walked into the lab incensed because he had been told, "Treat the patient, not the lab." She said, "No wonder nobody listens to us!" However, he had been given good advice. How you feel as a whole person, physically and mentally, is what counts, more than any test results. Learn to take test results and some of what medical professionals tell you with a grain of salt. Having a positive attitude and defusing the feeling of helplessness are two of the best and most essential things you can do to help yourself.

The major focus of our current medical system as a whole is profit.[8] Helping patients is a lower priority for the system. Some individual medical professionals want to help and are well intentioned, but medical education and the medical profession as a whole are based on pharmaceutical treatments that mostly manage rather than cure diseases. Nutrition education is not taught in most medical schools and barely touched on in residency programs.[9] Natural and nutritional health information will come from your family and friends, the internet or the library because the professionals rarely know about these things.

The rest of this chapter is about "help" you might receive from the medical system. Some of the more commonly prescribed drugs and medical treatments carry risks that you should be aware of so you can make informed decisions about using them. This section also contains information about natural remedies that you might try using with or instead of conventional treatment. I don't want you to get bogged down in negativity, so I suggest that you glance at the headings and only read the sections that apply to you.

Mosquito repellents

This section applies to everyone because I suspect that none of us has escaped mosquito bites. The standard way to prevent mosquito bites is to apply a mosquito repellent containing DEET (diethylmetatoluamide) which was originally developed as a pesticide.[10] A study done on Everglades National Park employees in the 1980s reported that one-fourth of the employees using repellents had adverse effects such as rashes, skin irritation, numb or burning lips, nausea, headaches, dizziness and difficulty concentrating.[11]

---

7 For more information about dysbiosis see http://www.food-allergy.org/root3.html .
8 Rosenthal, 1.
9 Blaylock, Russell L., MD. *Natural Strategies for Cancer Patients.* (New York: Kensington Publishing Corp., 2003), 128.
10 Wikipedia article on DEET. https://en.wikipedia.org/wiki/DEET
11 *Scientific American*, DEET. www.scientificamerican.com/articles-is-it-true-that-deet.

Many years ago a nurse told me about a non-toxic, inexpensive alternative to DEET. One to two hours before you expect to encounter mosquitoes, take 100 mg of vitamin B-1 (thiamine) and you will not be bitten. Mosquitoes dislike the smell of the vitamin emerging from the skin. One 100-mg tablet of B-1 is good for the whole day unless the day is extremely long. When I expected to be gardening most evenings last summer, I took a B-1 tablet every morning and never had a bite. However, this summer I got a bite at 9 pm when I had taken B-1 at 6 am. I moved taking vitamin B-1 to lunchtime and was not bitten again.

If you are going to take B-1 daily for an extended period of time, be sure you also take a multiple vitamin or multi-B supplement daily so your B vitamins do not get out of balance. If B-1 seems to not be working for you, smell the tablets. I once had a bottle of B-1 that did not work, bought another brand, and when I opened the new bottle I could smell the slightly-unpleasant odor of B-1. Make sure each new bottle of vitamin B-1 has the B-vitamin odor that mosquitoes dislike.

Cancer Treatments

Like most doctors, oncologists rarely receive training in nutrition. Instead they learn about radiotherapy and pharmaceuticals including the latest cancer drugs. However, in spite of what we hear about new drugs and "cures," there has been little change in the death rate for the major cancers in the last thirty years. All that has changed is that earlier diagnosis is possible due to better screening, meaning that patients may live a few years longer. This may take some patients past the five-year survival mark, and five years is the point at which one is counted as a "survivor."[12] Yet, although there has been progress in nutritional treatment for cancer, most oncologists are unaware of it and/or refuse to believe it. They often tell patients to discontinue all supplements during chemotherapy because they might interfere with the effectiveness of the cancer treatment. Actually, the opposite is true. Most oncologists do not even tell their patients that they can improve the outcome of their treatment by eating more fruits and vegetables.[13] (I searched to find an oncologist who sounded more holistic, and she does encourage her patients to improve their outcomes with diet).

There is ongoing data manipulation to convince the public that chemotherapy is more effective now than it was in the past. Improved early detection of cancer makes it seem as if patients are living longer, and studies in which current data is compared to older studies give the impression that the increased survival time is due to new treatments. Another misleading strategy is to compare high-dose to low-dose use of a chemotherapeutic drug. The high-dose patients live longer because they are the patients who are in better shape to begin with. (The sickest patients may not tolerate the toxicity of

12 Blaylock, 129-130.
13 Blaylock, 132-133

the high dose). Furthermore, if a patient is started on the high dose and must drop down on dosage or drop out of the study, that patient is not counted. [14]

The decision about what type of treatment to pursue after the diagnosis of cancer is very personal, unique to each individual. I cannot and do not want to appear to be telling you what to do. In the first chapter of this book I wrote about agreeing to take chemotherapy, if needed, in reaction to my husband's despair, so I realize that personal circumstances are factors in the decision. However, I would urge you to choose your oncologist carefully. Be sure he or she is willing to let you pursue natural strategies along with conventional treatments. In addition, check the track record of any doctor you are considering. There are doctors who over-treat, and may actually seem to eradicate the cancer, but the patient then dies of side effects like heart failure.[15] Although there is always a feeling of urgency to get started on treatment, you would do well to take a little time and choose your oncologist wisely.

Chemotherapy is very effective in saving lives with some kinds of cancers. For example, there is a greater than 90% cure rate for children with T-cell acute lymphocytic leukemia (ALL) when treated with chemotherapy. Our great-nephew took a three and one half year course of chemotherapy for ALL and is doing very well. In the case of cancers which have a high cure rate from chemotherapy, if your personal circumstances make it reasonable, you might consider taking it. **There are other types of cancer, often solid tumor cancers, for which chemotherapy is not likely to save your life.** Oncologists speak of chemotherapy bringing about "tumor response." This means the tumor shrinks or stops growing. It may or may not buy you a little time, but it is not a cure, although it might be implied that it could be.[16]

Chemotherapy is toxic; the hope is that it is more toxic to dividing cancer cells than it is to normal cells. Patients who are not well nourished are more likely to suffer toxic effects and are more likely to suffer a relapse of the cancer later on. [17]

Chemotherapy may be given when the lymph nodes are clear and there is no indication that the cancer has spread. A friend who had a mastectomy was told by her oncologist that she needed to have a genetic test, and if she was at high risk for cancer genetically, should take chemotherapy. (I suggested that she insist on having a PET scan that showed evidence of metastasis before considering chemotherapy). Thankfully, her genetic tests results were good. It made no sense for her to take chemotherapy without some indication of spread because a study showed that breast cancer patients who were given chemotherapy had earlier relapses of their cancer than women given hormone

---

14 Blaylock, 75-76.

15 Quillin, Patrick, PhD, RD, CNS. *Beating Cancer with Nutrition*, (Carlsbad, CA,, Nutrition Times Press, 2005), 16, 26.

16 Blaylock, 73-74.

17 Blaylock, 77.

therapy alone.[18] Dr. Russell Blaylock reports that it is his clinical impression, backed up by medical literature dating back to 1987, that chemotherapy makes cancer more aggressive and likely to metastasize.[19] When I agreed to take chemotherapy if needed because of my husband's despair, I did not have the information in this paragraph. Now I would refuse to take chemotherapy no matter what the circumstances.

Chemotherapy can cause complications and side effects in every and any part of the body, some of **which can be lessened with nutritional support.** (See pages 82 to 106 of *Natural Strategies for Cancer* for more about this). Since a primary audience for this book is people with allergies, I must tell you that one of chemotherapy's side effects can be causing food allergies, even in previously non-allergic people. Chemotherapy kills the rapidly dividing cells that line the intestine, and can cause leaking of whole or partially digested food proteins into the bloodstream, thus inducing new food allergies. This diverts an already over-burdened immune system away from the more important job of fighting cancer cells. Chemotherapy can also cause an overgrowth of *Candida albicans* in the intestine or other parts of the body. Intestinal yeast can potentially lead to more or worsening food allergies.[20] Radiotherapy to the abdominal area also damages the intestinal lining, leading to food allergies, and also causes intestinal overgrowth with *Candida albicans*.[21]

Although they are much less problematic than chemotherapy or radiotherapy, the decision to take hormone drugs for reproductive cancers should be considered carefully before you begin treatment. My cousin suffered a complex tibial plateau fracture after being on hormone drugs for breast cancer for a short time. Several months later she broke her pelvis in a fall that was minor enough that got up from it and didn't get an X-ray until the next day. After the first fracture, she was given a bone density test that showed osteopenia. I told her that she should have her vitamin D blood level checked and get on the *correct* dose of vitamin D *for her*, plus take not just calcium, but magnesium and critical bone-building trace minerals and vitamins.[22] See the PDF *20 Key Nutrients For Bone Health* footnoted here for more about what nutrients are needed and "Sources," page 271, for a hypoallergenic bone supplement.

Although my breast cancer was hormone receptor negative and would not be influenced by hormone drugs, my oncologist discussed them with me so I would know all the options. She said if I were to take the drugs, they would not prevent a recurrence of the same cancer, but could prevent a new breast cancer. She also told me that hormone

---

18 Blaylock, 78. Also Houston, S.J. 'The Influence of Adjuvant Chemotherapy on Outcome After Relapse in Patients with Breast Cancer." Proc Ann Meet ASCO 11: A108, 1992.

19 Blaylock, 78-79. Also McMillan, T.J. and I.R. Hart. "Can Cancer Chemotherapy Enhance Malignant Behavior of Tumors?" *Cancer and Metastasis*. Rev 6:503-520, 1987.

20 Blaylock, 97.

21 Blaylock, 116.

22 Brown, Susan E. PhD. 20 Key Nutrients For Bone Health. http://www.betterbones.com/wp-content/uploads/2016/11/20keybonenutrients.pdf

drugs can cause ovarian cancer. We agreed that I would skip the drugs and practice every possible natural strategy instead.

Allergy Drugs

The most profitable drugs for allergies have historically been asthma inhalers with their continually rising prices (at least until 2016 when the price of the life-saving Epi-Pen™ for anaphylaxis was raised 600%!) There is a captive audience for inhalers because asthma can be life-threatening and the feeling of being unable to breathe is frightening. People will pay whatever the drug companies demand in order to be able to breathe. However, there are dark secrets about asthma inhalers which I learned the hard way.

I had asthma when I was young but outgrew it and had no trouble with it for over 40 years until viral pneumonia and undetected mold in our house brought it back. I was treated with inhalers which helped for a few days and then became ineffective. Then I was put on a series of more and more potent inhalers, none of which really worked. When I took an LDA shot (see page 49 for more about this treatment), I had to avoid inhalers as part of the protocol. The evening of my first day without them, I felt as if a tremendous allergy burden had been lifted. The only change I had made, and had not made with previous shots, was eliminating the inhalers. I Googled "allergy to asthma inhalers" and read the experiences of bloggers who had problems with inhalers. One mother wrote about her daughter being helped by Albuterol™ administered by a nebu-lizer[23] at home, but whenever she used an Albuterol™ inhaler when they were out, she got much worse. They had to rush home to stop her reaction by using the same drug with a nebulizer. Another blog told of a man whose asthma had been getting worse and his inhalers were ineffective. Then he used an old inhaler that had been stored in an exercise bag in his hot car, and it worked like magic. See "Sources" page 272 for where online to read these and other stories of life-threatening reactions to asthma inhalers in the last several years.

In January, 2009, the FDA banned the propellant which had been used in asthma inhalers for many years ostensibly because it might affect the ozone layer adversely. It was replaced with hydrofluroalkane (HFA) in all propellant activated asthma inhalers and nasal sprays. The well-kept secret of asthma inhalers is that HFA is made with corn-derived ethanol. The official position is that there is not enough corn or yeast residue in HFA to cause problems. This may be true for most people, but some corn and/or yeast sensitive patients do react to the propellant. Dry powder inhalers contain lactose and traces of milk protein, so milk-allergic patients cannot use them. The only safe way to administer inhaled medications to some asthma patients is with a nebulizer.

---

23 A nebulizer is a device that turns the asthma drug solution into an aerosol which the patient then inhales for five to ten minutes.

A "side effect" of the FDA mandated change in propellants is that there likely will be no generic inhalers for twenty years after the 2009 propellant change which caused all asthma inhalers to be reclassified as new drugs. (Twenty years is how long some of the patents on the new inhalers will be in effect). An online *Consumer Reports* article found that the price of non-generic inhalers nearly doubled in the first three years after the propellant change.[24] Although the inhaled steroid drug I used was generic (because it was taken with a nebulizer and did not contain the new propellant) and had been around for decades, its cost was over $500 for a month's supply without insurance, and it cost about $120 per month with insurance.

In 2013, *New York Times* writer Elizabeth Rosenthal wrote about the massive hikes in the price of asthma inhalers. The fact that the FDA would not have been forced by the CFC regulations to change the propellant came to light. However, the drug companies spent a tremendous amount of money lobbying for the change so they could have new patents and a free hand in raising prices for a long time.[25] Rather than becoming even more negative here, I will let you read the articles footnoted online.

I am not advising anyone to discard their inhalers because that could create a potentially life threatening risk. However, I think everyone should know about the natural treatments for asthma that may reduce or eliminate dependence on inhalers. There are effective natural bronchodilators that are free. One is nitric oxide (NO) which is made in the paranasal sinuses and is in every breath taken through your nose.[26] A second and more important natural bronchodilator is carbon dioxide (CO_2). Asthmatics lack these for two reasons: (1) many breathe mostly through their mouths, and (2) asthmatics breathe a much higher volume of air per minute, up to five or six times as much as normal people. This lowers the CO_2 level in their blood and the alveoli of their lungs which reduces the ability of hemoglobin to release oxygen into the tissues where it is needed. Over-breathing also resets the CO_2 trigger that tells us when to breathe to a lower level, which perpetuates the vicious cycle of over-breathing, bronchoconstriction and asthma.[27] The cycle can be broken by practicing the Buteyko breathing method. It is not a quick fix and requires work, discipline, and commitment, but it is worth the effort to avoid the unpleasant side effects and expense of bronchodilator drugs, which you should need less as you make progress with the method. Studies in Australia and New Zealand

---

24 Inhaled Steroids, *Consumer Reports.* https://www.consumerreports.org/health/resources/pdf/best-buy-drugs/Inhaled SteroidsFINAL.pdf, page 6.

25 Rosenthal, Elizabeth. "The Soaring Cost of a Simple Breath." *New York Times*, October 13. 2013 http://www.nytimes.com/2013/10/13/us/the-soaring-cost-of-a-simple-breath.html?pagewanted=all& r=0 Also see http://www.motherjones.com/kevin-drum/2013/10/heres-why-your-asthma-inhaler-costs-so-damn-much

26 Cardell, Lars Olaf. The Paranasal Sinuses and a Unique Role in Airway Nitric Oxide Production? *American Journal of Respiratory and Critical Care Medicine,*166:2 (202) pp.131-132.

27 McKeown, Patrick, MA, H Dip. *Asthma-Free Naturally.* (San Francisco, CA, Conari Press 2008), 20-21.

found that after three months of using Buteyko breathing, patients used reliever inhalers 90% less often and used 50% less inhaled steroids.[28] When patients using Buteyko breathing become symptom-free and the set-point of the CO_2 trigger reaches a high enough level, under a doctor's supervision, the amount of inhaled steroids can slowly and gradually be reduced, possibly eliminating the need for all inhalers.[29]

In *The Allergy Solution*, Dr. Leo Galland tells about a respiratory therapist who got asthma. When he told her about Buteyko breathing, it made wonderful sense to her, and she wondered why, as a respiratory therapist, she had never heard of it.[30] That is something we might wonder about every alternative to a Big Pharma high-profit-making drug in this chapter and alternatives for some conventional treatments.

An exhaustive discussion of the Buteyko breathing method is beyond the scope of this book. However, you can read more about it and the natural bronchodilator CO_2 on pages 70 to 73. Also see page 273 of "Sources" for how to get books, a CD and a DVD that you can use to learn this technique and for sources of more information about the Buteyko breathing method. See pages 246 to 248 for my experiences with Buteyko breathing.

Allergy Shots

With conventional allergy shots, patients are injected with gradually increasing amount of extracts of the pollens, dust, molds, etc. to which they are allergic. Individuals make IgG antibodies to the extracts, which compete with the IgE antibodies involved in allergic reactions, thus offering some protection from reactions.

I took allergy shots from age 10 to 39, and although they did help some, they did not eliminate my inhalant allergy problem. They also are not effective for and thus are not used for food allergies. Since there is a risk of anaphylaxis after a conventional allergy shot is given, shots must be given in a doctor's office where the patient is observed for a half hour after the shot.

In the 1960s, a new type of allergy shots was developed in England. It then was used in the United States in the 1990s through 2001 and was called EPD for Enzyme Potentiated Desensitization. This treatment employs very low doses of allergens and many more allergens than are in conventional shots. The American version of EPD which is currently used in the United States is called LDA (Low Dose Allergens). These shots are effective for food allergies and chemical sensitivities as well as inhalant allergies. They cover essentially all foods and everything an individual might breathe. They are very effective for inhalant allergies, which may take just a few shots to eliminate. My hayfever went from "I hate spring" to nonexistent at twenty days after my first EPD shot. The

---

28 McKeown. *Asthma-Free Naturally*, 18.

29McKeown, Patrick, MA, H Dip. *Close Your Mouth*. (Loughwell, Buteyko Books, 2004), 88.

30 Galland, Leo, MD. *The Allergy Solution*. (Carlsbad, CA, Hay House, Inc., 2016), 231.

response for food allergies and chemical sensitivities can take up to two years, but it is worth the extra time and work.

With EPD and LDA, all of the patient's problems are treated at once, so an improvement in general health should occur. Because LDA exploits a natural phenomenon, it can be diverted by high-dose exposures to allergens at the time of the injection and for three weeks afterwards while the lymphocytes induced by the treatment are maturing. Therefore, patients must exercise strict control of their environmental and dietary exposures to allergens as well as avoiding many medications at the time of their treatments and for up to three weeks after a treatment.[31] For this reason, LDA has the reputation of being an ordeal to take. Indeed, it does involve much participation on the part of the patient. If you do not have chemical sensitivities or major inhalant allergies and dietary manipulation is sufficient to solve your problems with food allergies, you may want to work with your diet rather than taking LDA.

LDA injections are usually taken at two month intervals initially. As the patient progresses, the interval between injections is gradually extended until they are taken at intervals of a year or more. In my opinion, LDA comes closer to a cure for allergies than any other treatment, and for some people it really is a cure. My son Joel is one of those people. He started EPD at age 11. Since pre-adolescent children respond more quickly than adults, his eczema from food allergies cleared up ten days after his first shot. Two weeks later, when he was allowed to try his problem foods, he could eat everything without the eczema returning. It returned about five weeks later when it was almost time for another shot. In a few years he reached the point that one shot a year was enough. He did things he would not have done as easily with food allergies like attend college and graduate school far from home and travel for his job. He is now in his 30s and takes one shot a year. However, to be realistic, patients with very severe food allergies and dysbiosis may not have the experience he did. I still don't eat "normally," but I have plenty to eat and a very nutritious diet that may have contributed to my breast cancer not spreading. I started EPD because I literally did not have any safe foods to eat. Considering how far I have come, it has been worthwhile to take this treatment.

So why have you never heard of LDA? Part of the reason is that those who give it keep a low profile. EPD was used in the United States in the 1990s as part of an Investigational Review Board study. When the IRB expired, the use of EPD continued for a year or two. Then the political climate changed and in 2001 the FDA shut down EPD. It was on the FDA's import alert list so it could not be brought into the country under the "compassionate use" designation for use by an individual, a provision which is allowed for many other treatments, drugs and products.

Aside – Here is an interesting tidbit of information about import alert. The herb stevia was on the import alert list in the 1990s. Now it is sold as a supplement rather

---

31 Shrader, W.A., MD. *Low Dose Allergen Immunotherapy Patient Instruction Booklet.* 8th Edition, May, 2014, 18, 20, 38.

than a sweetener. It has a record of hundreds of years of safe use as a natural non-caloric sweetener in South America and Japan. Could putting a safe herb on import alert have been due to fear of competition with aspartame?

After the FDA shut-down of EPD, LDA was developed. As an American-made product, using the same type of allergen extracts as in conventional allergy shots, it is legal, but the FDA has harassed the makers of LDA to the point that the first one quit. Considering the constraints of the protocol that must be followed at shot time, I can't realistically see that it can be that much of a threat to Big Pharma, but....

For more information about LDA visit www.drshrader.com, www.food-allergy.org/epd, and see *The Low Dose Immunotherapy Handbook* as described on the last pages of this book.

Bone "Building" Drugs

Our bodies continually remodel our bones to keep them strong. Bone cells called osteoclasts resorb old bone, and osteoblasts replace these areas with new bone. Drugs that are given for osteoporosis, such as Fosamax,™ Actonel,™ Boniva,™ Reclast,™ and Prolia™ suppress the activity of osteoclasts, so resorbtion of the bone doesn't occur. Although this makes bones look denser on bone density tests, unfortunately the normal remodeling of the bone does not occur. As time goes by, the bone becomes composed of more and more old, brittle, worn out bone. **Taking these drugs actually increases your risk of fractures, the problem they are supposed to prevent.** These fractures often occur with no injury that would cause a fracture, just during normal use.[32]

Fosamax™ has also been linked to **esophageal cancer.** One bone building drug, Forteo,™ stimulates osteoblasts, so although it really does build bone, the stimulus can result in osteosarcoma, a form of **bone cancer,** in patients who take it. [33]

One side effect of biophosphonate bone-building drugs is that if a tooth is extracted, the extraction cavity might not heal, and the **jaw bone may die** (osteonecrosis), leading to infection and exposed bone. Even with extensive dental surgery, the condition may be painful for the rest of one's life.[34] The only action taken was that these drugs currently carry a black box warning which says that they may cause osteonecrosis of the jaw.

Natural treatments for osteopenia and osteoporosis include participating in a weight-bearing exercise such as walking and making sure blood vitamin D levels are high enough, namely, at least above 50 ng/ml, not the low amount considered normal on most lab tests. Individuals also should take a complete supplement designed for these

---

32 Simpson, Lani. Fractures Caused by Osteoporosis Drugs? Is Anyone Listening? http://www.lanisimpson.com/blog/fractures-caused-by-osteoporosis-drugs-is-anyone-listening)

33 The Top 5 Reasons You Should Never Take Osteoporosis Drugs https://saveourbones.com/top-5-reasons-why-you-should-never-take-osteoporosis-drugs/

34 Roberts, Barbara H., MD. *The Truth About Statins.* (New York, NY, Pocket Books, Simon & Schuster, 2012), 159-160.

conditions such as a supplement which contains calcium, magnesium, critical bone-building trace minerals such as chromium, boron, manganese, and silica, and vitamins A, D, B6, B12 and folic acid. For more information on nutrition for your bones, see the PDF *20 Key Nutrients For Bone Health* (http://www.betterbones.com/wp-content/uploads/2016/11/20keybonenutrients.pdf). See "Sources," page 271, for a hypoallergenic bone supplement that contains a broad spectrum of needed nutrients.

Proton Pump Inhibitor Drugs

Everyone, but especially those prone to food allergies, should be wary of taking proton-pump inhibitor (PPI) drugs, or stomach acid suppressing drugs such as Nexium™, Prilosec™, and Prevacid™. Stomach acid is essential for proper digestion of food. Without it, partially digested food ferments in the intestine. This leads to leakage of food fragments into the bloodstream thus contributing to food allergies.[35]

Stomach acid is essential for proper digestion and absorption of food. Since minerals are especially difficult to absorb without sufficient stomach acid, suppressing stomach acid can lead to nutritional deficiencies. **PPI users are more likely to have bone fractures due to reduced absorption of calcium and other minerals**. There is a higher incidence of **pneumonia** and other infectious diseases among those taking PPIs. This is because stomach acid is the first line of defense against bacteria entering our bodies by way of the digestive system. These drugs also lead to increased risk of heart problems, kidney disease, and dementia.[36]

Two of the more serious side effects of PPIs have been reported in the *Journal of the American Medical Association*. A data analysis study was done on elderly people who were initially free of dementia. After seven years, those who had taken PPIs were 52% more likely to have developed **dementia** than those who did not take PPIs.[37] Chronic **kidney disease** also increased 20 to 50% with PPI use. The incidence was higher in those who took PPIs twice daily than those who took them once daily.[38]

PPIs are frequently prescribed for gastro-esophageal reflux disorder (GERD) which occurs when the irritating contents of the stomach enter the esophagus. Sufficient stom-

---

35 Kresser, Kris. Proton Pump Inhibitors: So Dangerous That Prescriptions Border on Being Criminal. June 14, 2016. https://www.sott.net/article/320501-Proton-Pump-Inhibitors-So-dangerous-that-prescriptions-border-on-being-criminal

36 Kresser, Kris. Proton Pump Inhibitors: So Dangerous That Prescriptions Border on Being Criminal. June 14, 2016. https://www.sott.net/article/320501-Proton-Pump-Inhibitors-So-dangerous-that-prescriptions-border-on-being-criminal

37 Gomm, W., Von Holt, K., et al. "Association of Proton Pump Inhibitors With Risk of Dementia: A Pharmacoepidemiological Claims Data Analysis." *JAMA Neurology*, 2016 Apr;73(4):410-6. doi: 10.1001/jamaneurol.2015.4791.

38Lazarus, B, Chen, Y, et. al. "Proton Pump Inhibitor Use and the Risk of Chronic Kidney Disease." *JAMA Internal Medicine.* 2016 Feb;176(2):238-46. doi: 10.1001/jamainternmed.2015.7193.

ach acid is necessary to signal the pyloric valve between the stomach and the esophagus to close. What is needed for GERD is not acid-suppressing drugs, but a hydrochloric acid supplement taken with every meal and snack so the pyloric valve closes well.

Heartburn commonly occurs when we age because of the decline in the ability to make enough hydrochloric acid (HCl) after a big meal when it is most needed. Since the signal to "make acid" persists for hours, we end up with too much stomach acid several hours later, often in the middle of the night. Although it seems counterintuitive, the natural treatment for heartburn is to take hydrochloric acid with meals to cause the pyloric valve to close, facilitate digestion, and turn off the "make acid" signal that causes secretion of HCl much later, thus producing heartburn.

Consult your holistic medical practitioner about whether and how you should take hydrochloric acid supplements. This is not intended to be advice but rather is an account of how I started taking HCl. I had several stool tests for dysbiosis with undigested food in them and was not making progress. Therefore, I was instructed to take a hydrochloric acid supplement to see if it would help the dysbiosis. I was told to start with one 300 mg tablet per meal for a few days. Then I was to increase to two tablets per meal for a few days and to continue increasing to six tablets. If I felt any burning sensation in my stomach after meals, I was to decrease the dosage to the previous level and stay there. I took six tablets with every meal, and smaller amounts with snacks, for several years. As my health improved, my ability to make stomach acid improved, and I began to notice a burning sensation after meals. Therefore I gradually decreased the dosage. When my health became worse again recently I had to return to six tablets per meal. Other supplements such as slippery elm can increase comfort while in the process of adding HCl, or if you forget to take sufficient HCl. Slippery elm is most effective when taken as the powder mixed into water so it can coat the esophagus.

Over-the-Counter Pain Medications

Over-the-counter pain medications such as nonsteroidal anti-inflammatory drugs (NSAIDS) and acetaminophen (Tylenol™) can be problematic for individuals with food allergies or liver problems. The NSAIDS include aspirin, ibuprofen (Motrin™, Advil™), celecoxib (Celebrex™), naproxen (Aleve™), the prescription arthritis drug indomethacin (Indocin™), and others. Although most are sold without a prescription, these medications can harm some people.

A single dose of aspirin or other NSAIDs can increase intestinal permeability tremendously in individuals with possibly compromised intestinal health. This includes people with food allergies as well as intestinal diseases such as Crohn's disease, other inflammatory bowel disease (IBD) or irritable bowel syndrome (IBS). This increased permeability can lead to worsening food allergies especially if the drug is taken long-term.[39] The *Physician's Desk Reference* warns about the possibility of gastrointestinal bleeding, ulceration and perforation when using nonsteroidal anti-inflammatory drugs and reports that a NSAID arthritis drug can lead to the development of inflammatory bowel disease.[40] Dr. W. A. Shrader, Jr. says that all nonsteroidal anti-inflammatory drugs cause some degree of mucosal atrophy in the intestine.[41]

Acetaminophen (Tylenol™) also can be problematic because the liver can be challenged by the task of detoxifying it. It should be avoided by those with liver disease or who consume alcohol.[42]

What can we do for pain instead of using drugs? The most effective treatment is to treat the problem causing pain. Dr. Leo Galland reports that having patients avoid all foods to which they are allergic can eliminate arthritis pain and the need for drugs.[43] For other types of joint and muscle pain, seek treatment from a physical therapist who pays attention to the whole body, not just the painful area. Sometimes postural problems or issues with neighboring joints can affect the painful area even if the original problem was due to an injury. Then diligently do the exercises the therapist prescribes.

There are many natural remedies for pain; this list is not exhaustive. For sore muscles or injuries, application of cold (initially) or heat can help. A half-hour soak in a bathtub of warm water with one cup of Epsom salts relaxes achy muscles and soothes joints. Herbal remedies taken regularly, such as feverfew for migraine headaches, can reduce dependence on drugs. Acupuncture is also effective for pain.

I have found homeopathic arnica to be very effective. Before my mastectomy, I told a nutritionist about my desire to avoid drugs. She told me that when she had surgery, she had her family slip her arnica beginning as soon as possible after surgery. She said arnica could be used as often as every half hour and then less frequently when the pain did not return in a half hour. She also told me what drug to ask for instead of the more "potent" narcotics if needed. (It wasn't needed). I did very well with the arnica, an intravenous form of ibuprofen which was started at the conclusion of the surgery and continued through my twenty-two hour hospital stay, and Tylenol for about two weeks at home. Since then I have used arnica for muscle and joint pain and arthritis.

Homeopathic remedies come in different strengths depending on how they are diluted; which strength is needed may vary between individuals and with the condition

---

39 Galland, Leo, MD. "Leaky Gut Syndromes," http://mdheal.org/leakygut.htm .
Also an interview with Leo Galland, MD by Marjorie H. Jones, RN., "Leaky Gut – What Is It? What Factors Cause It? What Can Be Done?" *Mastering Food Allergies Newsletter,* #86, July/August 1995, 4.
Also Jenkins, R.T., et al.," Increased intestinal permeability in patients with rheumatoid arthritis: a side-effect of oral nonsteroidal anti-inflammatory drug therapy?" *Br J Rheumatol,* 1987.26(2): 103-7.
40 1996 *Physician's Desk Reference,* 817, 862, 1619, 1681, 2579. (On page 1681, it says of indomethacin, "The development of ulcerative colitis and regional ileitis have been reported to occur rarely.")
41 Personal communication from W. A. Shrader, Jr., MD, April, 1997.
42 "Tylenol™ Precautions,"http://www.webmd.com/drugs/2/drug-7076/tylenol-oral/details#precautions
43 Galland, Leo, MD. "Leaky Gut" interview, 2.

treated. I tried homeopathic arnica for surgical-type pain when I had a 2½ hour needle biopsy to remove all calcifications from the non-affected breast to determine if it also needed to be removed. The 200C strength was effective then so I took it for my surgery. Now I use the 30C strength for aches and pains. Homeopathic combinations for pain or arthritis also are helpful.

Finally, consume anti-inflammatory foods and supplements regularly. Omega-3 fatty acids and boswellia taken daily can reduce inflammation and chronic pain. See the list of anti-inflammatory foods on pages 227 to 229, the "Ginger Tea" recipes on pages 191 to 192 and the high-omega-3 seed milk and smoothie recipes on pages 188 to 189.

Thyroid Drugs

Our thyroid glands make two main hormones, triiodothyronine (T3) and thyroxin (T4). T4 is often called a storage hormone. It has four iodine atoms and loses one of them to make the more active, shorter-lived T3. Sometimes it loses the wrong iodine atom and makes a mirror image of T3 called reverse T3. Reverse T3 ties up the receptors for T3 on cells, so the normal T3 molecules cannot exert their effect. This basically neutralizes the normal T3 that is present. Individuals on too high a dosage of synthetic T4 may convert some of it to reverse T3, thus making them more tired, etc.

The most commonly prescribed drug for hypothyrodism is Synthroid,™ a synthetic form of T4. It is the fourth most commonly prescribed drug in the United States at more than 70 million prescriptions annually.[44] Its sales come to over one billion dollars annually.[45] Some hypothyroid patients can adequately convert this to T3, but many cannot. Those who can't never get adequate relief from their symptoms, yet their TSH (thyroid stimulating hormone) blood test returns to normal, so they are told that they are fine, and just have to stay tired, cold, depressed, and having weight or cardiac problems.[46]

Why is thyroid disease so often mismanaged? Dr. Jeffrey Dach says, "Follow the money trail." The pharmaceutical companies which have made Synthroid™ over the years pay for meetings, research, speakers, etc. to support their position, and most doctors are influenced by the companies' advertising.[47]

If you are taking synthetic T4 and not experiencing relief from your symptoms of hypothyroidism, try to find a holistic doctor who will prescribe **natural desiccated thyroid**, such as Armour™ thyroid. If a person is allergic to pork or if the ratio of T4 to T3

44 Bowthorpe, Janie A, M.Ed. *Stop the Thyroid Madness II: How Thyroid Experts are Challenging Ineffective-Treatments and Improving the Lives of Patients.* (Dolores, CO, Laughing Grape Publishing, 2014),103.

45 Pulse of Nat Health Newsletter, "Natural Thyroid Medications at Risk," March 22, 2016 http://www.anh-usa.org/natural-thyroid-medications-at-risk/

46 Bowthorpe, Janie A, M.Ed. *Stop the Thyroid Madness: A Patient Revolution Against Decades of Inferior Thyroid Treatment.* (Dolores, CO, Laughing Grape Publishing, 2012),168-169.

47Bowthorpe, Janie A, M.Ed. *Stop the Thyroid Madness II,* 103.

in natural thyroid is not correct for that individual, he or she will need a combination of **synthetic T4 and synthetic T3 (Cytomel™) in the correct ratio.** To find such a doctor, consider members of the American Academy of Environmental Medicine (AAEM) who have taken courses in thyroid disease at AAEM meetings. These doctors will do testing that is more helpful than the TSH test, and which may show that a patient has a high amount of reverse T3, anti-thyroid antibodies, etc. See "Sources," page 272, for a searchable physician database for the AAEM.

Statins

Statins are cholesterol-lowering drugs which came into use in the 1990s and include Lipitor™, Lescol™, Lescol XL™, Mevacor™, Altoprev™, Crestor™, Zocor™, and others. The use of statins is based on a false premise called the "lipid hypothesis" which says high cholesterol causes heart disease. The truth is that it does not, and that statins accelerate the progression of heart disease.[48]

Cholesterol is essential for life. It makes up 25% of the weight of our brains and is especially important for mental function. Low cholesterol levels are associated with increased mortality from all causes.[49] Those with lower blood cholesterol levels have higher death rates from cancer, stroke, violence, and suicide.[50] Cholesterol is vital for making vitamin D and hormones, including sex hormones. It also is an essential molecule for the structure of the cell membrane of every cell in our body. The normal blood values for cholesterol and other blood fats have decreased from the levels they were forty years ago[51] when I worked as a medical technologist. How "normal" changed baffles me. Do the new normal values exist to support the sales of more statins?

While statins do decrease the levels of cholesterol on a patient's blood test, this does not mean the patient's heart health is better. Rather, it means that there is an increased risk of dying from a heart attack. In a study published in *Atherosclerosis*, 6,673 users of statins who had no previously known coronary artery disease (i.e. they were taking statins preventatively) had coronary CAT scan angiography (CCTA) which enabled the researchers to see their coronary arteries and determine the composition of plaque in the

---

48 Mercola, Joseph, DO. The Cholesterol Myths That May Be Harming Your Health. October 21, 2011. http://mercola.ebeaver.org/2011/10/22/the_cholesterol_myths_that_may_be_harming_your_health/

49 Iribarren, C., Reed, DM, et. al. "Low serum cholesterol and mortality. Which is the cause and which is the effect?" *Circulation*. 1995 Nov 1;92(9):2396-403.

50 Fallon, Sally with Mary Enig, PhD. *Nourishing Traditions.*, (Brandywine, MD, NewTrends Publishing, 2001), 6.

51 When I worked as a medical technologist n the 1970s, the normal blood range for cholesterol was 150 to 280 ng/dl (from my copy of *Interpretation of Diagnostic Tests* by Jacques Wallach, MD, copyright 1970). Now, in 2017, the normal range on a test done by LabCorp is 110-199 ng/dl.

arteries. Patients taking statins had a 52% increase in presence and extent of calcified coronary plaque compared to those not taking statins.[52]

A study in *Diabetes Care* showed that diabetics with advanced artery disease and taking statins had significantly more calcification in their arteries than non-statin taking diabetics. In those who began taking statins during the course of the study, progression of coronary and abdominal aorta calcification increased significantly when they began using statins. Calcification is dangerous in major arteries; they become stiff and inflexible when lined with calcium deposits and individuals are more likely to experience a blockage (heart attack) or abdominal aortic aneurysm, which is usually fatal.[53]

Diets that contain more cholesterol and naturally saturated fat such as butter do not increase cardiac risk. The Framingham Heart Study, which has been monitoring the heart health of over 6,000 people every five years since 1948, does not support the lipid hypothesis. After 40 years, the study director admitted that the people who ate the most saturated fat and cholesterol had lower rates of heart disease and weighed less.[54]

In a British study of several thousand men, half of them reduced saturated fat and cholesterol in their diets, increase consumption of unsaturated oils and margarine and stopped smoking. The other half continued to eat and smoke as they pleased. After one year, those on the "good" diet had twice as many deaths as those who did not change their eating habits and even continued smoking.[55]

The purpose of stains is to reduce the amount of cholesterol in one's blood. They do improve blood test numbers, which does not improve heart health. At what risk of serious side effects are patients taking statins to improve their blood tests? The number of side effects caused by statins is staggering. Here is a partial list:[56]

Statins interfere with the synthesis of CoQ10, essential for our mitochondria to produce energy. This affects every cell in the body because CoQ10 is required by the electron transport chain, which is how we get most of the ATP (adenosine tri-phosphate) "energy molecules" from our food most efficiently.

Statins create problems with muscle weakness, cramping, and pain. Dr. Barbara Roberts estimates that in her practice she sees this side effect in 20% of patients on sta-

52 Nakazato, Ryo, Gransar, H., et al. "Statins use and coronary artery plaque composition: results from the International Multicenter CONFIRM Registry." *Atherosclerosis*. 2012 Nov;225(1):148-53. doi: 10.1016/j.atherosclerosis.2012.08.002. Epub 2012 Aug 24.

53 Saremi, Aramesh, Bahn, G, et al "Progression of vascular calcification is increased with statin use in the Veterans Affairs Diabetes Trial (VADT)." *Diabetes Care*. 2012 Nov;35(11):2390-2. doi: 10.2337/dc12-0464. Epub 2012 Aug 8.

54 Fallon with Enig, 5.

55 Fallon with Enig, 5.

56 Roberts, 46-71. Also The Grave Dangers of Statin Drugs, Pulse of Natural health newsletter, July 14, 2016 http://www.anh-usa.org/the-grave-dangers-of-statin-drugs-and-the-surprising-benefits-of-cholesterol/

tins. A severe form of this problem is rhabdomyolysis, which affects muscles all over the body and can be fatal.

Statins can cause joint and tendon problems, including tendonitis.

Statins can cause liver damage.

Statins cause cognitive problems in many patients, including the inability to concentrate and remember.

Statins can cause nerve damage, including painful neuropathy.

Statins cause a 25% increase in the incidence of cancer.

Statins also cause a 25% increase in the incidence of new cases of diabetes.

Statins increase the risk of hemorrhagic stroke.

Statins can cause depression.

Statins can increase appetite and block the beneficial effect of exercise, thus encouraging weight gain.

In spite of the fact that **statins do not prevent the dire consequences they claim to treat**, one in four Americans over the age of forty five take statin drugs.[57] Why are so many people taking statins? Cardiologist Dr. Barbara Roberts explains that there are clinical practice guidelines determining when a person should be taking them. If a doctor neglects to prescribe them according to these guidelines and the person suffers a heart attack, the doctor can be sued.[58] (I wonder who wrote the guidelines, and if they were influenced by drug companies).

If you are being pressured to take statins, I would suggest telling your doctor that you would like to try changing your diet instead. In the 1980s, the Lyon Diet Heart Study showed that eating a Mediterranean diet lowers the LDL "bad" cholesterol and CRP (C-reactive protein) blood tests as much as statin usage.[59] Those eating a Mediterranean diet had an approximately 70% decrease in risk for both heart attacks and mortality from heart disease.[60] If you decrease your blood cholesterol level naturally with diet, you will avoid the risks of statins and lower your risk of heart attack. The anti-cancer diet on pages 25 to 27 is a Mediterranean diet with the addtional benefit for blood fats of glycemic control.

YOU are the person who is in charge of your health. You do not have to take treatments that are risky or that you do not want to take. Use your mind, think about all your options, make wise decisions, and use whatever natural strategies you can to optimize your health.

---

57 Wehrwein, Peter. "Statin Use is Up, Cholesterol Levels are Down." *Harvard Health Publications*, April 15, 2011. http://www.health.harvard.edu/blog/statin-use-is-up-cholesterol-levels-are-down-are-americans-hearts-benefiting-201104151518

58 Roberts, 44.

59 Roberts, 113.

60 Roberts, 107-114.

The Foundation of True Health

Diet is a modern concept. We analyze our food for nutrient levels and decide what to eat based on the current, but ever changing, recommendations for certain nutrients by federal agencies or popular diet "experts." Conventional dieticians assume that the nutrients we can measure are the only ones that are important. Do we really know about *everything* we need that can be provided by our food?

The isolated tribes studied by Dr. Price ate what their ancestors ate, namely, the traditional foods they enjoyed, which were made from whatever grew or could be hunted or fished nearby. They ate what was satisfying to them, exercised as they worked, breathed naturally, and didn't experience modern types of stress. Their lives were built on the foundational cornerstones of true health – satisfaction with their food, healthy breathing, and peace.

I hope that you will find the next few chapters of this book helpful in building the best foundation for your health.

Satisfaction With Food

What makes a meal satisfying? Having enough to eat is important. The food also should be tasty and some variety is pleasing. However, the major factor in achieving lasting satisfaction may be the nutrients in the meal. I suspect that we are most satisfied when we get all the nutrients we need in the correct balance. If you eat a thousand-calorie portion of chips or sweets, by the numbers, you will have eaten enough. However, your blood sugar level will have risen dramatically and then plummeted, leaving you hungry again in an hour or two.

My husband never liked having soup for dinner. "It's too much water," he'd say. Even if he ate three bowls of soup, he didn't feel satisfied. Then when he had minestrone-type vegetable soup made with homemade bone broth, he was satisfied.

On pages 12 to 13, this book discussed cattle having a healthy 1:1 ratio of omega-3 to omega-6 fatty acids in their body fat if 5% linseeds was added to their food. A series of experiments[61] was done in which volunteers ate meat and dairy products from linseed-fed cattle vs. cattle fed only corn, wheat and soy.

In the first experiment, for three months the volunteers ate meat and dairy products either from cattle fed 5% linseeds or cattle fed the standard fare. Then they were given blood tests to measure the ratio of omega-3 to omega-6 fat in their blood. The volunteers who had eaten standard meat and dairy products had an unhealthy 1:15 ratio. Those who ate meat and dairy products from the linseed fed cattle had a healthy 1:5 ratio.

The second experiment involved overweight diabetics. Those who ate meat and dairy products from the linseed fed cattle lost three pounds on average. The volunteers who had eaten standard meat and dairy products did not lose, in spite of the fact that both groups were given the same amount of food.

In the final experiment, an independent laboratory conducted taste tests in which the tasters sampled all the foods but did not know the source of each food. The vast majority of tasters said that meat and dairy products from the linseed-fed cattle tasted better than the standard meat and dairy products. Dr. David Servan-Schreiber's interpretation of this was, "It's as if our taste buds recognize what is good for our bodies' cells and translate this message for us by reacting differently to healthy food."[62] This supports the idea that food that gives us the nutrients we need tastes better and thus will be more satisfying.

This chapter will help you return to the easily digested, highly nutritious foods of the isolated tribes Dr. Price studied. The first step is to begin with whole foods such as

---

61 Servan-Schreiber, David, MD, PhD. *AntiCancer: A New Way of Life.* (New York: Penguin Group, Inc., 2009), 78-80.

62 Servan-Schreiber, 80.

naturally raised plants and grass-fed animals. Then enjoy them prepared in ways that make them even more nutritious and easy to digest so you absorb more nutrients. Foods prepared in traditional ways include fermented vegetables, cultured dairy products, bone broth and soups made from it, legumes and grains that have been soaked and/or fermented so their natural phytates don't keep us from absorbing their nutrients, and nuts which have been soaked and dried to make them easier to digest. If the thought of much cooking exhausts you, don't despair. See pages 251 to 257 for where to purchase commercially prepared cultured vegetables and dairy products, bone broth, etc.

Season these foods with whole sea salt, healthy fats, herbs, spices and love to lead yourself and your family to the best health. The recipes on pages 108 to 192 will guide you in making the types of food discussed here. On pages 193 to 207 there are recipes for healthy treats to provide edible love on special occasions. Then savor the goodness and real flavor of your food as you improve your health.

Cultured Vegetables

I have a friend who told me about how her German family enjoyed their harvest of cabbage year-round as sauerkraut. Every year her father sliced the cabbage and layered it in crocks with salt. The crocks were kept in the basement, and when her mother wanted to include sauerkraut in a meal, my friend was sent to downstairs to bring some up. She enjoyed a sample for herself while she was there as well.

This happened in the 1940s before pesticides were widely used, so the cabbage they grew was populated with a bountiful supply of *Lactobacillus* and other lactic-acid producing bacteria. Thus the fermentation went well and turned the cabbage into sauerkraut every time without fail.

Then I told my friend about taking a food and dairy microbiology class in college and spending one of the lab sessions making sauerkraut just the way her father had, by slicing the cabbage and layering it with salt in a crock. We weighted the tops of the crocks down well, and left them to ferment for the next week. I don't remember where the crocks were put to ferment. Maybe the temperature there was a little off. I also don't know where our professor got the cabbage. Maybe he was given leftover heads that the food service for the dormitories didn't want. He may not have been able to choose perfect heads of cabbage with no bad spots, and I'm sure the cabbage was not organic. This was in the early 1970s and there was no health food store in the small college town.

With eight students taking the course, and each of us having a lab partner to work with, we prepared four crocks. At the next lab session, only one of the crocks had sauerkraut in it. The other three contained horribly rotten cabbage that released a stench I will never forget. Having seen this fermentation go wrong is part of the reason every fermented recipe in this book uses a freeze-dried starter culture so you are sure that you have the correct bacteria working for you. It's a waste of time and food to end up with a rotten mess, plus for health reasons, I like to know that the correct bacteria gets a head start on anything unfriendly that might be on the vegetables or in the milk.

In addition to using a culture to ferment vegetables, you should use the best organic produce you can find. Pesticides are not friendly to the bacteria you want to grow. Any rotten spots on the vegetables may contain bacteria you don't want. I've cut bad spots off with a wide margin, but those batches didn't seem to keep as long as the ones that I made with perfect produce. Furthermore, use purified water and sea salt. Chlorinated water and salt that contains anti-caking agents, iodine, etc. are not friendly to the desired bacteria. Use organic spices and herbs if you wish to add seasonings to cultured vegetables.

Some cultured vegetable recipes online and in other books call for homemade whey instead of a culture. I have not used whey because it is a byproduct of making yogurt and I am allergic to dairy products. However, if you are making your own yogurt as well as cultured vegetables and find a recipe that calls for whey, give it a try. The microbiologist in me hopes you used a starter for the yogurt within the last few weeks so your whey contains just the bacteria you need.

All jars, lids, knives, peelers, food processor parts, measuring spoons and cups, cutting boards, weights, airlocks, and any other equipment you use to make cultured vegetables should be scrupulously clean. Although I always wash all my jars and culturing equipment after use before putting them away, the next time I make cultured vegetables, I re-wash them, in the dishwasher if possible, right before I use them again. This could be "took too much microbiology in college" paranoia, so you might want to try just one washing between uses.

Along with being organic and unblemished, your vegetables should be very clean. Wash them in several changes of water until there is absolutely no dirt left. I tried fermenting Swiss chard stems once, and they all rotted very quickly. I must not have succeeded in removing all the dirt, although I tried. Do not use soap or anything other than water to wash the vegetables. Sprays and soaking solutions for washing vegetables can inhibit the desired bacteria.

Fermented vegetables are partially digested by the bacteria that make them, so they are very easy to digest. In this state, you may be able to eat some vegetables that you cannot eat raw or cooked. They also contain enzymes to help with the digestion of your meal and vitamins such as B vitamins including vitamin B-12, vitamin C, and vitamin K.

Fermented vegetables are a very effective probiotic for intestinal problems. (But don't give up your probiotic supplements). In traditional cultures, they are often eaten as condiments, in small quantities with each meal. If you eat a teaspoon to a tablespoon of cultured vegetables twice a day, or even with every meal, it will do your intestinal flora a world of good.

Specific instructions for the various kinds of fermented vegetables are found in the recipes on pages 110 to 119. To purchase cultured vegetables containing live health-promoting bacteria already made, see "Sources," page 257 or visit a well-stocked health food store.

Cultured Dairy Products

My friend whose father made sauerkraut also told me about her grandmother's yogurt. Whenever there was extra milk left over after milking the cows, it was set on the cozy top of the back of her wood-burning stove. The next day, that milk was yogurt. Without pasteurization or refrigeration, milk from healthy cows[63] contains bacteria that will produce a healthy fermentation. It contains *Lactobacillus* and other lactic-acid pro- ducing bacteria that break down the lactose and milk protein (casein) and produce acid to sour and thicken the milk.

There are several types of cultured milk in addition to yogurt, including acidophilus milk, kefir, buttermilk, and pima. All of them can be made with cow milk and the right culture. I haven't tried to make all of them with milk from other animals, but I have made goat milk yogurt, acidophilus milk and kefir and camel milk yogurt. Since I have never had access to sheep milk, I haven't made any cultured products using it. We can buy sheep milk yogurt in health food stores here and it is thick, rich and delicious. See "Sources," page 256, to purchase sheep yogurt or ask your health food store to carry it..

The last time I made kefir was about twenty years ago. It worked well only when I used the Good Life™ kefir bug and culture which are no longer available. This is one reason I am not including a kefir recipe in this book. A second reason is that one of the organisms that is part of the kefir fermentation is a species of the yeast *Saccaromyces* closely related to bakers' and brewers' yeast, so kefir is often not tolerated by those with food allergies.

Several factors influence the quality of homemade fermented milks such as yogurt and acidophilus milk. The most important are the temperature at which they are made, the milk used, and the culture used. There are several yogurt makers on the market. Cur- rently, all of them keep the milk at about 110°F, which is good for making cow milk yogurt quickly, but not good for alternative milks. Alternative milk products do not thicken as quickly as cow milk products, and therefore require longer incubation and can not be rushed by the higher temperature.

My favorite inexpensive incubator for yogurt and acidophilus milk is a homemade "proofing box" incubator which I originally made to incubate sourdough bread. To make a homemade incubator, you will need a Styrofoam cooler (mine cost about $5), a shop light, preferably with plastic rather than metal casing (costing about $10-15), a 25-watt incandescent light bulb, and a thermometer. Install the light bulb into the shop light. Discard the lid of the cooler. Make a small hole in the bottom of the cooler near one end and thread the cord of the shop light through it until the base of the shop light

---

63 Modern cows are often not healthy enough to produce milk containing the *Lactobacillus* required for yogurt fermentation. This is due to treatment with antibiotics required because giving cows recombinant bovine growth hormone (rBGH) to increase milk production leads to infections in the milk glands. See page 13 for more about rBGH.

touches the inside of the cooler. Tape the cord on the outside of the cooler to keep it from slipping. Use wire or tape to attach the hook end of the shop light to the bottom of the cooler near the other end of the cooler. Turn the cooler upside down on a table or counter top and plug in the light. Put the thermometer in the proofing box. After about an hour, read the temperature on the thermometer. If it is between 90°F and 98°F, your proofing box is ready to use. If it is higher, experiment with propping one end of the box up a half inch or so until you find how much you need to prop it up to maintain the temperature in the proper range. I use the ring from the lid of a canning jar to prop up the end of my box, thus maintaining the temperature at about 95°F. If the temperature is lower than 90°F, check it in another hour or two; the temperature will almost certainly have risen into the right range by then. If it has not, change the light bulb to one with higher wattage. The first few times you use your proofing box, it is a good idea to check the temperature every hour or two to be sure that the temperature is staying at about 95°F. Don't lose sleep watching the box, however. If the temperature drops a little over-night, the fermentation will still work, just correct the temperature when you rise in the morning.

A homemade proofing box is very versatile. It can be used to make sourdough bread as well as fermented milks. (Mine was even used as an incubator for science projects years ago). If you are making more than one kind of fermented milk at a time, you can incubate several jars of different kinds of milk at the same time. You can also make larger batches of fermented milk using a proofing box than you can using a yogurt maker. You do not need special containers when making yogurt in a proofing box, so you can store your yogurt in the same jars in which you made it.

If you wish to purchase a proofing box, Brod & Taylor™ makes one which is sold in the King Arthur Flour™ Bakers' Catalogue and on their website. It folds to less than three inches thick for convenient storage. It has a digital temperature control which does not keep the temperature totally stable. The temperature actually varies at different times of day or night and different seasons of the year. Put a small jar of water in the box and take the temperature of the water after it's been on about an hour or two. I find that I need to set the temperature at 85 to 90°F for the temperature of the water to be 95°F. Experiment to determine where to set the digital temperature control to get the actual temperature that you want, which is about 95°F. When you use the box, it is a good idea to check the temperature every hour or two during non-sleep hours to be sure that the temperature is staying at about 95°F.

The type of milk used also influences the character of your yogurt or acidophilus milk. Cow and sheep milk, being relatively high in fat and protein, make thick, creamy yogurt and acidophilus milk. Whole goat milk makes thinner fermented milk than cow milk. Yet when the culture is at its peak, cultured goat milk products are quite creamy. Non-fat goat milk makes very watery fermented milk and contains less fat soluble vita-mins, so use whole milk.

Camel milk makes thin yogurt, but once I had very thick camel yogurt. I was getting raw camel milk from a family locally. The husband was out of town, the kids got sick, just as they were getting better, the wife got sick, so the camels didn't get milked for about three days. When the husband returned home and milked the camels, I received some of that milk, and it was concentrated enough to make thick yogurt. Camel milk yogurt is delicious even when thinner, and all homemade yogurt is great for your health.

The type of organisms in the culture and age of the culture you use also affect your fermented milk. Yogurt cultures free of cow milk and starch can be purchased from GI ProStart™. To make acidophilus milk, I use Klaire Laboratories Therbiotic Factor 1™ supplement as a starter. See "Source," pages 261 to 262, for information on ordering these cultures.

The consistency of acidophilus milk will vary with the age of the culture. The batch made from the powdered acidophilus culture will be creamy but not extremely thick. Then as the culture reaches its peak with successive batches, your acidophilus milk will become much thicker. When the acidophilus milk becomes thinner again with subsequent batches, it is time to start a new culture from the acidophilus supplement, Therbiotic Factor 1™.

Cultured dairy products have many health benefits. If you are lactose intolerant and the milk is allowed to ferment a full 24 hours, you will most likely tolerate it. Fermented milks contain enzymes that help us digest and absorb the nutrients in the milk more easily, and possibly help with the digestion and absorption of other foods eaten at the same time. People who eat cultured dairy products regularly have less bone loss as they age. Additionally, the lactic acid bacteria they contain are great for intestinal health.

Recipes for cultured dairy products are found on pages 120 to 125, or purchase cow milk yogurt with live bacteria at health food or grocery stores. Information about where to purchase goat and sheep yogurt is found in the "Sources" section on page 256 or shop at a health food store.

Easily Digested Grains, Legumes and Nuts

Grains, legumes and nuts are seeds of the plants that produced them. When you consider that seeds germinate in damp soil, it makes sense that they need some protection from becoming decomposed by the bacteria around them during the germination process. Therefore, these foods contain enzyme inhibitors and/or phytic acid that make them harder for us as well as soil bacteria to digest. These substances interfere with our absorption of the minerals and other nutrients that they contain. However, with long pre-soaking in water or water plus an acidic ingredient and properly cooked, or when fermented before cooking, these foods become easy to digest and are very nourishing

Oatmeal boxes used to contain instructions that said to soak the oatmeal overnight before cooking it for breakfast. That was good advice, but not what today's impatient consumers want to hear. Grains contain both enzyme inhibitors and phytic acid. The phytic acid combines with minerals such as calcium, magnesium, iron, copper and zinc in the intestine and prevents us from absorbing those minerals. Because of this, a diet high in unsoaked, unfermented whole grains can lead to serious mineral deficiencies and bone loss.[64] Soaking grains in warm water for twelve to twenty four hours neutralizes the enzyme inhibitors and enables the grain's enzymes, *Lactobacillus* and other bacteria to break down the phytic acid.[65]

The fermentation that occurs when we make sourdough bread, and to a lesser extent with yeast bread, allows for the breakdown of phytic acid and makes digestion and absorption of nutrients easy. However, conventionally made quick breads, crackers, and granola remain hard to digest and it is difficult for the body to derive their nutrients. If these items are baked at home, the flour can be soaked for twelve to twenty four hours before baking. The best nutrition is obtained if the flour is soaked in buttermilk or other cultured milk products or with an acidic ingredient.[66] Recipes for grains and baked goods made more digestible and nourishing are found on pages 141 to 153. For yeast and sourdough bread recipes, see pages 153 to 173.

Sprouting grains also neutralizes phytic acid and enzyme inhibitors.[67] Recently I noticed that the King Arthur Flour™ Baker's Catalogue now sells sprouted whole wheat flour. An online search led to the To Your Health Sprouted Flour Company™. They produce a wide variety of sprouted flours including amaranth, quinoa, sorghum, and rice. To find a store that carries their products, search here: https://healthyflour.com/store-locator/ .

I baked twice with King Arthur™ sprouted flour and it produced very good 100% sprouted wheat yeast buns and muffins. I do not hesitate to recommend this flour in spite of my brief experience with it because I know King Arthur™ has a large test kitchen where new products are thoroughly tested before the are accepted for sale on their website and in their catalogue. As I have found true in my brief experience, they write that their sprouted whole wheat flour can be used in baking like their other whole wheat flour and substituted in equal amounts. If you tolerate wheat, you might want to consider baking with this flour.

If you're low on energy, baked goods made from sprouted flour can be purchased from Food for Life™. They offer both standard and gluten-free breads, English muffins, tortillas, buns, pocket breads and cereals. You will be amazed at the variety on their website here: http://www.foodforlife.com/products . Also see "Sources," page 252 to 253.

----

64 Fallon, Sally with Mary Enig, PhD. *Nourishing Traditions*. (Brandywine, MD, NewTrends Publishing, 2001), 452.

65 Cottis, Halle. Are Soaking Grains & Legumes Necessary & How To Properly Soak & Prepare Them. https://wholelifestylenutrition.com/health/is-soaking-grains-and-legumes-necessary-and-how-to-properly-soak-and-prepare-them/

66 Fallon with Enig, 476.

67 Fallon with Enig, 112-113.

Legumes are high in protein, minerals, B vitamins and essential fatty acids. However, they also contain enzyme inhibitors and phytic acid that must be neutralized for us to absorb the nutrients, especially the minerals. Beans should be soaked in warm water at least overnight and preferably for 24 hours before cooking to break down the enzyme inhibitors and phytic acid and to allow indigestible carbohydrates to be broken down and poured off in the soaking water. Rinse the beans with three changes of water after soaking and before cooking them. I find a crock pot ideal for cooking beans. Some traditional cultures added acidic ingredients to the soaking water for some beans and used just water for others. The beans that were often cooked with acidic ingredients such as whey, vinegar, or citrus juice include black beans, small white beans, garbanzo beans (chickpeas), and lentils. Legumes contain several anti-cancer agents.[68] Legume recipes are found on pages 174 to 180.

Nuts and seeds are foods that many people have trouble digesting and so must eat very sparingly. However, once made easier to digest, they are a very satisfying, non-perishable, convenient between meal snack for glycemic control diets and are good sources of many minerals, healthy fats and protein. Nuts from large trees with very deep roots, such as pecans, are high in trace minerals.[69]

Nuts contain many enzyme inhibitors, some of which can be irritating to the mouth. The large number of enzyme inhibitors is what makes them so hard to digest. Soaking nuts enables their own enzymes to break down enzyme inhibitors.[70] To be easily edible and nourishing they should be soaked in salted water for twelve to twenty four hours and then dried in a slightly warm oven or dehydrator until crisp.

Cashews have a toxic oil called cardol between their inner and outer shells, so they are cracked and roasted twice to eliminate the cardol before we purchase them. What are sold as "raw" cashews are not really raw and need to be soaked for only six hours.

Grain recipes are found on pages 141 to 173. Legume recipes are on pages 174 to 180. Recipes for nourishing nuts and seeds are found on page 182. Recipes for foods made using soaked nuts are found on pages 181 to 184, 187 to 189 and 193 to 196. To find where to purchase baked goods made from sprouted flour, including wheat- and gluten-free products, see "Sources" page 252 to 253 or visit a health food store.

Bone broth

A generation or two ago, when we bought meat, we got the bone too. Frugal cooks got the most out of their meat purchase by saving bones, small pieces of meat and scraps of vegetables and making them into nourishing broths and soups.

---

68 Fallon with Enig, 495.
69 Fallon with Enig, 514.
70 Fallon with Enig, 512.

Broth made from bones and meat scraps is extremely nutritious. An acidic ingredient is added to the broth to draw the minerals out of the bone and into the broth, especially calcium, magnesium and potassium. The protein from the collagen on the bones is broken down and goes into the broth also, in the form of gelatin. Gelatin from bone broth (not the commercially made highly processed white powder) is very healing for intestinal disorders, and may also be helpful for other chronic diseases. The way to tell if you cooked your broth long enough is to see whether it gels when cooled. The longer you cook the broth, the more nutrients are drawn into it, so some authorities recommend cooking it for up to twenty four hours. A crock pot is ideal if you wish to do this. However, people with allergies who are sensitive to monosodium glutamate may have trouble tolerating long-cooked broths because the longer they are cooked, the more natural glutamates are in the broth. If you are reacting to bone broth, try cooking it for only six to eight hours.

Now that butchering is done in large plants and the bones are discarded, you may have trouble finding bones for bone broth. If there is a large health food store with a butcher counter near you, ask there. The Weston Price Foundation local groups may also be able to direct you to local sources.

Most of the broth recipes in this book are made from game animals and less common fowl and are found on pages 128 to 140. Beef and chicken bone broth are found on pages 131 and 137. See pages 264 to 265 for sources of bones and meat from game animals and fowl and also for sources of bones from more common animals such as chicken and beef. If you're low on energy, consider purchasing bone broth already made. See "Sources," page 254, for contact information of companies which make real bone broth or look in the frozen food section of your health food store.

Whole Sea Salt

Most of the salt we eat is highly refined, even sea salt. I have been using sea salt for many years and didn't realize this until recently. When I first read *Asthma-Free Naturally*, a natural remedy given for help with asthma was to drink warm water with ¼ teaspoon of sea salt in it.[71] I tried it and it didn't seem to help. Some time later, I was introduced to Celtic sea salt. Since I was not used to sprinkling the moist chunks of salt, I greatly over seasoned some summer squash I was cooking. When I ate the salty squash, my airways became more open. I learned that there is sea salt, and then there is real whole sea salt with all the minerals in the ocean in it. It's gray and not as pretty, but it contains what we really need.

---

71 McKeown, Patrick, MA, H Dip. *Asthma-Free Naturally*. (San Francisco, CA, Conari Press 2008), 122.

I find it helpful to drink a mug of hot (slightly cooled tea temperature) water with ¼ teaspoon of fine Celtic™ sea salt or a scant ¼ teaspoon of coarse Celtic™ sea salt added. Especially if using the coarse salt, stir until it is dissolved before drinking. The salt supports adrenal function and the production of cortisol. If I am having a reaction, this amount of salt in the water does not taste salty. If I'm doing well, it tastes slightly salty. I think if I do not taste saltiness, just pleasantly mineralized water, it is an indication that my body needs more salt.

The federal government recommends limiting sodium intake to 2300 milligrams per day, an amount which is easily met or exceeded without ever touching a salt shaker if you eat processed foods. Consuming only this amount is supposed to lead to lower blood pressure and lower cardiac risk. Unfortunately, sodium is only part of the story. Many minerals are needed to promote good cardiac health as well as to maintain a healthy fluid balance between intercellular and extracellular fluids. The potassium to sodium ratio needs to be high enough, so the amount of potassium you consume is critical. This is especially true now because potassium intake has declined as fruits and vegetables have become less prominent in our diets.

Consuming too little sodium makes your body work hard to conserve salt, which actually causes higher risk of having a fatal heart attack than consuming too much. A 2011 study published in the *Journal of the American Medical Association* showed that low sodium intake was not predictive of low blood pressure and was associated with increased risk of hospitalization and death from cardiac problems.[72]

For best health, consume all of the minerals you need in adequate amounts, rather than only restricting sodium. Eat foods that are good sources of magnesium and potassium, such as avocados, dark leafy greens, sweet potatoes, winter squash, yogurt, and many fruits. Avoid processed foods. If you are eating a good whole foods diet that supplies enough of all the minerals you need and use whole unrefined sea salt, your body will tell you the right amount of salt for *you* to eat by what tastes good to you, in my opinion. Individuals with impaired adrenal function may need more than the federal recommended amount. Those with heart or kidney disease should consume the amount of salt their doctor recommends.[73] Please consult your medical practitioner before you implement the suggestions in this chapter or book.

Gray sea salt contains only 82% sodium chloride. The remaining 18% is magnesium and over 80 trace minerals.[74] Some people feel better with this, and some feel better with

---

72 Katarzyna Stolarz-Skrzypek, MD, PhD; Tatiana Kuznetsova, MD, PhD; Lutgarde Thijs, MSc; et al. Fatal and Nonfatal Outcomes, Incidence of Hypertension, and Blood Pressure Changes in Relation to Urinary Sodium Excretion. *JAMA*. 2011;305(17):1777-1785. doi:10.1001/jama.2011.574 http://jamanetwork.com/journals/jama/fullarticle/899663

73 Kresser, Chris. Shaking Up the Salt Myth: The Human Need for Salt, April 13, 2012.   https://chriskresser.com/shaking-up-the-salt-myth-the-human-need-for-salt/

74 Fallon with Enig, 49.

red sea salt from Hawaii. You may find that your food not only seems more flavorful with these complete salts, but that you also appreciate these salts for their health benefits.

In spite of the nutritional benefits of unrefined salt, I still use refined sea salt for making cultured vegetables. When I first begin using unrefined (Celtic™) sea salt for all other cooking, I found that at least one jar in each batch of cultured vegetables made with unrefined salt went bad fairly frequently, as opposed to almost never. Therefore, I went back to using the Natural Grocers™ store brand of pure refined sea salt (with nothing added, no iodine or fillers) for cultured vegetables. If you cannot find pure refined sea salt with no additives, use kosher salt. I suspect that there are a few more bacteria present in unrefined salt than in refined salt.

I hope the information in this chapter enables you to make your food truly satisfying and that the superior nutrition they provide will help your health.

The Breath of Life

Breathing is the essence of life. Before there was medical equipment that monitored heartbeats and brain waves, a life was defined as the span of time between the first breath a baby took and the last breath of the elder. Healthy breathing continues automatically: we are only aware of our breathing when there is something wrong. However, even when our breathing seems just fine, we may not breathe as healthily as did our ancestors who were farmers, manual laborers, and appliance-less housewives

Most of us spend much of our time sitting at computers, often slouched over the desk. Then in the evening, we watch TV slouched in our favorite over-stuffed chair. Poor posture and lack of movement encourage breathing with the upper chest muscles, which only ventilates the upper lobes of the lungs.[1] Chest breathing is less-than-ideal and is often done with the mouth open.

Diaphragmatic breathing is the most efficient way to breathe because it uses the lower lobes of the lungs which have the most blood vessels for exchanging gasses. Nasal breathing is healthier than mouth breathing because the nose is designed to thoroughly warm and moisturize air before it gets to the lungs. In addition, particulates and allergens are filtered out by the nose and never reach the lungs if you breathe nasally. These particulates are cleared from the body in fifteen minutes if you breathe through your nose. If you breathe through your mouth, it can take from two to four months for all of them to be removed from the alveoli of the lungs.[2] Nasal diaphragmatic breathing tends to be more regular and relaxed than upper chest breathing. Mouth breathers in general have poorer health than nasal breathers.[3]

It is essential for cancer patients to breathe nasally using the diaphragm for maximun oxygenation of all of their tissues. Cancer cells prefer to metabolize anaerobically (with without oxygen) so keeping tissues fully oxygenated will give stray cancer cells less ability to grow and begin a metastasis.[4]

Asthmatics have an additional problem with their breathing, which is that the volume of air they breathe per minute is too large. A healthy person breathes between three and five liters of air per minute. Asthmatics breathe from ten to twenty liters per minute routinely and over twenty liters per minute during an asthma attack. This overbreathing causes the level of carbon dioxide (CO_2) in their blood and the alveoli of their lungs to be too low.[5] After the level has been low for long enough, which can be as little as 20 or

1 McKeown, Patrick, MA, H Dip. *Asthma-Free Naturally*. (San Francisco, CA, Conari Press 2008), 89.

2 McKeown. *Asthma-Free Naturally*, 30-31.

3 McKeown. *Asthma-Free Naturally*, 33.

4 Wilder, Bee. Breathing Through Your Nose is Essential: Benefits of Nose Breathing & Nitric Oxide. http://healingnaturallybybee.com/breathing-through-your-nose-is-essential/#a5

5 McKeown. *Asthma-Free Naturally*, 20-21.

more hours in one 24-hour period, the respiratory control center in the brain re-sets to maintain a lower level. This new set point makes asthmatics continue to overbreathe and keeps their CO_2 level low.[6] Since CO_2 is a natural bronchodilator, this is the opposite of what asthmatics need. Thus, the way asthmatics breathe worsens and perpetuates their problem. If the asthma initially was caused by allergies, eliminating the offending substances may not improve breathing because the respiratory center in their brain is now maintaining a low CO_2 level that leads to constricted airways.

Buteyko Breathing for Asthma

The Buteyko breathing method is a training system that uses breathing exercises to temporarily raise CO_2 levels in the blood and lungs. If the exercises are done often (usually three times a day) and the higher level of CO_2 is not breathed off excessively, (which may require successful treatment of asthma symptoms) this gradually resets the CO_2 trigger to cause the asthmatic to breathe a smaller volume of air. Resetting the trigger raises the level of CO_2 in the blood consistently, which dilates airways, reduces blood pressure (if needed), and warms cold fingertips by dilating arteries and capillaries and thus improving circulation.

The Buteyko breathing method employs a self-test called the control pause (CP) which is used to monitor progress. It is an indicator of the level of CO_2 in one's blood and the alveoli of the lungs. If performed first thing in the morning when breathing has not been influenced overnight by activity or conscious efforts to breathe correctly, it indicates the level of the CO_2 trigger that dictates when to take a breath. As you practice the exercises, over time, your morning control pause should increase. When it reaches 20 seconds, symptoms should improve. With a CP of 40 seconds, you should be free of asthma.[7] Patrick McKeown states on his Buteyko breathing training DVD that when your control pause reaches 20 or above, you will be free of asthma symptoms unless exposed to your triggers. At 40 or above, he says triggers no longer cause symptoms.

Everyone, not just asthmatics, will be sharper mentally when breathing exercises or activity significantly increase the CO_2 level in the blood and alveoli of the lungs, even if it is a temporary increase. Asthmatics will also feel better physically. The reason is that oxygen is carried to all of the organs and tissues in the body by the hemoglobin in red blood cells. The ease of release of oxygen from the hemoglobin is dependent on the CO_2 level in the blood. (This is called the Bohr effect and was discovered by Dr. Christian Bohr in 1908).[8] If the CO_2 level is low, oxygen binds to the hemoglobin molecule more

---

6 McKeown. *Asthma-Free Naturally*, 236.

7 McKeown. *Asthma-Free Naturally*, 55-56..

8 Bohr, Christian, K. Hasslebalch and August Krogh, "Concerning a Biologically Important Relationship: The Influence of the Carbon Dioxide Content of Blood on its Oxygen Binding." Translation of article from *Skand. Arch. Physiol.* 16, 401-412, 1904. https://www.udel.edu/chem/white/C342/Bohr%281904%29.html Also see "The Bohr Effect." http://en.wikipedia.org/wiki/Bohr_effect

tightly. If it's very low, as in asthmatics, tissues will be low in oxygen even while fully oxygenated blood travels through them over and over.[9]

Reduced CO_2 also causes constriction of arteries and capillaries, thus reducing the ease of blood flowing around the body and to the brain.[10] Decreasing the CO_2 concentration in the blood by breathing heavily significantly reduces the flow of blood to the brain.[11] Between this effect and the tight binding of oxygen to hemoglobin, anyone who is over-breathing due to anxiety or being in a rush may have less than optimal levels of oxygen both in the brain and in all tissues of the body. When Buteyko breathing or meditative breathing (on the next page) is practiced, even non-asthmatics will notice that they feel calmer and their minds are clearer due to better brain oxygenation.

One of the Buteyko breathing exercises is a nose-unblocking exercise which is based on increasing your CO_2 level. Nitric oxide (NO) will also unblock the nose and is a natural bronchodilator, an antimicrobial agent for the nose and sinuses, and reduces pulmonary vascular resistance. When I learned that the release of NO from the paranasal sinuses could be stimulated by humming, I tried humming.[12] For me, humming is also an effective way to unblock my nose and is easy to do, which helps me get on with breathing exercises more quickly and easily. If you hum a tune, you can do it in public without anyone wondering about your sanity, unlike using Buteyko nose unblocking exercise.

When I first heard about Buteyko breathing from a friend, I was about to visit my son in the Washington DC area. She urged me to find out if there were any Buteyko breathing practitioners near his home. (There were not; nor are there any within several hundred miles of where my friend and I live in Colorado). She had trained with a Buteyko breathing practitioner in California when she went to visit her mother while suffering from uncontrollable coughing due to a respiratory infection. I appreciated her good advice and wish I could have taken it.

If you begin Buteyko breathing and there are training courses or a practitioner near you, you should seriously consider taking advantage of them. If there is no one near, you

---

9 McKeown. *Asthma-Free Naturally*, 230.

10 McKeown. *Asthma-Free Naturally*, 230-231.

11 McKeown, Patrick, MA, H Dip. *Close Your Mouth*. (Loughwell, Buteyko Books, 2004), 11.

12 Cardell, Lars Olaf. The Paranasal Sinuses and a Unique Role in Airway Nitric Oxide Production? *American Journal of Respiratory and Critical Care Medicine*,166:2 (202) 131-132. http://www.atsjournals. org/doi/full/10.1164/rccm.2205014

Also Lundberg, J O and E Wietzberg. Nasal nitric oxide in man. *Thorax*. 1999; 54: 947-952. https:// www.ncbi.nlm.nih.gov/pmc/articles/PMC1745376/pdf/v054p00947.pdf

Also Cardell, Lars Olaf. Nitric Oxide and the Paranasal Sinuses. *Anatomical Record*. 2008 Nov;291(11):1479-84. http://www.ncbi.nlm.nih.gov/pubmed/18951492

Nitric oxide production in the sinuses is why breathing through the nose is beneficial. In addition to the benefits mention in this abstract, nasally breathed air puts nitric oxide into the lungs where it causes bronchodilation.

can purchase a set containing a DVD of a training session taught by Patrick McKeown, the book given to participants at the training session, as well as a CD that provides coaching for reduced breathing. The book that libraries often have, *Asthma-Free Naturally*, is another useful resource. It is possible to teach yourself with these resources. See page 273 for where to purchase them.

In addition, McKeown has written a book about breathing for relaxation and relief of anxiety, *Anxiety Free: Stop Worrying and Quieten Your Mind*.

For more about my experiences with Buteyko breathing see pages 246 to 248.

Meditative breathing

Breathing is useful for more than exchanging gasses in your lungs. Controlled breathing is the basis of meditative practices used in many religions, qigong, yoga, and similar practices. However, as Dr. David Servan-Schreiber says in *AntiCancer*, you do not have to believe in anything to profit from its health benefits for relaxation and for helping overcome cancer.[13] Meditative breathing uses the same biological phenomenon to produce relaxation as Buteyko breathing does. When I read about meditative breathing, I was impressed with how similar the two methods are. The differences are that Buteyko breathing has you consciously try to reduce the volume of air you breathe, and meditative breathing does not have you try to influence your breathing nor are there tests of any kind. It is pure pleasure.

Here is Dr. Servan-Schreiber's beautifully written description of how to practice meditative breathing:

"Begin by sitting comfortably, in what the Tibetan master Sogyal Rinpoches calls a 'dignified' posture. It gives full freedom to the flow of air that slips down through the nostrils toward the throat, then the bronchi, and finally to the bottom of the lungs, before reversing its route. With your attention focused, take two deep, slow breaths to begin relaxation. A sensation of comfort, lightness, and well-being will settle into your chest and shoulders. As you repeat this exercise, you will learn to let your breathing be led by your attention, and to let your attention rest on your breath. As you relax, you may feel your mind become like a leaf floating on water, rising and falling as waves pass underneath. Your attention accompanies the *sensation* of each intake of breath and the long exhalation of air leaving the body gently, slowly, gracefully, all the way to the end, until there is nothing more than a tiny, barely perceptible breath left. Then there is a pause. You learn to sink into this pause, more and more profoundly. It's often while resting briefly in it that you feel in the most intimate contact with your body. With practice, you can feel your heart beating, sustaining life, as it has been doing indefatigably for so

---

13 Servan-Schreiber, David, MD, PhD. *AntiCancer: A New Way of Life*. (New York: Penguin Group, Inc., 2009), 166.

many years. And then, at the end of the pause, notice a tiny spark light up all by itself and set off a new cycle of breath. What you feel is the spark of life, which is always in us and which, through this process of attention and relaxation, you may discover for the first time.

"Inevitably, your mind is distracted from this task after a few minutes and is drawn toward the outside world: the concerns of the past or the obligations of the future. The essential art of this 'radical act of love,' consists of doing what you would do for a child who needs undivided attention. You recognize the importance of these other thoughts, but while patiently promising to attend to them when the time comes, you push them to the side and come back to the person who really needs you in the present moment, that is, yourself."[14]

By practicing this daily for at least ten minutes, cancer patients can bring coherence to their biological rhythms. That means their heart rate, blood pressure, respiration, and other functions all cycle in synchronization with each other. This results in better immune function, less inflammation, and better regulation of blood sugar levels.[15] Patients may also achieve a level of calmness and mellowness that they have never experienced before.

On the Buteyko breathing CD, Patrick MeKeown says, "Relaxation, stilling my mind and quieting my breathing, is the best thing I've ever done." Taking charge of your breathing is a very basic way to help yourself and something only you can do for yourself. It is a special gift that you give to yourself.

---

14 Servan-Schreiber, 164-165. I hope that including this quote inspires every cancer patient who reads it to get and read *Anti-Cancer*.
15 Servan-Schreiber, 168.

Peace

In the chapter about helping yourself, we discussed how a positive attitude and banishing feelings of helplessness was good for health. (See pages 40 to 42). For optimal health, it is also essential to pursue peace.

Writing this chapter was daunting. I don't have all the answers. There are so many things in our lives that contribute to a lack of peace.

Way too many things to do each day
Irritating people
Whiny children
Incessant phone calls
Impossible bosses
Uncooperative co-workers
Malfunctioning computers, washers, furnaces...
Waiting two weeks for a repairman to come
Exhaustion
Pain
Hunger
Poor health

The list of peace-breakers seems endless.

Each of us will pursue peace in her or his own way. However, I hope the list of suggestions below contains a some things that might help you.

1. Slow down. Try to decrease the number of commitments you have. Some, such as earning a living and taking care of one's family, are essential. However, try to eliminate as many as possible of your non-essential commitments, starting with the least important.

2. Introduce some times of solitude into your life. (I hear mothers of small children asking, "Are you crazy?) Watch the sun set. Go outside and look at the stars for a few minutes after the kids are asleep. Take a walk in a natural area.

3. Unplug. Spend much less time on the internet, doing emails, using cell phones, and watching TV. Consider turning all these devices off for a certain period of the day or certain day(s) of the week. They are such time-consumers that they can easily make the rest of life rushed and thus interfere with more important things that you should do.

4. Practice meditative breathing as described in the previous chapter. If you are doing Buteyko breathing for asthma, listen to the Buteyko CD at least once a day. I find it very relaxing. The exercises that have you take your control pause repeatedly, while good for re-setting your CO_2 trigger, may not be relaxing but rather like taking a test.

5. Listen to music while you work or any other time you can.

6. Get some exercise every day, outdoors if possible. Walk, run, swim or bicycle. The rhythm of these forms of exercise is calming.

7. Release grievances and personal conflicts. Forgive those who have hurt you, whether they "deserve" it or not. Whatever they did is not worth ruining your peace of mind or health. Unless they are immediate family members, you don't have to get chummy with them (Why ask for more trouble?), but forgive them deep in your soul. You are only hurting yourself and letting them control you by holding on to and mentally rehearsing how you have been wronged

8. Give up worrying. If doesn't accomplish anything except for draining your energy. Don't ignore the problem. Think about it; if things can be done to remedy it, make a "to do" list. Work through the list, but don't fret. Commit the problem to God.

9. Talk to friends who are positive people and are givers, not takers only. Avoid people who drain you and drag you down with negativity as much as possible.

10. Cut yourself some slack. You are not, and don't have to act as if you are responsible for the world. You can't do it all, so don't try. Prioritize what you have to do by level of importance and accept having to let some of the things at the bottom of the list go.

11. Keep breathing. When tense or rushed, we often tend to hold our breath or breathe shallowly and erratically. If you notice yourself doing this, take a good diaphragmatic breath in, allow a relaxed exhale, and then try to get into a normal breathing rhythm with relaxed exhales.

12. Give it all to God. Lay it at His feet and *leave it there*. He IS in charge of the world.

See the next chapter for more about a higher level of peace.

Ultimate Peace

Until now, this book has been about how to improve physical health. However, we are not only bodies; we also have minds and spirits. No part of us is unaffected by the other parts.

When I was young, I received advice for getting along with people that included avoiding conversation about potentially controversial topics such as politics and religion. This seemed like good advice to me unless I knew that the other person was likely to share my views on such subjects.

Then I spent over three and a half years struggling to breathe with asthma that was not relieved by medication. I felt as if my life were threatened on a near-daily basis for much of that time. Two years ago, while the asthma was still uncontrolled, I experienced another threat to my life when I was diagnosed with cancer.

These experiences have made me think about more than just the health of my body. The cancer could limit the time I have to convey any message, so I feel compelled to say important things I want to say *now*. I am about to break the old rule about what subjects to discuss. I am going to write about religion in contrast to *the real thing*.

It seems to me that religion is often an artificial man-made system that touches only the surface of life, sometimes detrimentally. It offers us no real connection, no personal relationship with God. It usually offers a formula, a system of what we must do and not do to achieve heaven. It may make us feel better mentally, but doesn't really cure what ails the soul or spirit. Sometimes adhering to formulas of rules, rituals, special days, etc. makes us think that we are as close to God as is humanly possible. This then serves as an immunization against *the real thing*. I have known people who persistently follow the formula and go through the motions in this kind of situation even though they find them meaningless. Amazingly, a few people in "rules" religions understand *the real thing* and it doesn't bother them that much of what their belief system teaches is at odds with *the real thing*.

Often people who realize that their religion is artificial and meaningless throw away the whole system with both hands. This is what I did at a young age. As a young child, I liked Sunday school where we heard about Jesus. In junior high school, we learned the rules. It was all so artificial that I felt I could not stand it. Finally, after listening to many complaints, my mother said I didn't have to go to the classes or church any more.

In high school I met new friends who were unusual in a way that I liked. For instance, my friend Leslie had such a sweet, calm spirit, she just exuded the peace that I wanted. My friends explained their beliefs to me, gave me things to read and prayed for me. In John 6:44, Jesus says, "No one can come to me unless the Father who sent me draws him." I've heard that the Greek word translated "draw" can also mean "drag." At age 17, I was easy to draw, as my friends were praying and waiting. I watched my father dragged at age 68 in response to my prayers of almost nineteen years. Cancer was the rope around his neck that dragged him. That he finally came to knowledge and acceptance of *the real thing* was a gift of God's mercy to him and to me.

What is the diagnosis of what ails our minds and spirits? There are a myriad of symptoms – guilt, depression, anxiety, etc. – all manifestations of a lack of peace. A peaceful spirit is needed for true physical health and mental health.

I once heard that a psychiatrist said, "If I could get rid of my patients' guilt, I soon would have no patients." We all know that we have failed in many ways, ranging from being irritable at our family and friends to more serious offenses against people. We have fallen short of what our consciences tell us we should do.

There is a difference between true guilt and guilty feelings, or false guilt.[1] With true guilt, we really are guilty. For example, my friend does not deserve me lashing out when I am upset about something that she isn't responsible for. I rightly feel guilty because I am guilty. I have wounded my friend and my conscience tells me this should not happen. *The real thing* gives the solution for true guilt.

Religion is what we try to do for God to earn his favor. *The real thing* is what God does for us, with no merit on our part. There is nothing that we have to do except admit our need and inability to do anything for ourselves and accept what He has done for us. When I hurt my friend, it is also an offense against God who tells us to "Love one another." (John 13:34). To achieve inner peace, I need to make amends with my friend and ask for forgiveness. Forgiveness from God has already been bought for us by Jesus, we only have to admit our need for it and accept it.[2]

The real thing brings us into a personal relationship with God. How can this be with our burden of guilt blocking the path? The answer to this question is that God bears the burden of our guilt Himself in the person of Jesus. Since relationships are two-sided, we must respond by confessing our need and asking Him to take the guilt upon Himself and grant us forgiveness and closeness with Him. Each of us has free will to make this decision. Once we admit that we need His forgiveness, he transforms us. "If anyone is in Christ, he is a new creation: old things are passed away; behold, all things have become new." (II Corinthians 5:17).[2]

To learn more about this relationship, receive forgiveness, and experience true peace with God (the most basic kind of peace), I suggest that you do what I did. Go straight to the source. Ask God to reveal Himself if He really exists. You can be totally honest with Him. Tell Him your hang-ups with religion and doubts about Him. (I heard a man say he used many swear words when he did this. It must have been all right because he found *the real thing*. See the books listed below for the experience of others who did

---

1 Guilty feelings can come from false guilt, as in a child whose parents have unreasonably high standards that they can never meet, or someone who is molested and feels shame and thinks that they did something to cause it.

2 Stott, John R.W. *Basic Christianity*. (Grand Rapids, MI, Willian B. Eerdmans Publishing Company, 1971), 107-136.

this.[3]) Get a Bible,[4] a version that fits you language-wise, and read it with a blank-slate mind to find out whatever you can, even if you disagree.

Be willing to be drawn or to find out the whole thing is bunk. You may find *the real thing*. Then "the peace of God, which passes all understanding, will keep your hearts and minds." (Philippians 4:7)

The ultimate cure is Jesus.

Additional Information

Stott, John R.W. *Basic Christianity*. Willian B. Eerdmans Publishing Company, Grand Rapids, MI, 1971. Stott was a British theologian who was greatly respected for over 65 years before his death in 2011. This book is short but complete and is for adults of all ages.

Bethke, Jefferson. *Jesus > Religion: Why He Is So Much Better Than Trying Harder, Doing More, and Being Good Enough*. Nelson Books, a division of Harper-Collins Christian Publishing, Nashville, TN, 2013. This book is written by a young man and directed at young adults but may speak to older adults as well.

The Seeker's Bible, New Testament with notes and helps by Greg Laurie. Tyndale House Publishers Inc., Wheaton, IL, 2000.

Stern, David H. *The Complete Jewish Bible*. Messianic Jewish Publisher, Clarksville, MD, 1998, 2016. Available online here with free shipping: https://www.barnesandnoble.com/w/complete-jewish-bible-david-h-stern/1102359994?ean=9781936716845

---

3 For the experiences of two people who asked questions, see these books:
    McDowell, Josh. *Evidence that Demands a Verdict, Volumes I and II*. Here's Life Publishing, San Bernardino, CA, 1989.
    Strobel, Lee. *The Case for Christ*. Zondervan, Grand Rapids, MI, 1998.

4 There is a variety of advice given to a person reading the Bible for the first time. Most often the New Testament, usually the Gospel of John, is recommended as the place to start. However, the first chapter of John contains a great deal of symbolic language that can be confusing. Those of Jewish heritage might start with the Old Testament and learn about their Messiah there before moving on to the rest of the Bible. (See where to get *The Complete Jewish Bible* above). When I, at age seventeen, went to a bookcase in my parents' house and removed a twenty-six year old Bible which still had pages stuck together, I read the book of Ecclesiastes first. I recently read about an Iraqi Christian who was drawn by a passage in the book of Amos. Ask God for direction on where *you* should begin.

Internet Resources

Smith, Colin, M.P. "Meet Jesus" sermon series. UnlockingTheBible.org, 2017.

http://unlockingthebible.org/sermon/he-brings-life/

http://unlockingthebible.org/sermon/he-wants-you-to-be-saved/

http://unlockingthebible.org/sermon/he-is-the-savior/

http://unlockingthebible.org/sermon/he-is-god/

http://unlockingthebible.org/sermon/he-can-be-trusted/

http://unlockingthebible.org/sermon/he-gives-strength/

http://unlockingthebible.org/sermon/he-knows-you-completely/

Each of these webpages contains a video of the sermon as well as a text copy. At the top of this list is a sermon that is very basic, yet complete and should not be missed. The rest give information about who Jesus is and our relationship with Him.

Putting Good Nutrition into Practice

In previous chapters of this book we discussed how to optimize health by practicing good nutrition and breathing, pursuing peace, and making wise choices of treatments. More pages were devoted to nutritional ways to help yourself than to anything else. Now it is time to put the information about good nutrition into practice.

Readers of this book have a variety of health problems that can make cooking difficult. Cancer patients often have extremely low energy or are incapacitated by chemotherapy. Those with food allergies and gluten intolerance may also experience limitations of energy and time yet realize that they have best control of their diets and health if they prepare most foods themselves.

The question that arises is, "How can I do what is best health-wise with no energy to cook?" A simple change to address problems of low energy or insufficient time is to use commercially prepared healthy foods rather than preparing everything at home. See pages 251 to 257 for sources of healthy prepared foods, including foods for allergy and gluten-free diets. If you have someone who can shop for you or are able to shop yourself, check grocery and health food stores for healthy prepared foods and read labels of foods that seem promising. Then see "When Cooking is Difficult" on the next page for easy meal ideas and for more advice about how to eat well when low on energy.

If you are able to cook or have a friend or family member who will do some cooking for you, see "Easy Dinners" on pages 94 to 107 and the other recipe chapters that follow. At the end of each chapter you will find suggestions for foods featured in the chapter that you can purchase already made as well as sources of related recipes.

Enjoy the healthy foods in the following chapters. I hope that much improved health accompanies better nutrition.

When Cooking is Difficult

Some readers of this book may be recovering from surgery, undergoing chemo-therapy or suffering from incapacitating illness. In spite of their misery, they have read about ways to improve their health. Some ways, such as meditative breathing, require little energy. However, even thinking about making cultured vegetables or bone broth may be exhausting. Here are some ideas for what to do when cooking is difficult that I hope will be helpful.

One suggestion is to let major food preparation tasks be done by companies which make and sell bone broth, cultured vegetables or dairy products, or even bread, Eng-lish muffins and cereal made with sprouted grains. See pages 252 to 257 for a list of companies that make health promoting-foods and search their websites to find where their products are sold nearby or how to order them online. Although pricey, if you are searching for bone broth, cultured vegetables, sprouted grain bread, and nut butters made from soaked nuts, Wise Choice Market carries all of these for one-website shop-ping. See "Sources," page 251 for ordering information.

My hope is that you have family members or friends who will help you with meals, laundry, and shopping. The "Easy Dinners" chapter that follows will provide ideas for oven or crockpot meals that can cook while the helper is away.

Another option is to hire help. In the Denver, Colorado area, there is a caregiver agency called Elderlink™ that is considerably less expensive than other agencies because the caregivers are self-employed. Elderlink™ screens caregivers, has them bonded and insured, connects them with clients, and helps with schedules. The caregivers will help with anything from an occasional four-hour shift to 24-7 care. If there is a moderately priced agency such as Elderlink™ nearby, and especially if you will need help for a short time only, hiring a caregiver may be something to consider.

Cooking, even when done by a family member, friend, or paid caregiver, can and should be kept simple. See the recipes on pages 95 to 98 for whole meals that can be cooked in the crockpot, or try crockpot bean soup for dinner. (Several types of easy legume soup recipes are on pages 178 to 180). One-dish meals baked in the oven are found on pages 98 to 100. Another option is to plan an oven meal, which is an oven entrée (pages 101 to 102), oven vegetable (pages 103 to 105) and oven grain (pages 146 to 149) baked in the oven at the same time. Perhaps you or the cook will even make an easy and comforting warm oven fruit dessert (pages 105 to 107).

Use frozen vegetables and pre-washed salad greens to save on washing and chopping. Frozen vegetables are just as nutritious as fresh and may even contain more nutrients if the fresh vegetables have been stored for some time or shipped long distances.

Here is an example of how home care can work, especially for those on special diets. In her older years, Marjorie Hurt Jones, author of *The Allergy Self-Help Cookbook*, had a stroke that left her with mobility problems. Her husband, Stan, was legally blind. She told me they had "assisted living at home." They had a caregiver come most mornings to cook, do laundry and take them to appointments. Marge taught her helper about allergy cooking. Her helper was then able to prepare a wide variety of wheat-free baked goods, dinners that could be put in the oven in the afternoon, and other easily warmed or ready-to-eat foods. The Joneses did quite well, ate healthily, enjoyed being in their own home, and escaped problems of institutional living such as over-medication and infections.

There is quite a contrast between what Marge and Stan ate and what my 93-year old aunt is served in the assisted living center where she ended up after a fall. I listen to her and her diabetic friend complain about the biscuits and gravy for breakfast, white flour and sugar laden baked goods at every meal, sloppy Joe sandwiches on Wonder Bread™-style buns, and especially the Tex-Mex food served several times a week, which is too spicy for both of these ladies in their 90s. This illustration makes it obvious that I would prefer to age at home, but as with medical decisions, *you* must make the decision that is best for *you*.

What I am about to write is my opinion biased by living with inhalant allergies from early childhood and food allergies from my mid-20s to the present in my mid-60s. A second disclaimer is that I am assuming the audience for this discussion is people of adequate mental condition to read this book. In my opinion, *each person* should be allowed to make *his or her own decision* about relinquishing control of aspects of life such as what to eat and where to live. All of us should be allowed to control our diet and the quality of the air we breathe because these can have a tremendous impact on health. We should have the right to breathe and eat in a way that improves our health rather than to have medical professionals apply unwanted "bandaids" (usually drugs) to health problems that can be treated by diet and environmental control.

Current law gives us the right to refuse any medical treatment. However, when my aunt had an eye treatment for macular disease that she had taken many times while living at home, the assisted living facility nurse brought osycodone and insisted that my aunt take it. Each of us must realize that we are not helpless and be assertive about our rights if necessary. Knowing that we have rights and fleeing from helplessness is good for both mental and physical health. See pages 40 to 42 for more about the benefits of dispelling helplessness.

With good nutrition and loving help, I hope you will be much better very soon! For now, read the easy dinner recipes starting on page 94 and the prepared food section of "Sources," pages 251 to 257, and decide what you would like to eat.

About the Recipes and Ingredients

Hippocrates said, "Let your food be your medicine and your medicine be your food." The purpose of the recipes in this book is to offer you food to enhance and improve your health, as well as being delicious and enjoyable.

The recipes in this book apply the preparation techniques used by the primitive cultures Dr. Price studied that make foods both easy to digest and highly nutritious. Most of them are also allergy-friendly. A list of recipes from other sources is found at the end the recipe chapters to offer non-allergic readers more variety. For example, the last sentence in the cultured vegetables chapter refers readers to pages 93 to 102 in *Nourishing Traditions* for cultured vegetable recipes containing more allergenic ingredients such as garlic and corn.

Allergy cooking, especially baking, is more exacting than cooking with more forgiving "normal" ingredients. In allergy cooking and bread-machine baking, the measurements often cannot be rounded off to the nearest half teaspoon or fourth cup without changing the quality of the completed food. Therefore, some of the recipes in this book use less common amounts of ingredients, such as $1/16$ teaspoon or ⅙ cup. A chart is included on page 249 to help you measure such amounts. It is worthwhile to invest in a liquid measuring cup that has eighth cup markings, an ⅛ cup coffee measure for dry ingredients, and a set of measuring spoons that has an ⅛ teaspoon. If you are measuring very small amounts of dry ingredients such as stevia in measuring spoons, you can fill the ⅛ teaspoon, level it off, and then used a knife to divide it down the middle and scrape half of it out.

Many of the recipes contain ingredients that may be unfamiliar to some readers. Therefore, these less common ingredients are discussed below.

Ingredients

Cultures

About one fifth of the recipes in this book are for cultured foods. Several decades ago, all that was required to ensure a successful outcome of fermentation was to make sure the food had the correct environmental conditions. The skin of grapes was populated with the right yeast to make wine, cabbage contained the right bacteria to make sauerkraut, and unpasteurized milk contained *Lactobacillus* to produce yogurt. In San Francisco, the air would populate bread dough with the right yeast and bacteria to produce sourdough bread. These organisms, producers of fermentation that would preserve food, made the food tasty and enriched it with nutrients. These bacteria also populated our bodies with beneficial flora and thus were good for our health.

However, now milk often is laced with antibiotics, vegetables are covered with pesticides, and we live in a world of multiple antibiotic resistant "super bugs." Therefore, I recommend always using the correct culture when you make cultured foods. It ensures that the fermentation will go well (rather than having the food spoil as described on pages 60 to 61) and that the food benefits one's health. Information about the cultures used here follows.

Yogurt cultures contain the friendly bacteria *Lactobacillus bulgaricus* and *Streptococcus thermophilus*. Some cultures and commercially made yogurt also contain *Lactobacillus acidophilus*. However, this organism will be present in the final yogurt in very low numbers because the other organisms in the yogurt culture will eventually make the milk too acidic for *Lactobacillus acidophilus* to thrive. Yet, if other species of *Lactobacillus* such as *Lactobacillus bulgaricus* temporarily make a home in the intestine, they can enable *Lactobacillus acidophilus* from probiotic supplements to implant and grow.

Most yogurt cultures contain cow milk. However, GI Pro Start™ makes a yogurt culture that does not. It is gluten-free, casein-free, and acceptable on the Specific Carbohydrate (SCD) and GAPS diets. See page 261 for ordering information.

Acidophilus milk cultures contain only *Lactobacillus acidophilus*. Like commercial yogurt cultures, the starters sold for the purpose of making acidophilus milk contain cow milk so are not used in the recipes in this book. Instead, some dairy-free probiotic supplements can be used for making acidophilus milk. The supplement that I recently have used in reasonable quantities is Klaire Therbiotic Factor 1™. Four capsules of Therbiotic Factor 1™ (about one teaspoon of the powder) will make a quart of excellent acidophilus milk. Klaire also makes a probiotic called *L. acidophilus* SCD Compliant™ that works but requires twelve capsules to make a quart of acidophilus milk. To order these supplements, see "Sources," page 262.

Cultures for making fermented vegetables contain lactic acid-producing bacteria that, before pesticides, were normal flora of vegetables. These organisms include *Lactobacillus plantarum, Leuconostoc mesenteroides* and *Pediococcus acidilactici*. I use Caldwell Starter Culture for Fresh Vegetables™. (See "Sources," page 261). When I first chose it, it had the best hypoallergenic ingredient list of any vegetable culture on the market. This culture still says "lactose-free and vegan" on the box, but a few years ago added maltodextrin to their ingredient list. Although maltodextrin can come from corn, I have not noticed any allergy problems from using this culture. The box contains instructions and their website contains a video on how to make fermented vegetables using this culture. Instructions are also found in the recipes on pages 110 to 119.

Sourdough cultures which come as a small jar of dough or packet of freeze dried dough contain wild yeast and bacteria of the genus *Lactobacillus* that live in a symbiotic relationship. The *Lactobacillus* gives the bread its characteristic sour flavor, but the degree of sourness varies with the type and source of the culture. Because the yeast may be a different strain than commercial baker's yeast, some people who are allergic to bread made with baker's yeast can eat sourdough. (Ask your doctor whether this might be true for you before trying it). Wild yeast leavens bread much more slowly than baker's yeast.

These sourdough cultures almost always contain wheat flour. The cultures must be fed often, which is not a problem if you use them weekly for baking. If not using them often, I tended to forget to feed them and would find them growing green, pink or black scum, so they had to be discarded. See "Sources," page 262 for a gluten-free live sourdough culture.

Several years ago, the King Arthur Baker's Catalogue began selling a freeze-dried *Lactobacillus* culture that can be used to make sourdough bread, which they call **French-style sourdough starter**. It is wheat-free and gluten-free. When I asked them about other allergenic ingredients use to produce it, they said it could contain a trace of beef from the media which was used to grow the bacteria. To use this culture, a very small amount of the culture is added to water and flour and kept in a cozy place for 18 to 20 hours. Then a small amount of SAF instant yeast and the remaining bread ingredients are added. After kneading, the dough incubates for several more hours before shaping, rising, and baking. Using the freeze-dried culture makes the sourdough process predictable enough to make the bread in a programmable bread machine. It also eliminates the need to keep a live culture in your refrigerator and remember to feed it routinely. See "Sources," page 262 for the freeze-dried culture.

Baker's yeast is available in two varieties. **Active dry yeast** is yeast that has been freeze-dried to retain its activity. An expiration date is usually stamped on the package and the yeast should be good until that date if you store it in the refrigerator after opening it. Active dry yeast is available in one-fourth ounce (2¼ teaspoon) packets or four ounce jars in most grocery stores. In addition, you can purchase it in one pound bags and store the yeast in your freezer. Do not thaw and refreeze this yeast each time you use it. Instead, occasionally take out a small amount to use within a few weeks and keep it in a jar in the refrigerator. Leave the remainder of the yeast in the freezer. Red Star™ active dry yeast is free of grains and preservatives and works well for allergy and gluten-free breads made in a bread machine as well as by hand.

Instant or quick-rise yeast leavens bread more rapidly than active dry yeast. It is useful for making bread by hand more quickly. To use quick-rise yeast in your bread machine, use a quick cycle designed to be used with quick-rise yeast or a recipe developed for quick-rise yeast. This "fast" type of yeast is not recommended for most non-wheat bread machine breads because their gluten structure is more fragile. If quick-rise yeast is used, the bread may over-rise and then collapse during baking. However, quick-rise yeast does work well for white spelt bread and breads made with bread flour, which is a high-gluten white wheat flour. Because SAF Instant Yeast™ tolerates acid better than active dry yeast, it is used for all sourdough bread made with the freeze-dried starter discussed above. Quick-rise yeast also can be purchased in one pound bags and kept in the freezer except for a small refrigerated jar to be used in the immediate future. See "Sources," page 260, for where to purchase yeast.

Milks

To make the various fermented milks in the next chapter, you must begin with milk. All of the fermented milk recipes in this book can be made with cow milk but individuals with dairy allergy may want to try the alternative milks listed below. The higher fat milks will produce thicker fermented milk. Local chapters of the Weston Price Foundation (www.westonaprice.org) can help you find sources for the alternative milks listed here or for raw milk.

Goat milk is the most commonly available alternative animal milk. Most health food stores and some grocery stores sell fresh pasteurized goat milk. Goat milk is lower in protein than cow milk, so yogurt or acidophilus milk made from it form a very soft curd that liquefies if the cultured milk is stirred. Skim goat milk is commercially available. However, it is less nutritious than whole goat milk and makes very thin, watery yogurt and acidophilus milk, so I advise using whole goat milk instead.

Sheep milk is higher in protein and fat than goat milk so makes yogurt which is very thick and creamy. To get fresh sheep milk, you will have to find a nearby sheep dairy or a local farmer who milks sheep. Local Weston Price Foundation chapters may be able to help. Sheep yogurt is sold in health food stores near my home so I have purchased it rather than searching for sheep milk. See "Sources," page 256, for where to order sheep yogurt, or ask your health food store to carry it.

Camel milk has a delicious sweet mild flavor and makes soft-curd yogurt like goat milk. Amazingly, I live near a small family-owned camel dairy farm. Consult your local chapter of the Weston Price Foundation to see if you have a camel dairy nearby, or see "Sources," page 257, to purchase camel milk online.

If you have access to them, **other animal milks**, such as llama milk, also should work in the recipes in this book

Flours

Many different kinds of flour can be used instead of wheat flour in allergy and gluten-free cooking. The gluten-containing grain flours are the most allergenic; non-gluten grains may be easier to tolerate. Additionally, non-grain alternative flours are tasty and readily available. Since many individuals have never or rarely eaten alternative grains, allergy to them is not common.

Gluten-containing grain flours include spelt, kamut, rye, barley and wheat. Among the non-gluten grains are teff, rice, wild rice, millet, sorghum, and corn. Oats used to be classified as a gluten-containing grain, and do contain a protein very similar to gluten. However, now oats are considered acceptable in moderation for some gluten-sensitive individuals. Non-grain flours include amaranth, quinoa, buckwheat, tapioca, cassava meal, arrowroot, chestnut flour, water chestnut flour, and various legume flours and starches such as garbanzo flour, soy flour, carob powder, lupine flour, bean starch, and kudzu starch.

Gluten containing grains make the most "normal" baked goods. **Spelt, kamut,** and **rye** make good yeast breads. However, spelt and kamut are very closely related to **wheat,** being in the same genus but different species. (This, with recent misinformation from the government, has led to confusion about spelt. See the footnote about spelt on the next page). Baked goods made with **barley** flour are slightly more crumbly but still have good texture and flavor. The "crumbliness" of barley makes it especially well suited for making tender pie crusts. Oat flour also has a fine flavor, although some oat-based baked goods are quite dense and occasionally can be gummy.

Individuals who consume wheat, especially **cancer patients, should purchase organic wheat flour.** About two weeks before harvest, non-organic wheat is sprayed with Roundup™ (glyphosate) to desiccate the wheat, thus making it easier to harvest and process into flour. Since this occurs shortly before harvest, it accounts for 50% of the glyphosate on harvested wheat. The State of California has classified glyphosate as a probable carcinogen. In addition, it is an endocrine disruptor, damages DNA and thus is linked to birth defects, and harms beneficial intestinal flora.[1] If you cannot afford organic flour, seek out King Arthur™ white whole wheat flour. Although they have organic options for most types of flour, their "regular" flour is not certified organic. However, a customer care representative reassured me that they carefully choose the farmers who grow their wheat and most to all of them eschew pre-harvest spraying with Roundup™.[2] Because their white whole wheat flour is an identity preserved product,

---

1 Roseboro, Ken. "Why is Glyphosate Sprayed on Crops Right Before Harvest?" EcoWatch, March 5, 2016. https://www.ecowatch.com/why-is-glyphosate-sprayed-on-crops-right-before-harvest-1882187755.html

Also Benbrook, Charles M. "Trends in glyphosate herbicide use in the United States and globally." *Environmental Sciences Europe,* 28:3, 2016. https://enveurope.springeropen.com/articles/10.1186/s12302-016-0070-0 Benbrook writes, "Other factors contributed to rising glyphosate use. These include steady expansion in the number of crops registered for use on glyphosate product labels, the adoption of no-tillage and conservation tillage systems, the declining price per pound of active ingredient, new application method and timing options, and new agricultural use patterns (e.g., as a desiccant to accelerate the harvest of small grains, edible beans, and other crops).... Harvest-aid uses of glyphosate have become increasingly common since the mid-2000s in U.S. northern-tier states on wheat, barley, edible beans, and a few other crops, as well as in much of northern Europe [41, 42, 43]. Because such applications occur within days of harvest, they result in much higher residues in the harvested foodstuffs [42]. To cover such residues, Monsanto and other glyphosate registrants have requested, and generally been granted, substantial increases in glyphosate tolerance levels in several crops, as well as in the animal forages derived from such crops."

2 Quote from the customer care representative's email about King Arthur's white whole wheat flour, their first identity preserved product: "In addition to other requirements of this [identity preserved] program, our farmers are not permitted to use glyphosate as a pre-harvest application on the white winter wheat it's milled from. Our team is continuing to expand the level of control we have over aspects of growing practices to our other products, and we recognize that our work in this is never done. Although most of our flour is from wheat fields and farmers that do not use glyphosate pre-harvest, we're unable to offer a 100% guarantee of this except on our organic line of flours."

the farmers that grow this wheat are not permitted to use glyphosate as a pre-harvest application.

Be sure to purchase high-quality flour. Arrowhead Mills™ and Bob's Red Mill™ flours are good for most grains and grain alternatives. For spelt, I recommend using Purity Foods™ flour. All of the spelt recipes in my books were developed using Purity Foods™ flour because their flour is milled from a European strain of spelt that is higher in protein than other strains and consistently produces high quality baked goods. Purity Foods™ also sells a sifted spelt flour called "white spelt" flour. Ask your health food store to carry Purity Foods™ flour or search for VitaSpelt™ to purchase it online.

There is tremendous variability in other brands of spelt flour from brand to brand and bag to bag of the same brand. If you cannot purchase Purity Foods flour™ and must use another brand, you will need to add more spelt flour to recipes to achieve the right consistency in your non-yeast baked goods. Other brands of spelt flour are not recommended for yeast bread. All brands of spelt flour must display an erroneous "Contains wheat" allergen warning on the bag.[3] However, spelt is tolerated by many individuals who are allergic to wheat. It does contain gluten so should not be consumed by those on a gluten-free diet.

Non-gluten grains include **teff, rice, wild rice, millet, sorghum,** and **corn.** Baked goods made with these flours are more crumbly than those made with gluten-containing

---

3 **About spelt:** A great deal of confusion has risen concerning spelt. The United States government now requires that foods be labeled to indicate whether they contain any of eight food allergens. As part of the implementation of this law, the FDA has declared that spelt is wheat and bags of spelt products must be labeled "Contains wheat." Although spelt and wheat are indeed closely related, they are two different species in the same genus. Spelt is *Triticum spelta* and wheat is *Triticum aestivum*. When asked why they had decided that spelt is wheat, a FDA official said that it was because spelt contains gluten. (They had no answer to the question of whether rye would also be considered wheat because it contains gluten).

Spelt does indeed contain gluten and should not be eaten by anyone who is gluten-sensitive or has celiac disease, but the presence of gluten does not make spelt wheat. The gluten in spelt behaves differently than the gluten in wheat in cooking. It is extremely difficult to make seitan from spelt. When making seitan from wheat, a process of soaking in hot water is used to remove the starch from the protein. If the same process is followed with spelt, the protein structure also dissolves in the hot water. Spelt seitan must be washed by hand very carefully under running cold water.

Because the gluten in spelt is more soluble than wheat gluten, making yeast bread with spelt is also different from making it with wheat. The individual gluten molecules merge more readily to form long chains and sheets that trap the gas produced by yeast. This means that it is possible to over-knead spelt bread. There are some bread machines that work quite well for wheat and even other allergy breads but are unacceptable for spelt bread because they knead so vigorously that they over-develop the gluten. It is possible that the greater solubility of spelt protein makes it easier to digest than wheat. Undoubtedly, most people have had much less prior exposure to spelt than to wheat, resulting in less opportunity to become allergic to spelt. Whatever the reason, there are people who suffer allergic reactions after eating wheat but do not react to spelt. I have talked to many of them. Consult your doctor about your own food allergy test results and follow the diet recommended for you, but there is no need to unnecessarily restrict spelt consumption based on error-ridden government labeling requirements.

grain flours. Some recipes using these flours contain a starch for "glue," but still you have to expect some crumbs and heaviness. However, the flavor of the non-gluten grains is excellent. Millet and sorghum have an especially good flavor, and since they are not staples of most diets, may be tolerated better than rice.

Non-grain flours such as **amaranth, quinoa, buckwheat, tapioca starch, cassava meal, arrowroot** and various **legume flours** are surprisingly versatile. Their flavor may take a little getting used to, but given a little time, you will likely enjoy them. If quinoa is used with apple juice, sesame seeds, or carob, its distinctive flavor will be masked. My recipes which use amaranth and quinoa usually contain a starch to improve the texture of the final product. Most of the non-grains, especially if used with a starch, produce acceptable, non-crumbly texture in baked goods. However, an occasional batch of amaranth flour might yield gummy pancakes or yeast bread. Yet, if one cannot tolerate any grains, fussiness may be outweighed by hunger. When amaranth pancakes turned out gummy, I toasted them until crisp.

Nut flours or ground nuts also are used in a few recipes in this book. They contain no carbohydrates but are a good source of protein, healthy fat, vitamins and minerals. **Almond flour** has the added advantage of being available in a very finely ground form that is good for baking. Not all almond flour is suitable for baking however. It must be made from blanched (skinless) almonds and be very finely ground to produce consistently acceptable baking results. In addition, nuts and nut flours should be stored in the refrigerator or freezer to keep the fat from becoming rancid. Of the types of finely-ground blanched almond flour available, I prefer Honeyville™ almond flour because it is economical and excellent for baking. See "Sources," page 266, to purchase this flour.

Sweeteners

The recipes in this book are sweetened without sugar. Instead, most of them are made with sweeteners allowed on the anti-cancer diet. These include agave, coconut sugar and stevia. **Agave** and **coconut sugar** have very low glycemic index scores so do not provoke the release of much insulin. Some of the recipes provide options for sweetening with **fruit sweeteners** of various kinds to give individuals on allergy rotation diets more sweetening options for every day of their rotation diet. See "Sources," page 267, for information about purchasing these sweeteners.

Stevia is a natural non-nutritive sweetener that has no impact on blood sugar. In fact, the herb it comes from is promoted as a supplement helpful for diabetics. This herb is *Stevia rebaudiana* and is a member of the composite (lettuce) family. It has been used in Japan, Paraguay, Brazil, and other parts of the world for hundreds of years. Furthermore, it is approved by the FDA for use as a supplement and as an "additive" in soda pop, although they have ruled against labeling it as a sweetener. It is available in several forms such as finely crushed leaves, liquid, and white powder.

Most stevia has a slight licorice-like taste which may be noticeable in bland recipes but is almost undetectable in recipes containing strongly flavored ingredients. However, several years ago a new more neutral tasting white stevia powder was developed which is treated during production with an enzyme that reduces the licorice taste. Some brands of this "next generation" stevia powder are cut with allergenic ingredients such as malto-dextrin, which usually comes from corn. The stevia recipes in this book were developed using the most neutral, purely-sweet tasting of the new stevia powders which contains no fillers and also is the most economical. It may be ordered from Berlin Seeds.™ See "Sources, page 267, for ordering information.

Stevia is a good sweetener for cooking as well as for health. Unlike some man-made non-nutritive sweeteners, stevia can be heated to any cooking temperature and for any length of time without breaking down. Expect your stevia sweetened desserts to be light colored; baked goods made with stevia do not brown much. A great baking combination is stevia and chocolate or carob because the chocolate or carob masks any licorice-like taste and contributes a rich brown color. The amount of stevia in a recipe may be given as a range because the perception of how sweet stevia tastes varies from person to person. Until you know how much stevia you prefer, use the smaller amount in the recipe the first time you make it. Then increase the amount gradually, if desired, until it tastes best to you. If you prefer more than the largest amount given in the recipe, that is fine. It will not affect how the recipe rises, etc.

Leavening Ingredients

The principle of leavening is the production of gas which is trapped in the structure of a baked product in the form of small bubbles. These bubbles solidify as the food bakes. In yeast bread, the gas is produced by the metabolism of **yeast.** (For more about yeast turn back to page 86). Non-yeast baked goods are leavened by the reaction of **baking soda** with an **acidic ingredient** to produce carbon dioxide gas that forms bubbles.

In this book, the acidic ingredient used in baking may be a liquid such as lemon juice, lime juice or rhubarb concentrate (recipe on page 190) or a dry powder such as cream of tartar or unbuffered vitamin C powder or crystals. When the baking soda and acidic ingredient become wet, they react with each other to release gas into the batter or dough, thus making it rise. Commercial baking powder contains both components plus a starch (usually cornstarch) to keep the acid and basic components dry so they do not react until shortly before baking. Featherweight™ baking powder contains potato starch instead of cornstarch. Since potato should be rotated, if you are on a rotation diet, use this baking powder only on your potato day. See "Sources," page 258 to order this baking powder.

Baking soda is a simple, pure chemical which individuals on rotation diets need not rotate. The various acidic ingredients that can be used with it to produce leavening include unbuffered vitamin C powder, cream of tartar, vinegar, citrus juices, pineapple juice, rhubarb concentrate, yogurt and buttermilk. (See page 190 for a recipe for rhubarb concentrate). Except for hypoallergenic non-corn source vitamin C, these acidic ingredients should be rotated if you are on a rotation diet.

Most of the recipes in this book call for **unbuffered vitamin C powder or crystals** as the acidic component of leavening. (Powder and crystals are used in equal amounts). The powder is available in a very hypoallergenic form which usually does not require rotation. I use Ecological Formulas™ brand which is a tapioca source vitamin C powder. Commonly, vitamin C is made from corn, so seek out a brand not made from corn. Also, take care to purchase unbuffered vitamin C because buffered vitamin C will not provide the acid needed for the leavening process. Unbuffered vitamin C powder and unbuffered vitamin C crystals may be used interchangeably in the same amounts. See "Sources," page 259, for ordering information for tapioca source vitamin C powder.

Cream of tartar comes from grapes as a byproduct of wine making. If a person is on a rotation diet, cream of tartar should be rotated on the same day as grapes. If you wish to substitute cream of tartar for the vitamin C called for in a recipe, use about the same amount of cream of tartar as the recipe calls for of baking soda, or about four times as much vitamin C as is called for. For example, if a recipe calls for 1 teaspoon of baking soda and ¼ teaspoon of vitamin C, use 1 teaspoon of baking soda and 1 teaspoon of cream of tartar. You may have to experiment with the amounts a little to produce the best results.

Vinegar, citrus juices, or **rhubarb concentrate** can be substituted for vitamin C as the acidic component in leavening. Use about three times as much of these liquids as the amount of baking powder the recipe calls for. For instance, if a recipe calls for 1 teaspoon of baking powder and ¼ teaspoon of vitamin C, use 1 teaspoon of baking powder and 3 teaspoons of vinegar, citrus juice, or rhubarb concentrate. In some recipes, you may need to decrease the amount of other liquids to compensate for the volume of vinegar, citrus juice, or rhubarb concentrate you are using. **Yogurt** and **buttermilk** may also be used as the acidic component of leavening. Use recipes for baked goods made with buttermilk or yogurt such as found in *Nourishing Traditions* for the correct amount of these acid ingredients and baking soda.

The acidic leavening ingredients mentioned above also can be used to make salad dressings. If you cannot use vinegar due to yeast allergy, substitute citrus juices in an amount equal to the vinegar or rhubarb concentrate in a slightly greater amount. You can also substitute ½ teaspoon to 1 teaspoon of a tart-tasting brand of unbuffered vitamin C powder mixed with ¼ cup water for the vinegar in your favorite salad dressing recipe. Ecological Formulas™ tapioca-source vitamin C is great tasting in salads. (See "Sources," page 259, for information on ordering this brand of vitamin C). Adjust the amount of vitamin C to your taste preference. For a few salad dressing recipes using these ingredients, see pages 125 to 127.

Although **guar gum** and **xanthan gum** do not contribute to the leavening process by producing gas, they are types of soluble fiber that can help to trap leavening gases in breads and other baked goods made from low- and non-gluten flours. When used in yeast breads, they help to strengthen bread's structure so it can rise well. They can also be used to thicken oil-free salad dressings. Guar gum is derived from a legume and therefore should be rotated on the same day as beans. Xanthan gum is derived from the bacteria, *Xanthomonas compestris*. Unfortunately, this bacteria is usually grown in corn-containing media, so xanthan gum may cause reactions in individuals who are allergic to corn. Guar and xanthan gum can be substituted for each other in equal amounts.

The type of **water** used might seem to have no effect on the leavening process but it does affect yeast. Do not use distilled water in yeast bread; yeast needs the minerals that are in tap water, purified water and spring water to thrive. In addition, **do not drink distilled water**. It can leach minerals out of the body with continued use.

Game Meats

Game meats are used in the bone broth recipes in this book. As discussed in a previous chapter, game is higher in omega-3 fatty acids than conventionally raised commercially produced meat. In spite of the health benefits of game, some people are reluctant to try it because they expect it to taste "gamey" or to be expensive and hard to find. Indeed, if your neighbor goes hunting and gives you some game, it may taste "gamey" because of the way it was handled. Proper cooking can usually overcome this problem. If hunted game has a wild taste, rub the frozen meat with salt before you put it in your refrigerator to thaw. Trimming the fat before cooking also reduces the gamey taste. A final suggestion is to educate the hunter. Meat from animals that are frightened and run and then are killed does not taste as good as meat from animals that are not startled and are killed with the first shot. Furthermore, the animal should be refrigerated and butchered as soon as possible.

Commercially produced game has a better flavor than some home-hunted game and may not be any more expensive than grass-fed beef. Call around for prices when you are shopping for game. Game animals graze and have very healthy lives. They get much exercise throughout their lives and are not given hormones or other drugs.

Game meat tends to be tougher and less well marbled with fat than most of the meat in your grocery store. Long slow cooking with liquid, such as in a crockpot, tenderizes game meat. You can also grind game to overcome toughness and use the ground meat in casseroles and burgers.

Now that we have discussed new foods you might use, the next chapters provide recipes which tell how to make these foods into delicious meals and snacks that will help optimize your health.

Easy Dinners

Meals can be easy to prepare or to have a family member, friend or helper prepare using appliances you probably already have such as an oven and a crockpot. When one is short on energy or time, a crockpot can be a lifesaver. With a crockpot, dinner can be started in the morning and a delicious meal will be ready at the end of the day. A crockpot also saves money because less expensive cuts of meat are flavorful and tender when cooked all day and because dried beans are easily prepared in a crockpot.

The recipes in this chapter are for a three-quart crockpot. If your crockpot holds five or six quarts, you can still use these recipes. If you are cooking for one or two people, cut the recipes in half for smaller size crockpots. However, I would suggest investing about $25 in a no-frills six-quart crockpot to make the best use of your time. If you cook a larger quantity of crockpot meals than will be eaten immediately, freeze the leftovers for future meals. When you remove the leftovers from the freezer, you will be glad that the meals are already made, ready to heat and eat. The best way to use a crockpot to simplify your life is to own a six-quart crockpot, double the recipes in this chapter, and freeze enough leftovers for several meals.

The crockpot bean soups on pages 178 to 180 take little time to make, but you must plan ahead and start the recipe the day before the soup will be served for dinner. Put the beans to soak the morning of the day before you plan to serve the soup or at least soak them overnight. If you will be pressed for time the next morning, also prepare the vegetables and other ingredients the evening before serving the soup. In the morning, rinse the beans, add the other ingredients to the pot, turn it on, and you will have a delicious, wonderful-smelling dinner ready to eat by late afternoon.

Conventional ovens usually are not considered time-saving appliances, but you will save time using your oven and the recipes here if you count *your* time rather than how much time it takes food to cook. Although the food will cook slowly, allowing time for the flavors to blend deliciously, the amount of time you or a helper spends working on the meal can be brief. The recipes in this chapter include a few for a whole meal cooked in one baking dish and many for entrées or side dishes which cook in separate baking dishes at the same time as the rest of the meal.

Oven meals usually consist of a main dish, a starchy side dish such as a grain or starchy vegetable, a non-starchy vegetable, and possibly a dessert all baked together in the oven at the same time. When I first made oven side dishes, I was amazed at how delicious and easy-to-make oven grains and oven vegetables were – much tastier than their stove-top counterparts. The side dishes and desserts are more flexible than some oven-baked foods such as pies and cakes. They can cook at a range of temperatures and for a range of times. Whatever time and temperature the main dish needs, the side dishes usually will take also. However, you may need to add a little more water to the side dishes if they will cook for a longer-than-usual time or at a higher temperature.

With your entire dinner in the oven, you can rest or catch up on other activities during the hour or two before dinner. The side dishes, and sometimes even the main dish, can be served directly from the casserole or baking dish they cooked in, thus also saving time and energy on washing dishes.

Enjoy the spare time and simplicity of these meals.

Crockpot Dinners

Crockpot Roast Dinner

This recipe makes inexpensive, less-tender cuts of beef taste like gourmet fare. It's so easy and delicious that it makes a great meal if you have visitors. With most of the meal in your crockpot, you will have time to visit with your friends.

> 1 2 to 2½ pound chuck roast, rump roast, or pot roast of beef, buffalo,
>   or other red game meat
> 2 large or 3 small potatoes, scrubbed or peeled and cut into chunks (optional)
> 3 carrots, scrubbed or peeled and cut into 2-inch pieces
> 1 onion, peeled and sliced or cut into eighths (optional)
> ½ cup purified water, bone broth, or red wine[1]
> 1 tomato, chopped, 1 tablespoon tomato paste or 2 to 3 tablespoons sugar-free
>   catsup[1] (optional)
> Dash of unrefined salt
> Dash of pepper (optional)

Scrub or peel and cut up the vegetables and put them into the bottom of a three quart crockpot. Set the roast on top of the vegetables. Stir together the water, broth, or wine with the tomato, tomato paste or catsup. Pour the liquid over the roast. Sprinkle the roast with the salt and pepper. Cook on low for 10 to 12 hours or on high for 5 to 8 hours. This recipe is very tasty when made with a sweet red wine such as Marsala. The alcohol evaporates during cooking leaving just its flavor, but if you are allergic to yeast, do not use the wine. If you prefer more juice with your roast, increase the amount of water, broth or wine to 1 cup and double the amount of tomato, tomato paste or catsup. Makes 4 to 6 servings.

---

1 If you are on a low-yeast diet for *Candida* or are allergic to yeast, do not use the wine or vinegar-containing catsup.

Corned Beef Dinner

This easy meal offers a change from the ordinary.

> 1 2 to 3-pound corned beef or bison brisket
> 2 to 3 potatoes, scrubbed or peeled and cut into large chunks
> 3 to 4 carrots, scrubbed or peeled and cut into 2-inch pieces
> Purified water
> 1 head of cabbage (optional)
> ½ teaspoon unrefined salt
> Dash of pepper (optional)

Scrub or peel and cut up the carrots and potatoes and put them into the bottom of a three quart crockpot. Place the corned beef on top of the vegetables. If the corned beef spices come in a separate package, sprinkle them over the meat. Add water to the crockpot until it is almost to the top of the meat. Cook on low heat for 10 to 12 hours or on high heat for 5 to 8 hours. About a half hour before dinner time, cut the cabbage into wedges. Fill a large saucepan about ⅔ full of water and bring it to a boil. Add the cabbage wedges, salt, and pepper and boil until the cabbage is cooked to your preference. Drain the cabbage. Remove the brisket from the crockpot and slice it against the grain. If you have guests, arrange the meat and vegetables on a dish or platter to serve. Makes 4 to 6 servings.

Sauerbraten

This is an impressive dish although it involves more work than the previous crockpot recipes. Serve it with mashed or baked potatoes.

> 1 2 to 3-pound rump roast of beef, bison, elk or venison
> 1¼ cups purified water, divided
> 1 cup wine vinegar or use lemon juice if yeast-sensitive
> 1 tablespoon unrefined salt
> 2 tablespoons agave or Fruit Sweet™ or ¼ cup apple juice concentrate, thawed
> 1 medium onion, sliced (optional)
> 1 unpeeled lemon, sliced
> 10 whole cloves
> 4 bay leaves
> 10 whole peppercorns
> 3 tablespoons tapioca starch or arrowroot or ¼ cup white spelt or unbleached flour (optional – for gravy)

A day or two before you plan to serve this recipe, stir together 1 cup of the water, the vinegar, salt and sweetener in a deep bowl or casserole dish. Add the meat, onion, lemon, cloves, bay leaves, and peppercorns to the liquid. Refrigerate for 24 to 36 hours, turning the meat once or twice during the marinating time. The morning of the day you plan to serve this, remove the meat from the liquid and put the meat in a 3-quart crockpot. Add 1 cup of the marinating liquid to the crockpot. Discard the rest of the marinating liquid. Cover the pot and cook it on low for 8 to 10 hours or on high for 5 to 8 hours. Remove the meat from the pot and put it on a serving dish or platter. If you wish to have gravy with this meal, in a saucepan stir the starch or flour thoroughly into the remaining ¼ cup of water until any lumps are gone. (Lumps will not be a problem with the **starch** which **is gluten-free**; if you use either type of flour, both of which contain gluten, a hand blender will get rid of the lumps). Pour the liquid from the crockpot into the saucepan and cook it on the stove over medium heat for a few minutes until it comes to a boil and thickens. Serve the gravy with the meat and mashed potatoes. Makes 4 to 6 servings.

Crockpot Stew

Omit the potatoes if you plan to freeze this stew. It can be served with or over baked or mashed potatoes instead.

> 2 pounds stew meat or round or chuck steak of any kind - beef, buffalo, lamb,
>   or red game meat
> 5 carrots (about 1 pound)
> 3 stalks of celery
> 1 onion (optional)
> 1½ pounds of potatoes (about 3 or 4, optional)
> ½ cup quick-cooking granulated or minute tapioca
> 2 bay leaves (optional)
> 2 teaspoons unrefined salt
> ¼ teaspoon pepper (optional)
> 2¼ cups purified water OR 1 28-ounce can peeled tomatoes

If you are using steak rather than stew meat, trim the fat and gristle from the meat and cut it into one or two inch cubes. Scrub or peel the carrots and potatoes. Cut the carrots into one inch pieces and cut the potatoes into two inch chunks. Slice the celery into one inch slices. Put the meat, vegetables, tapioca, seasonings, and water or tomatoes into a 3-quart crockpot. Stir the stew thoroughly to evenly distribute the tapioca. Cook it on low for 8 to 12 hours or on high for 5 to 6 hours. If you like your stew juicy, check the stew about 1 hour before the end of the cooking time and add a little boiling water if needed. Makes 6 to 8 servings. If made without the potatoes, this stew freezes well. The potatoes may become mushy if they are frozen.

Chicken Fricassee

This meal is delicious served over leftover cooked grain and freezes well. If lacking in energy or time, use the boneless skinless chicken.

> 1 2 to 3-pound chicken, skinned and cut into pieces or 2 to 2½ pounds
>   skinless boneless chicken breasts or thighs
> 1 teaspoon unrefined salt
> ½ teaspoon paprika (for color – optional)
> 1 small onion, sliced (optional)
> 3 stalks of celery, sliced
> 3 to 5 carrots, peeled and sliced (about 1 pound)
> 1 bay leaf
> 2 cups purified water or bone broth
> ¼ cup additional purified water
> ¼ cup tapioca starch or arrowroot

Put the onion, celery, carrots, and bay leaf in a 3-quart crockpot. Place the chicken pieces on top of the vegetables and sprinkle them with the salt and paprika. Pour the 2 cups of water or broth into the pot. Cover and cook on low for 8 to 12 hours or on high for 4 to 5 hours.

Remove the chicken pieces. Thoroughly combine the ¼ cup water with the starch, stir the mixture into the vegetables and liquid in the pot, and turn the pot up to "high." If using the whole chicken, remove the chicken meat from the bones. Discard the bones. Cut any large pieces of chicken into bite-sized pieces.

Stir the liquid in the pot occasionally. When it has thickened, return the chicken meat to the pot and cook for a few minutes more to reheat the chicken. Add more boiling water to the pot if you like your fricassee more juicy. Serve over cooked rice or other grain. (See recipes on pages 142 to 149). Makes 6 to 8 servings. Leftovers freeze well.

Oven One Dish Meals

Oven Stew

> 2 pounds beef stew meat or beef or buffalo round or chuck steak cut into
>   1 to 2 inch cubes
> 1 onion cut into eighths (optional)
> 4 carrots, peeled or scrubbed and cut into quarters
> 4 celery stalks cut into sixths
> 1 green bell pepper, seeded and cut into one-inch squares

¼ cup quick-cooking (minute) tapioca

1 to 2 cups fresh or 1 8-ounce can of mushrooms, drained[2] (optional)

1 teaspoon unrefined salt

¼ teaspoon pepper

1 28-ounce can of peeled tomatoes with the liquid

1 cup dry red wine or purified water

Thoroughly stir together all of the ingredients in a large casserole dish with a tight fitting lid such as a Dutch oven, or if you don't have a dish that is large enough, divide the ingredients into two 2½ to 3-quart casserole dishes with lids. Bake at 300°F, covered, for 4 hours. Resist the impulse to open the oven and uncover the stew to check it until near the end of the cooking time. Do check it at about 3 hours after you put it into the oven and add a little more water if needed. Makes 8 to 10 servings. Leftovers freeze well. If your Dutch oven is large enough, you can double the recipe or make a 1½ size batch to have more leftovers to freeze.

Lemon Chicken

Use skinless chicken pieces in this recipe if lacking in energy or time.

About 2 pounds of chicken pieces (breasts, thighs or legs) or a 2 to 2½-pound
  chicken, cut up

3 to 4 potatoes, about 1½ pounds of potatoes

2 tablespoons lemon juice

2 tablespoons oil, divided, plus more for oiling the dish

¼ teaspoon unrefined salt

Dash of pepper (optional)

Dash of paprika (optional)

Dash of lemon pepper (optional)

Lightly oil a 13-inch by 9-inch baking dish, preferably glass. Scrub the potatoes and cut them in half lengthwise; then cut each half into three lengthwise wedges. Place the potato wedges skin side down on one half of the dish. Brush the potatoes with about 1 tablespoon of oil and sprinkle them with paprika, salt and pepper if desired. Remove the skin from the chicken and lay the chicken pieces on the other end of the baking dish. In a small bowl, mix together the remaining 1 tablespoon of the oil and the lemon juice. Brush the chicken pieces with the lemon-oil mixture. Sprinkle the chicken with the remaining salt, paprika, and pepper and/or lemon pepper. Bake the dish at 400°F for 1½ hours, brushing the chicken with the remaining lemon-oil mixture after one hour of baking. Makes 4 servings.

---

2 If you are on a low-yeast diet for *Candida*, do not use the mushrooms.

Fish in Papillote

This is a delicious, no-dirty-dishes meal. Don't let the length of the recipe text deter you from trying it. To make it most healthfully, cook the fish and vegetables in a parchment paper pouch. In spite of the detailed directions for making the pouch, it's quick and easy to do and results in great flavor. If you must, you can wrap the food in aluminum foil.

⅓ to ½ pound fish fillets per serving, preferably a mild tasting fish such as
    orange roughy, tilapia, etc.
Vegetable of your choice, such as 8 to 10 spears of asparagus, a piece of
    broccoli or 1 to 2 carrots per serving
1 teaspoon oil per serving
1 teaspoon lemon juice per serving (optional)
Dash of unrefined salt
Dash of pepper (optional)
Dash of paprika (optional)

For each serving, cut a piece of parchment paper about twice as long and four times as wide as the fillet of fish. Fold it in half (so it is now twice as long and twice as wide as the fish) and cut it so it will be the shape of a plump heart when opened. Rub the center of the paper with a little of the oil. Preheat the oven to 400°F.

Peel the carrots, if you are using them. Cut each carrot into about six thin strips lengthwise. If you are using the broccoli, cut it into thin lengthwise strips. Break off the woody stem ends of the asparagus. Soak and swish them in water to remove any dirt from the tips.

Lay the fish on the parchment paper about ½ inch from the fold. Sprinkle the fish with the optional paprika. Lay the vegetable strips on top of the fish. Drizzle the fish and vegetables with the oil and lemon juice and sprinkle them with the salt and pepper.

Fold the top half of the parchment paper over the fish and vegetables along the crease that you made to cut the heart shape. Starting at the top center of the half-heart, hold the two cut edges of paper together, fold ½ inch of the edge toward the center of the heart and crease it. Fold this small section of the edge toward the center of the heart and crease it again. Then move a little farther along the edge of the half-heart and fold another small section of the edge of the paper toward the center of the heart twice in the same manner. Each double-folded section should overlap the previous section a little. Keep moving around the heart and folding small sections so that each section anchors the previous section until you reach the point at the bottom of the heart. Twist the paper at the point to lock the whole edge in place.

Put the parchment pouches on a baking sheet. Bake them for about 25 to 30 minutes if you are using thin fillets of fish. If you are using thick fillets, open one pouch and make sure the fish is opaque and flakes easily with a fork before serving it; if it is not done, cook the pouches a few minutes longer and then check again. Serve each person's fish and vegetables in the pouch.

Oven Main Dishes

Roast Beef, Bison, Lamb, or Pork

Roasting should be used as a cooking method only with tender cuts of meat. Less tender cuts may be cooked in a crockpot for good results. See "Crockpot Roast Dinner" on page 95.

Roast of beef, bison, lamb, or pork, a tender cut such as a rib roast
Dash of unrefined salt (optional)
Dash of pepper (optional)

Place the roast fat side up on a rack in a roasting pan. (A rack is not needed for rib roast with the rib side down). Turn the oven on to 350°F and put the roast into the center of the oven. Estimate the cooking time at 20 to 30 minutes per pound for beef, depending on how well done you like it, at 30 to 35 minutes per pound for lamb, or at 40 minutes per pound for pork. (In my opinion, pork should always be cooked well-done to kill any eggs of the parasite *Trichinella*). The actual roasting time depends on the shape of the roast and the fat content of the meat. Therefore, you will need to test your roast with a meat thermometer to see when it is cooked to your preference. Insert the thermometer into the center of the thickest part of the roast, but don't let it touch bone. The final thermometer readings should be:

Beef - rare: 140°F
Beef - medium: 160°F
Beef - well done: 170°F
Lamb: 160 to 180°F
Pork: 170 to 180°F

Remove the roast from the oven when it has reached the right internal temperature. Season the meat if desired. Allow it to stand for about 10 to 15 minutes for easier carving.

Oven Fried Chicken

3 pounds of skinless chicken breasts, thighs, legs or wings or a cut-up chicken
½ to ¾ cup flour, any kind – rice, sorghum, cassava meal, barley, spelt, etc.
¼ teaspoon unrefined salt
⅛ teaspoon pepper

Combine the flour, salt, and pepper in a plastic bag. (Rice, sorghum, and cassava are gluten-free). If needed, skin the chicken. Put the chicken pieces into the flour one or two at a time and shake the bag to coat the chicken thoroughly. Place the chicken pieces in a baking dish in a single layer. Turn the oven on to 375°F. Bake the chicken, uncovered, for one hour. Remove the pan from the oven and tilt it to allow the fat to run to one corner of the pan. Use a spoon or baster to pick up the fat and dribble it over the poultry. (If you wish, you can baste the chicken with oil instead of pan drippings). Return the chicken to the oven and bake it for another hour or so, for a total cooking time of about 2 hours. Remove it from the oven when it is browned and crisp. Makes 6 to 8 servings.

Pepper Steak

1 pound beef or game round steak, cut into serving-size pieces
1 to 2 bell peppers
Dash of unrefined salt
Dash of pepper
Purified water

Remove the stems and seeds from the peppers and slice them into strips. Place the steak pieces into a glass baking dish in a single layer. Add water almost to the top of the meat. Sprinkle the meat with salt and pepper and top it with the bell pepper strips. Cover the dish with its lid or with foil and bake it at 350°F for 2 hours. As the baking time nears completion, check the steak as it is cooking and add more water if necessary to keep it from drying out completely. The water should have almost completely evaporated by serving time. If it seems to be evaporating too slowly, remove the lid during the last 15 minutes of baking and turn up the temperature if necessary so that the water evaporates and the meat browns. Makes about 4 servings.

Basil Roughy

This dish is tasty, tender and will be on the table in nearly no time.

1 pound orange roughy fillets
1½ to 2 tablespoons oil or melted butter
1 tablespoon lemon juice (optional) or ¼ teaspoon unbuffered
    vitamin C powder plus 1 tablespoon purified water (tasty but optional)
⅛ teaspoon unrefined salt, or to taste
Dash of paprika (optional)
½ teaspoon dry sweet basil

If you are using the vitamin C, mix it with the water in a corner of a 9-inch by 13-inch glass baking dish until it is dissolved. Combine the oil or melted butter with the vitamin C solution or lemon juice in the baking dish. Put the fillets into the dish and turn them over so they are coated with the oil mixture on both sides. Sprinkle them with the salt, paprika, and basil. Bake at 350°F for about 15 minutes, or until the fish flakes easily with a fork. Makes 2 to 4 servings.

Oven Vegetables

These side dishes can cook with the main dishes on the previous pages at the same time and temperature. Instead of a starchy vegetable on pages 104 to 105, consider the oven grains on pages 146 to 149 for more side dish options. Leftover cooked grains can be eaten with chicken fricassee, page 98, or saved for future meals.

Oven Carrots

This dish will make you a cooked carrot lover especially if made with whole organic carrot sticks.

> 2 to 2½ pounds whole carrots or pre-peeled mini carrots
> ⅓ cup purified water
> ½ teaspoon unrefined salt
> 2 to 3 tablespoons oil

If you are using pre-peeled mini carrots, bake them at 350°F in a covered casserole dish for an hour. Drain off the water at this point in the recipe.

If you are using whole carrots, peel or scrub them and cut them lengthwise into quarters or into eighths if they are very large. Lay the carrot sticks parallel to each other in a 2 to 3 quart glass casserole dish with a lid.

To the partially cooked mini carrots or the raw whole carrot sticks, add the salt and water and drizzle the oil over the top of the carrots. Cover the dish with its lid and bake carrot sticks at 350°F for about 1 to 1½ hours or mini-carrots for an additional hour, or until they are browning and becoming caramelized. Makes about 8 servings.

Oven Peas or Beans

Because you start with frozen vegetables, this is very quick and easy to prepare.

> 1 10-ounce package frozen peas, cut green beans, or lima beans
> ⅓ cup purified water
> ⅛ teaspoon unrefined salt
> 1 tablespoon oil

Combine all of the ingredients in a 1 to 1½ quart glass casserole dish. Cover the dish with its lid, and bake at 350°F for 1 to 1½ hours for the beans or 20 minutes to 1 hour for the peas. Makes 2 to 4 servings.

Oven Cabbage

1 head of cabbage weighing about 1½ to 1¾ pounds
½ teaspoon unrefined salt
¼ teaspoon pepper (optional)
¼ cup purified water
3 tablespoons oil

Core and coarsely chop the cabbage and put it into a 3-quart glass casserole dish with a lid. Add the salt, pepper, and water. Drizzle the oil over the top of the cabbage. Cover the dish with its lid and bake at 350°F for 1 to 2 hours, stirring every 30 to 45 minutes. Makes 6 to 7 servings.

Baked Potatoes or Squash

White potatoes, white or orange sweet potatoes, or winter squash

Scrub and pierce the potatoes. Cut the squash in half and remove the seeds. Place the squash cut side down on a baking dish or a baking sheet with an edge. You may place white potatoes directly on the oven rack. Traditional yams (orange sweet potatoes) and white sweet potatoes may ooze sticky liquid so you may wish to use a baking dish for them. Bake with the rest of your oven meal for 1 to 2½ hours at 350°F to 450°F or until they are tender when squeezed and your main dish is done. (Use a longer cooking time with the lower temperatures. Potatoes take longer to bake than squash). An average serving size is one-half pound of squash or one potato per person.

Oven Onions

1½ pounds of small onions
Purified water
Unrefined salt
1 tablespoon of oil

Peel the onions and put them into a 3-quart casserole dish. Add water to ¼ inch depth and cover the dish with its lid or aluminum foil. Bake at 350°F for 40 to 50 minutes or up to 1½ hours until they are tender or done to your preference, or cook them until the rest of your oven meal is done. (For longer baking times, add water to ½ inch depth). Drain off the water. Season with salt and drizzle with a little oil before serving if desired. Makes about 6 servings.

Special Oven Squash

The easiest way to prepare winter squash in the oven is to cut it in half, remove the seeds, and bake it cut side down. (See page 104). However, if you have a little extra time and would like a change from plain squash, this is very tasty.

2½ pounds butternut squash
¼ teaspoon unrefined salt
2 tablespoons oil

Peel the squash. Cut it in half lengthwise and remove the seeds. Slice it into ¼-inch slices. Put the slices into an 11 inch by 7 inch baking dish, sprinkle them with the salt, and drizzle them with the oil. Stir to coat all of the slices. Bake at 350°F for 1½ to 2 hours, turning the slices after the first hour. Makes about 6 servings.

Crispy Oven Sweet Potatoes or White Potatoes

It is quickest to just scrub, pierce and bake potatoes, but if you want to make a special dish and have energy and time for slicing, these potatoes are delicious.

1½ pounds white potatoes or 2 pounds sweet potatoes
2 tablespoons oil
½ teaspoon unrefined salt
Pepper to taste (optional; it is great with the white potatoes)

Peel or scrub the potatoes and slice them into ¼-inch slices. (Sweet potatoes are best peeled). Put the slices into an 11 inch by 7 inch baking dish, sprinkle them with the salt and optional pepper, and drizzle them with the oil. Stir to coat all of the slices. Bake at 350°F for 1½ to 2 hours, turning the slices after the first hour. Makes 4 to 6 servings.

Oven Desserts

Warm-from-the-oven fruit desserts have a special place in the lives of those under duress. They are sweet and nutritious comfort food. On the following pages are easy fruit desserts that can be baked as part of an oven meal.

If it is summer or you prefer something cold, see the wide variety of easy-to-make fruit sorbets and frozen fruit treats in the "Simple Fruit Desserts" chapter of *The Ultimate Food Allergy Cookbook and Survival Guide* as described on the last pages of this book.

Baked Apples or Pears

This homey dessert is wonderful as part of an oven meal.

> 4 large baking apples* or pears*
> ½ cup thawed apple juice concentrate, apple juice, pear juice, or purified water
>   OR ¼ cup agave, Fruit Sweet™ or honey plus ¼ cup purified water
> ½ teaspoon cinnamon (optional)
> ¼ cup raisins (optional)

Core the apples or pears and put them in a 2½ quart glass casserole dish with a lid. Pour in the juice, sweetener, and/or water and sprinkle the cinnamon down the centers of the fruit. Stuff the fruit with raisins, if desired. Bake at 350°F for 40 to 50 minutes for the apples or 1 to 1½ hours for the pears or until the fruit is tender when pierced with a fork. Makes 4 servings.

Note on pears and baking apples: In my opinion, Bosc pears are the best variety for baking. Some varieties of apples hold their shape well when they are baked, such as Rome, Pink Lady, and Granny Smith. If you're planning to make this dessert for special occasions and will be buying the apples especially for baking, chose a baking apple or bosc pears. However, if you have old apples or pears in your refrigerator that you want to use up, any kind will be good in this recipe.

Quick and Easy Fruit Tapioca

This dessert is easy to make and a treat at the end of an oven meal. Cancer patients should use frozen fruit to avoid the chemicals from can linings. See "Sources," page 260, to purchase frozen pie cherries.

> 1 16 to 20-ounce package of frozen fruit or 1 16 to 20-ounce can of fruit,
>   such as juice-packed sliced peaches, pears or pineapple chunks, not
>   drained, OR 1 16-ounce can of water-packed pie cherries, drained
> ¼ cup quick-cooking (minute) tapioca
> 1 cup purified water or fruit juice for the peaches, pears, or pineapple, frozen
>   cherries, or blueberries, or ½ cup apple juice concentrate, agave or honey
> plus ½ cup purified water for canned cherries or tart frozen fruit such as
>   strawberries or raspberries

Combine all of the ingredients except the ½ cup water in a 1½-quart casserole dish. Taste the tart fruits and adjust the sweetness with more agave or honey if needed. Add the water if you did not add more sweetener to have added one cup of liquid total. Bake at 350°F for 40 to 60 minutes or until the tapioca is clear. Makes 4 servings.

Fresh Fruit Tapioca Pudding

Although this recipe is not quite as quick to prepare as the previous recipe, if you have fresh fruit you need to use up, this is the one for you. For an abundance of ripening fruit, double or triple the recipe and freeze the leftovers.

> 1½ to 2 pounds of apples, peaches, or nectarines
> ½ cup apple juice concentrate, thawed. or ¼ cup agave plus ¼ cup purified water
> 1½ tablespoons quick-cooking (minute) tapioca
> ¾ teaspoon cinnamon with apples or ⅛ teaspoon nutmeg with peaches or nectarines

Peel, core, and slice the fruit to produce about 9 or 10 cups of slices.

To cook this dessert on the stove top, combine ¼ cup of the apple juice concentrate or the agave, the fruit, and the spice in a large saucepan. Bring them to a boil over medium heat, reduce the heat, and simmer until the fruit is tender, about 15 to 25 minutes Near the end of the cooking time, combine the tapioca with the remaining ¼ cup apple juice concentrate or the water and allow it to stand for at least 5 minutes. Stir the tapioca mixture into the fruit when it is tender. Return the pan to a boil, and simmer for an additional 5 minutes. Let stand for at least 20 minutes before serving.

To cook this dessert in the oven as part of an oven meal, combine the peeled and sliced fruit, tapioca, juice or water plus agave and spice in a 1½-quart casserole dish. Bake at 350°F for 40 to 60 minutes, or until the tapioca is clear. Makes 4 servings.

For more easy dinner recipes, other easy recipes, how to save money and time on cooking, **and information about "cooking with ease"** see *Allergy and Celiac Diets with Ease* as described on the last pages of this book.

Cultured Vegetables

Cultured vegetables are extremely helpful for improving intestinal health. Good bowel flora is an essential defense factor for the intestine, and the best way to encourage healthy flora is to consume *Lactobacillus*-containing foods such as cultured vegetables. Cultured vegetables help us in other ways as well. The friendly bacteria in these foods partially digest the vegetables before we eat them, which in some cases makes them easier to tolerate if they are foods to which we are allergic. In addition, cultured vegetables are powerhouses of nutrition because they contain vitamins produced by the bacteria that ferment them. Also, the nutrients naturally present in the vegetables are more easily absorbed.

We add friendly organisms to our bodies when we eat cultured vegetables containing live *Lactobacillus plantarum*. This organism is a transient in our digestive systems like the *Lactobacillus bulgaricus* in yogurt. However, it creates a more acid environment in the intestine which enables the organisms in probiotic supplements to implant more easily and helps any *Lactobacillus acidophilus* already present in the intestine to thrive. It also inhibits unfriendly organisms in the intestine.[3] Do not heat these vegetables before eating them because heat will kill the beneficial organisms. By helping our intestinal *Lactobacillus* and *Bifidobacterium,* we help ourselves in many ways.

Individuals who have trouble tolerating cultured vegetables should begin by eating them in small amounts (less than a teaspoon, possibly a few shreds of cultured carrots) and very gradually and slowly increasing the quantity. The *Lactobacillus plantarum* in the vegetables may be doing some clean-up work on the intestinal environment and creating die-off of less friendly organisms. Once you get past the die-off symptoms, you should feel better and may be able to gradually increase the quantity to a teaspoon or two once or twice a day. Eventually you may be able to eat cultured vegetables with every meal and the enzymes provided by the vegetables will help digest your meals.

When making cultured vegetables, it is essential that only the desired bacteria added by the culture have a good chance of taking hold and growing. Read pages 60 to 61 to hear how to prepare the vegetables very hygienically so the right fermentation occurs. Wash your hands thoroughly before you start and then any time you touch something that hasn't been near-sterilized along the way.

Keeping the fermentation anaerobic (without oxygen entering the jars) is vital for successfully producing cultured vegetables. However, a tightly closed lid is problematic; if the fermentation is vigorous, the jar can become pressurized and break. Airlocks are the solution to this problem because they let gasses out without letting the room air in.

When I started culturing vegetables over three years ago, Kraut Kaps™ were the most common and economical airlocks and worked well. Now, while working on the

---

3 Chaitow, Leon, and Natasha Trenev, *Probiotics,* (Prescott, AZ, Hohm Press, 1995), 200.

"Sources" section for this book, I could not find the company that formerly was a one-stop website for all supplies needed for lactofermentation. In the process of looking for a new source for Kraut Kaps™ I found that the company had changed its name. I also found a new type of airlock made with silicone, the FermentEm™ airlock, which I purchased. They produce good cultured vegetables and have less parts so are easier to store compactly than Kraut Kaps™. The FermentEm™ lids are a slightly different shape, which makes it harder to place the lids on the jars with the silicone seal in position. With practice, I think the quick lid-placing technique can be mastered. I've used Ferment-Em™ airlocks for only two batches of cultured vegetables of at the time of this writing, so read reviews about how long cultured vegetables made with them last when the FermentEm™ airlocks are no longer new. Then make your own decision on which type of airlock to use. Kraut Kaps™ have produced many perfect jars of cultured vegetables for me during more than three years of frequent use. Currently I have jars of pickles made fourteen months ago using Kraut Kaps™ which are still good.

Glass weights such a Crock Rocks ™ and Pickle Pebbles™ are ideal for keeping your vegetables submerged under an inch of brine; they are non-porous, easy to wash, and chemically inert. However, I must admit that when I first started fermenting, I did not want to invest in a lot of equipment, so I searched for rocks of the right size in our yard and boiled them. Rather than purchasing airlocks, I tried loosely tightening the caps on the jars at first. However, the foam that escaped from the lids was a mess. After I got "hooked" on cultured vegetables for the health benefits and knew I'd keep making them for life, I invested in airlocks and glass weights.

Use plastic lids for wide-mouth canning jars for your cultured vegetables because the metal lids that come with the jars may leach metal into the brine which can inhibit fermentation. Plastic lids can be purchased at hardware stores with well stocked kitchen and canning sections. Silicone seals for plastic lids can be purchased online. However, if you order FermentEm™ airlocks, they come with the silicone seals. See "Sources," page 264, to purchase the lactofermentation supplies use in this chapter.

I have found that fine refined sea salt is best for making cultured vegetables. When I first begin using unrefined (Celtic™) sea salt for all other cooking, I found that one jar in each batch of cultured vegetables made with unrefined salt went bad fairly frequently, as opposed to almost never going bad when made with refined salt. Therefore, I went back to using the Natural Grocers™ store brand of pure refined sea salt for cultured vegetables. If you cannot find pure refined sea salt with no additives, use kosher salt. I suspect that there are a few more bacteria present in unrefined salt.

Cultured vegetables continue to ferment at a slow rate and develop more flavor during storage. Because the top shelf of the refrigerator tends to be the warmest spot, store them there if you have sufficient room.

Lactofermentation is creative fun and the vegetables produced are both delicious and wonderful for health. Enjoy these delicious condiments and the accompanying better health.

Cultured Carrots

4½ to 5 pounds of organic whole carrots (Avoid pre-peeled mini-carrots).
6 tablespoons fine refined sea salt
Purified water
1 envelope Caldwell Starter Culture for Fresh Vegetables™
Optional seasonings such as caraway seeds or celery seeds, about
    1 teaspoon per jar of carrots, or to your taste

Wash everything you will use to make cultured vegetables, preferably in a dish-washer if the items are dishwasher-safe. If hand washing, let the items air-dry. Wash six wide-mouth quart canning jars and six plastic lids (or two lids and four airlocks), six silicone seals for the lids and airlocks, a large glass bowl, a large non-metal spoon, mea-suring spoons and cups, a knife and cutting board, a large hole grater or the washable parts of a food processor (optional), weights for the tops of the vegetables, and anything you want to use instead of a spoon for tamping the vegetables into the jar. (I use a glass jar left from Cortas™ Pomegranate Molasses as a tamping instrument). Everything you use should be extremely clean.

To make enough brine to have a little remaining, heat two cups of purified water to warm but not boiling. Put 1 cup in each of two quart canning jars. Add 3 tablespoons of salt to each jar. Swirl the jars until the salt is totally dissolved. Add about three cups of room temperature purified water to each jar, filling it almost up to the brim. Cap with plastic lids and allow the brine to cool while you prepare the vegetables.

Wash the carrots in plain water and peel them. Trim off and discard any bruised or discolored spots. Thinly slice the wide end of two large carrots lengthwise to place on top of the shredded carrots. Shred the remaining carrots.

Add any desired seasonings to the bottom of each jar or intersperse them with the vegetables. (I add caraway to carrots). Pack the shredded carrots into the canning jars. Tamp them down as much as possible, leaving about 2½ to 3 inches of space at the top of each jar. Put a thin layer of large pieces of sliced carrots on top of the shredded veg-etables. Add a weight to hold everything down.

Dissolve the culture in one cup of room temperature purified water and allow it to stand for eight to ten minutes but no longer. Mix it with three cups of the prepared brine. Pour one cup of the mixture over the carrots in each jar. Add more brine to cover the carrots with about 2 inches of liquid, keeping the level of liquid at least 1 inch from the top of the jar. Cap the jars with plastic lids tightened loosely or use airlocks. Refriger-ate the leftover brine for possible use in a few days.

Place a pan to catch overflow under the jars and store the jars in a dark place at about 70°F for 5 to 10 days until the carrots taste quite tart. (Mine are usually ready at 7 days but can take 8 days in cold weather). Check the jars for overflow daily and clean up the mess if necessary. If too much brine is lost from the jars, add a little of the reserved refrigerated brine. Begin tasting daily at four days. When the carrots are tart enough, tighten the caps securely or replace the airlocks with plastic caps and silicone seals and refrigerate the jars. Makes four quarts.

Cultured Beets

Beets contain more sugar than most vegetables and can ferment vigorously. Keep close tabs on them and leave plenty of headspace in the jars to minimize overflows.

> 4 to 4½ pounds of organic beets including at least one beet that is large
>   enough to slice and use the slices as toppers in wide-mouth canning jars
> ½ cup (8 tablespoons) fine refined sea salt
> Purified water
> 1 envelope Caldwell Starter Culture for Fresh Vegetables™
> Optional seasonings such whole allspice, and/or whole cloves, about
>   1 teaspoon per jar of beets, or to your taste

Wash everything you will use to make cultured vegetables, preferably in a dishwasher if the items are dishwasher-safe. If hand washing, let the items air dry. Wash six wide-mouth quart canning jars and plastic lids (or two lids and four airlocks), six silicone seals for the lids and airlocks, a large glass bowl, a large non-metal spoon, measuring spoons and cups, a knife and cutting board, a large hole grater or the washable parts of a food processor (optional), weights for the tops of the vegetables, and anything you want to use instead of a spoon for tamping the vegetables into the jar. (I use a glass jar left from Cortas™ Pomegranate Molasses as a tamping instrument). Everything you use should be extremely clean.

To make enough brine to have a little remaining, heat two cups of purified water to warm but not boiling. Put one cup in each of two quart canning jars. Add ¼ cup of salt to each jar. Swirl the jars until the salt is totally dissolved. Add about three cups of room temperature purified water to each jar, filling it almost up to the brim. Cap with plastic lids and allow the brine to cool while you prepare the vegetables.

Wash the beets thoroughly in plain water and peel them. Thinly slice a large beet to place on top of the shredded beets. Shred the remaining beets.

Add any desired seasonings to the bottom of each jar or intersperse them with the vegetables. (I add both cloves and allspice to the bottom of each jar of beets). Pack the shredded beets into the canning jars. Tamp the vegetables down as much as possible, leaving about 3 to 3½ inches of space at the top of each jar. Beets require more head-space than most vegetables because they ferment quite vigorously. Put a thin layer of large pieces of sliced beets, possibly one slice large enough to cover most of the area in the jar, on top of the shredded beets. Add a weight to hold everything down.

Dissolve the culture in one cup of room temperature purified water and allow it to stand for eight to ten minutes but no longer. Mix it with three cups of the prepared brine. Pour one cup of the mixture over the beets in each jar. Add more brine to cover the beets with about 2 inches of liquid, keeping the level of liquid at least 1 inch or preferably 1½ inches from the top of the jar for ample headspace. Cap the jars with plastic lids tightened loosely or use airlocks. Refrigerate the leftover brine for possible use in a few days.

Place a pan to catch overflow under the jars and store the jars in a dark place at about 70°F for 5 to 10 days until the beets taste quite tart. (Mine have been ready at 5 to 6 days). Check the jars for overflow daily and clean up the mess if necessary. If too much brine is lost from the jars, which is not unusual with beets, add a little of the reserved refrigerated brine. Begin tasting daily at four days. When the beets are tart enough, tighten the caps securely or replace the airlocks with plastic caps and silicone seals and refrigerate the jars. Makes four quarts.

Cultured Dill Pickles

> About 4 to 4¼ pounds of pickling cucumbers
> ½ cup fine refined sea salt
> Purified water
> 1 envelope Caldwell Starter Culture for Fresh Vegetables™
> Fresh dill, a bouquet from the Farmers' Market or a 4-ounce package,
>   or to taste
> Dry bay leaves, one 0.15 ounce jar
> 4 cloves of garlic (optional, to taste)
> 4 fresh grape leaves[4] (optional)

Wash everything you will use to make pickles, preferably in a dishwasher if the items are dishwasher-safe. If hand washing, let the items air dry. Wash six wide-mouth quart canning jars and plastic lids (or two lids and four airlocks), six silicone seals for the lids and airlocks, a large glass bowl, a large non-metal spoon, measuring spoons and cups, a knife and cutting board, the washable slicing parts of a food processor (optional), weights for the tops of the pickles, and anything you want to use instead of a spoon for tamping the pickles into the jar. (I use a glass jar left from Cortas™ Pomegranate Molasses as a tamping instrument). Everything you use should be extremely clean.

To make the brine, heat two cups of purified water to warm but not boiling. Put one cup in each of two quart canning jars. Add ¼ cup of salt to each jar. Swirl the jars until the salt is totally dissolved. Add about three cups of room temperature purified water to

---

4 Grape leaves should be washed like homegrown lettuce to kill whatever insects might be present. Fill the sink with cool water and add a generous amount (about ¼ teaspoon) of salt. Swish the leaves in the water and let them soak for a few minutes. Then rinse the leaves in two or three changes of water.

each jar, filling it almost up to the brim. Cap with plastic lids and allow the brine to cool while you prepare the vegetables.

Wash the cucumbers in plain water, scrubbing them with a new (or dedicated) brush to remove all dirt. Cut off ¾ inch of the blossom end[5] of each cucumber because the blossom end contains enzymes that can cause the pickles to become mushy. Slice one or two large-diameter cucumbers lengthwise to place on top of the round slices. Slice the rest of the cucumbers crosswise. Put the dill and some of the bay leaves in the bottom of each of four quart jars. Reserve eight large bay leaves. Pack the crosswise-sliced cucumbers into the canning jars, tamping them down as much as possible, leaving 2½ inches of space at the top of each jar. Lay two of the reserved large bay leaves on top of the slices in each jar. Top them with two or more lengthwise slices of cucumber. If you have access to fresh grape leaves, also add a grape leaf. Bay leaves and grape leaves help to ensure crispness. Add a weight to hold everything down.

Dissolve the culture in one cup of room temperature purified water and allow it to stand for eight to ten minutes but no longer. Mix it with three cups of the prepared brine. Pour one cup of the mixture over the cucumbers in each jar. Add more brine to cover the cucumbers with about 2 inches of liquid, keeping the level of liquid at least one inch from the top of the jar. Cap the jars with plastic lids tightened loosely, or use airlocks.

Place a pan to catch overflow under the jars and store the jars in a dark place at about 70°F for 5 to 10 days until the pickles taste quite tart. (My pickles have been ready at 6 to 7 days). Check the jars for overflow daily and clean up the mess if necessary. Begin tasting daily at four days. When the pickles are tart enough, tighten the caps securely or replace the airlocks with plastic caps and silicone seals and refrigerate the pickles. Makes four quarts.

Sauerkraut

> 2 heads or about 4 to 4½ pounds of organic red and/or green cabbage
> ½ cup fine refined sea salt
> Purified water
> 1 envelope Caldwell Starter Culture for Fresh Vegetables ™
> Optional seasonings such as caraway seeds, celery seeds, or juniper berries, 1 to
>   2 teaspoons per jar

Wash everything you will use to make sauerkraut, preferably in a dishwasher if the items are dishwasher-safe. If hand washing, let the items air dry. Wash six wide-mouth quart canning jars and plastic lids (or two lids and four airlocks), six silicone seals for the lids and airlocks, a very large or two medium-size glass bowls, a large non-metal

---

5 The blossom end of a cucumber usually has a brown spot or there may be a brown spot with a bit or a lot of withered blossom attached. The opposite or stem end of the cucumber usually has a green wound from where the stem was removed or there may be a short stem attached.

spoon, measuring spoons and cups, a knife and cutting board, the washable slicing parts of a food processor (optional), weights for the tops of the jars and anything you want to use instead of a spoon for tamping the cabbage into the jar. (I use a glass jar left from Cortas™ Pomegranate Molasses as a tamping instrument). Everything you use should be extremely clean.

To make the brine, heat two cups of purified water to warm but not boiling. Put it into two canning jars. Add ¼ cup of salt to each jar and swirl it until the salt is totally dissolved. Add about three cups of room temperature purified water to each jar, filling them almost up to the brim. Cap with plastic lids and allow the brine to cool while you prepare the cabbage.

Remove and discard the outer leaves of each head of cabbage. Trim off and discard any bruised or discolored spots. Save four sturdy pieces of cabbage from the next layer which are a little larger than the diameter of your jars to cover the shredded cabbage inside the jars. Quarter and core the heads of cabbage. Thinly slice the quarters with a knife or use a food processor to slice them. Divide the cabbage equally between the large bowls.

Dissolve the culture in one cup of room temperature purified water and allow it to stand for eight to ten minutes but no longer. Mix it with three cups of the prepared brine. Divide the brine mixture between the bowls. Wash your hands very thoroughly. Using your hands, mix and massage the cabbage and brine in each bowl for 10 minutes to extract juice from the cabbage. This will soften the cabbage and should produce enough brine to cover or nearly cover it in the jars.

Pack the cabbage and brine into four canning jars. Add any desired seasonings to the bottom of each jar or intersperse them with the cabbage. Tamp the cabbage down as much as possible, leaving about 2½ to 3 inches of space at the top of each jar. Put a reserved large piece of cabbage on top of the sliced cabbage in each jar. Tamp the topper and sliced cabbage down as much as possible. Add a weight to hold everything down. Add more brine if needed to cover the cabbage with about 2 inches of liquid, keeping the level of liquid at least 1 inch from the top of the jar. Cap the jars loosely with a plastic cap, or use an airlock. Refrigerate the leftover brine for possible use in a few days.

Place a pan to catch overflow under the jars and store the jars in a dark place at about 70°F for 7 to 10 days until the sauerkraut tastes quite tart. Check the jars visually daily and clean up the mess of any overflow if necessary. If too much brine is lost from a jar, add a little of the reserved refrigerated brine. Begin tasting daily at four days. When the sauerkraut is tart enough, tighten the caps securely or replace the airlocks with plastic caps and silicone seals and refrigerate on the top shelf of the refrigerator if possible. The flavor will continue to develop during cold storage, so try not to eat the whole batch immediately. Makes four quarts.

Cultured Beans

About 4 pounds of organic green beans and two large-diameter organic carrots
6 tablespoons fine refined sea salt
Purified water
1 envelope Caldwell Starter Culture for Fresh Vegetables™
Optional seasonings such as sprigs of fresh dill or 1 teaspoon caraway seeds or
    celery seeds per jar or to taste

Wash everything you will use to make cultured beans, preferably in a dishwasher if the items are dishwasher-safe. If hand washing, let the items air dry. Wash six wide-mouth quart canning jars and plastic lids (or two lids and four airlocks), six silicone seals for the lids and airlocks, a large glass bowl, a large non-metal spoon, measuring spoons and cups, a knife and cutting board, the washable slicing parts of a food processor (optional), weights for the tops of the vegetables, and anything you want to use instead of a spoon for tamping the vegetables into the jar. (I use a glass jar left from Cortas™ Pomegranate Molasses as a tamping instrument). Everything you use should be extremely clean.

To make enough brine to have a little remaining, heat two cups of purified water to warm but not boiling. Put one cup in each of two quart canning jars. Add 3 tablespoons of salt to each jar. Swirl the jars until the salt is totally dissolved. Add about three cups of room temperature purified water to each jar, filling it almost up to the brim. Cap with plastic lids and allow the brine to cool while you prepare the vegetables.

Snap or trim the stem ends off the beans. Wash the beans in plain water and cut them to 4 inches in length. Cut off 3 to 4 inches of the wide end of the carrots and thinly slice them lengthwise to make "toppers" to place on top of the beans.

Add any desired seasonings to the bottom of each jar. (Fresh dill is great with beans). Tightly pack the beans into the canning jars standing on their ends. Top the ends of the beans with a thin layer of the carrot toppers. There should be about 3 inches of space at the top of each jar. Add a weight to hold everything down.

Dissolve the culture in one cup of room temperature purified water and allow it to stand for eight to ten minutes but no longer. Mix it with three cups of the prepared brine. Pour one cup of the mixture over the vegetables in each jar. Add more brine to cover the vegetables with at least one inch of liquid, keeping the top of liquid at least one inch from the top of the jar. Cap the jars with plastic lids tightened loosely or use airlocks. Refrigerate the leftover brine for possible use in a few days.

Place a pan to catch overflow under the jars and store the jars in a dark place at about 70°F for 5 to 10 days until the beans taste quite tart. (Mine have been ready at 6 to 7 days). Check the jars for overflow daily and clean up the mess if necessary. If too much brine is lost from the jars, add a little of the reserved refrigerated brine. Begin tasting daily at four days. When the beans are tart enough, tighten the caps securely or replace the airlocks with plastic caps and silicone seals and refrigerate the jars. Makes four quarts.

Cultured Broccoli or Cauliflower

> About 4 to 4½ pounds of organic broccoli or cauliflower
> 6 tablespoons fine refined sea salt
> Purified water
> 1 envelope Caldwell Starter Culture for Fresh Vegetables™
> Optional seasonings such as caraway seeds or celery seeds, 1 teaspoon per jar,
>   or to taste

Wash everything you will use to make cultured vegetables, preferably in a dish-washer if the items are dishwasher-safe. If hand washing, let the items air dry. Wash six wide-mouth quart canning jars and plastic lids (or two lids and four airlocks), six silicone seals for the lids and airlocks, a large glass bowl, a large non-metal spoon, mea-suring spoons and cups, a knife and cutting board, the washable slicing parts of a food processor (optional), weights for the tops of the vegetables, and anything you want to use instead of a spoon for tamping the vegetables into the jar. (I use a glass jar left from Cortas™ Pomegranate Molasses as a tamping instrument). Everything you use should be extremely clean.

To make enough brine to have a little remaining, heat two cups of purified water to warm but not boiling. Put one cup in each of two quart canning jars. Add 3 tablespoons of salt to each jar. Swirl the jars until the salt is totally dissolved. Add about three cups of room temperature purified water to each jar, filling it almost up to the brim. Cap with plastic lids and allow the brine to cool while you prepare the vegetables.

Wash the vegetables in plain water and cut them into florets. Thinly slice a stalk or two of broccoli or a piece of the core of a head of cauliflower to make slices to place on top of the florets in the jars.

Add any desired seasonings to the bottom of each jar or intersperse them with the vegetables. (I add celery seeds). Pack the florets into the canning jars. Tamp the veg-etables down as much as possible, leaving about 2½ to 3 inches of space at the top of each jar. Put a thin layer of large pieces of sliced stalks or core on top of the florets. Add a weight to hold everything down.

Dissolve the culture in one cup of room temperature purified water and allow it to stand for eight to ten minutes but no longer. Mix it with three cups of the prepared brine. Pour one cup of the mixture over the vegetables in each jar. Add more brine to cover the vegetables with about 2 inches of liquid, keeping the level of liquid at least 1 inch from the top of the jar. Cap the jars with plastic lids tightened loosely or use air-locks. Refrigerate the leftover brine for possible use in a few days.

Place a pan to catch overflow under the jars and store the jars in a dark place at about 70°F for 5 to 10 days until the vegetables taste quite tart. (Mine have been ready at 5 to 7 days). Check the jars for overflow daily and clean up the mess if necessary. If too much brine is lost from the jars, add a little of the reserved refrigerated brine. Begin tasting daily at four days. When the vegetables are tart enough, tighten the caps securely or replace the airlocks with plastic caps and silicone seals and refrigerate the jars. Makes four quarts.

Cultured Summer Squash

About 4½ pounds of organic yellow squash, such as crookneck or zephyr, or
    zucchini
6 tablespoons fine refined sea salt
Purified water
1 envelope Caldwell Starter Culture for Fresh Vegetables™
Optional seasonings such as caraway seeds, celery seeds, whole allspice, or
    whole cloves, about 1 teaspoon per jar, or to your taste

Wash everything you will use to make cultured squash, preferably in a dishwasher if the items are dishwasher-safe. If hand washing, let the items air dry. Wash six wide-mouth quart canning jars and plastic lids (or two lids and four airlocks), six silicone seals for the lids and airlocks, a large glass bowl, a large non-metal spoon, measuring spoons and cups, a knife and cutting board, a large hole grater or the washable parts of a food processor (optional), weights for the tops of the vegetables, and anything you want to use instead of a spoon for tamping the vegetables into the jar. (I use a glass jar left from Cortas™ Pomegranate Molasses as a tamping instrument). Everything you use should be extremely clean.

To make enough brine to have a little remaining, heat two cups of purified water to warm but not boiling. Put one cup in each of two quart canning jars. Add 3 tablespoons of salt to each jar. Swirl the jars until the salt is totally dissolved. Add about three cups of room temperature purified water to each jar, filling it almost up to the brim. Cap with plastic lids and allow the brine to cool while you prepare the squash.

Wash the vegetables in plain water and, if desired, peel them. Trim off and discard any bruised or discolored spots. Thinly slice 3 to 4 inches of the wide end of a large squash or two to place on top of the shredded squash. Shred the remaining squash.

Add any desired seasonings to the bottom of each jar. Pack the shredded squash into the canning jars. Tamp the vegetables down as much as possible, leaving about 2½ to 3 inches of space at the top of each jar. Put a thin layer of large pieces of sliced squash on top of the shredded squash. Add a weight to hold everything down.

Dissolve the culture in one cup of room temperature purified water and allow it to stand for eight to ten minutes but no longer. Mix it with three cups of the prepared brine. Pour one cup of the mixture over the vegetables in each jar. Add more brine to cover the vegetables with about 2 inches of liquid, keeping the level of liquid at least 1 inch from the top of the jar. Cap the jars with plastic lids tightened loosely or use air-locks. Refrigerate the leftover brine for possible use in a few days.

Place a pan to catch overflow under the jars and store the jars in a dark place at about 70°F for 5 to 10 days until the squash tastes quite tart. (Mine have been ready at 5 to 6 days). Check the jars for overflow daily and clean up the mess if necessary. If too much brine is lost from the jars, which is common with zucchini, add a little of the reserved refrigerated brine. Begin tasting daily at four days. When the squash tastes tart enough, tighten the caps securely or replace the airlocks with plastic caps and silicone seals and refrigerate the jars. Makes four quarts.

Cultured Asparagus

> About 5½ to 6 pounds of asparagus, preferably organic, but I have had positive
>   results using conventional asparagus in good condition
> 6 tablespoons fine refined sea salt
> Purified water
> 1 envelope Caldwell Starter Culture for Fresh Vegetables ™
> Optional seasonings such as peppercorns, 1 to 2 teaspoon per jar, or to taste

Shopping for organic asparagus can involve a major investment. One time I found only wilted organic asparagus so decided to purchase conventional asparagus that was in top-notch condition and on sale. The fermentation went well and the batch lasted over a year in good condition. Another money-saving option is making a half-batch of asparagus. To prevent wasting a half packet of the culture, possibly prepare two jars of another vegetable.

Before you begin making cultured asparagus, wash everything you will use to make it, preferably in a dishwasher if the items are dishwasher-safe. If hand washing, let the items air dry. Wash six wide-mouth quart canning jars and plastic lids (or two lids and four airlocks), six silicone seals for the lids and airlocks, a large glass bowl, a large non-metal spoon, measuring spoons and cups, a knife and cutting board, and weights for the tops of the asparagus. Everything you use should be extremely clean.

To make enough brine to have a little remaining, heat two cups of purified water to warm but not boiling. Put one cup in each of two quart canning jars. Add 3 tablespoons of salt to each jar. Swirl the jars until the salt is totally dissolved. Add about three cups of room temperature purified water to each jar, filling it almost up to the brim. Cap with plastic lids and allow the brine to cool while you prepare the asparagus.

Snap the asparagus spears and discard the woody ends. Wash the edible (tip) ends in plain water. If they contain much dirt, peel off a few of the small leaves near the tips and at the end opposite the tips. If there is dirt under them, you may want to protect your investment by peeling off all of the leaves along the spears. During spring rains here, I find most of the dirt accumulates under the small leaves near the tips; at other times I have found more dirt at the end opposite the tips. Consider this as you decide about removing all the small leaves. Trim the ends of the spears opposite the tips so each spear is about four inches long. Save the small pieces that have been cut off to culture.

Add the peppercorns to the bottom of each jar. Pack the asparagus into the canning jars tip down as tightly as you can pack them. If the last jar is not packed tight, pack the small pieces of asparagus that were trimmed off in the bottom of the jar to anchor the full spears as firmly as possible. Add a weight to each jar. Consume the jar containing the small pieces first.

Dissolve the culture in one cup of room temperature purified water and allow it to stand for eight to ten minutes but no longer. Mix it with three cups of the prepared brine. Pour one cup of the mixture over the asparagus in each jar. Add more brine to cover the ends of the spears with about 2 inches of liquid, keeping the level of liquid at least 1 inch from the top of the jar. Cap the jars with plastic lids tightened loosely or use airlocks. Refrigerate the leftover brine for possible use in a few days.

Place a pan to catch overflow under the jars and store the jars in a dark place at about 70°F for 5 to 10 days until one of the short asparagus ends tastes quite tart. (Mine have been ready at 5 to 7 days). Check the jars for overflow daily and clean up the mess if necessary. If too much brine is lost from the jars, add a little of the reserved refrigerated brine. Begin tasting daily at four days. When a short end of asparagus tastes tart enough, tighten the caps securely or replace the airlocks with plastic caps and silicone seals and refrigerate the jars. Makes four quarts.

For recipes for additional types of cultured vegetables see *Nourishing Traditions*[6], pages 93 to 102. **For where to purchase cultured vegetables already made,** see "Sources," page 257.

---

6 Fallon, Sally with Mary Enig, PhD. *Nourishing Traditions.*, (Brandywine, MD, NewTrends Publishing, 2001), 93-102.

Cultured Dairy Products and Salad Dressings

Cultured dairy products confer amazing health benefits similar to those described for cultured vegetables at the beginning of the last chapter. The bacteria they are made with improves our intestinal flora and inhibits the growth of unhealthy organisms in the intestine. Yogurt has a long history of being recommended for many benefits including long life. Cultured dairy products are also nutritionally superior to the milk from which they are made.

Yogurt has been credited with almost miraculous health enhancing properties. The Greek physician Galen prescribed it for stomach problems about A.D. 150. King Francis I of France paid a fortune for the formula for "the milk of eternal life." In 1902, Russian microbiologist Elie Metchnikoff published *The Prolongation of Life,* which claimed that yogurt was a veritable fountain of youth.[1] While yogurt and other fermented milks do not actually have miraculous powers, they can greatly contribute to our health and to the health and vitality of our unseen allies, *Lactobacillus* and *Bifidobacterium,* which are health-promoting intestinal bacteria.

Cultured milk is milk in its most tolerable, digestible, and absorbable form because it is predigested by the organisms that make it. The lactose-free specific carbohydrate diet for inflammatory bowel disease permits yogurt that has been fermented for twenty four hours because after twenty four hours of fermentation virtually all of the lactose has been predigested by the yogurt bacteria.[2] Furthermore, the calcium in fermented milks helps *Lactobacillus acidophilus* adhere and implant in the intestine.[3]

Yogurt is extremely nutritious. It is higher in B vitamins and vitamin K than the milk from which it is made. Its protein is predigested to short peptides and free amino acids which makes the milk less allergenic and highly bioavailable.[4] On a 100-point scale comparing the biological value of the protein in foods to that of human breast milk (at 100 points), cow milk scores 84.5, cow yogurt scores 89.3, and goat yogurt scores 90.5.[5]

Fermented milks are indeed marvelous foods for our health. But the problem is that cow milk is a major food allergen for some individuals. Even predigested, as it is in fer-

1 Alth, Max, *Making Your Own Cheese and Yogurt,* (New York, NY, Funk & Wagnalls, 1973, 12-16.

2 Gottschall, Elaine, BA, MSc. *Breaking the Vicious Cycle: Intestinal Health Through Diet.* (Baltimore, Ontario, The Kirkton Press, 1994), 133.

3 Mitsuoka, Tomotari. "Intestinal Flora and Aging." *Nutrition Reviews,* December, 1992. 50(12):442.

4 Chaitow, Leon, and Natasha Trenev, *Probiotics,* (Prescott, AZ, Hohm Press, 1995), 36.

5 Chaitow, Leon, et al,, 36.

mented milks, it is likely to cause allergic symptoms. How can we feed fermented milks to our intestinal *Lactobacillus* and *Bifidobacterium* without having reactions ourselves?

The solution is to eat fermented milks made from alternative milks. Goat and sheep yogurt are commercially available. In addition, acidophilus milk and yogurt can be made at home with goat, sheep, camel or any other available animal milk. Unfortunately, I have been unable to produce satisfactory yogurt from rice and nut milk at home.

When you make your own fermented milks, you know that they are fresh, that the organisms in them are alive, and that no additives have been used. It is a craft which is easy to master and may be one of the best things you ever do for yourself and your family. Dr. Gruia Ionescu, director of a large allergy clinic in Germany, has his patients eat at least a pint of yogurt a day in addition to taking probiotic supplements. He says, "The yogurt is milk in its most digestible form, and the *Lactobacillus* in it is just so beneficial that if they can handle the yogurt at all, we want them to eat it."[6] Do not give up on trying fermented milks until you have made them using alternative milks. If you are on a rotation diet for food allergies, try to find four alternative milks to ferment and rotate fermented milks from different animal sources if you eat them on a daily basis.

Good hygiene is important in all cooking, but when you are making fermented foods, it is paramount to the outcome of your recipe. Wash your hands thoroughly before you start and wash them again whenever they may have become contaminated with anything as you proceed with food preparation. Use scrupulously clean pans, spoons, and other utensils. I like to use a long-handled spoon to stir the milk as it is coming to a boil and just leave the spoon in the pot; it is then sterilized along with the milk. However, if you must remove the spoon from the pan, set it on a clean dish, and get a new spoon if it may have become contaminated. If you introduce organisms into the milk besides the "friendly flora" yogurt or acidophilus milk organisms you want to grow, the results of your fermentation may be compromised.

I have always sterilized milk by boiling it briefly to prevent any stray bacteria from affecting the fermentation. However, in the last few years I learned more about phytic acid (found in whole grains, legumes and nuts) and the importance of good nutrition for escaping its negative effects. Those consuming a diet high in vitamin C, vitamins A and D from animal sources and absorbable calcium are less likely to have bone loss and tooth decay if consuming much phytic acid.[7] Because the calcium in raw milk is more absorbable than in pasteurized milk, I re-thought boiling raw milk. In addition, individuals with good intestinal flora are less likely to be harmed by phytic acid because their intestinal flora can break it down, so we need to continue to consume yogurt and acidophilus milk which will improve intestinal flora. Therefore, to get the benefits of raw

---

6 Interview with Gruia Ionescu, Ph.D., "Candida – A Different Approach," *Mastering Food Allergies Newsletter*, #37, July/August 1989, 6.

7 Nagle, Ramiel. "Living with Phytic Acid." The Weston A. Price Foundation. https://www.westona-price.org/health-topics/vegetarianism-and-plant-foods/living-with-phytic-acid/

milk from cultured milk, the recipes in this chapter give the option of not sterilizing raw milk and thus preserving the enzyme that breaks down phytic acid.

Read more about cultured dairy products on pages 62 to 64, and then enjoy making and eating the foods below.

Acidophilus Milk

Acidophilus milk is fermented milk that tastes much like yogurt. It is made with a pure culture of Lactobacillus acidophilus. It does not get as thick as yogurt, especially if made with goat milk. It has traditionally been used as a treatment for gastrointestinal disorders.

> 1 to 1¼ quarts whole goat, camel, cow or other animal milk
> 1 teaspoon Klaire Labs Therbiotic Factor 1™ (empty out four capsules) or other culture which contains only *Lactobacillus acidophilus* (See "Sources," page 262, to order Therbiotic Factor 1™).

First Day

Immerse the metal tip of a digital thermometer in boiling water to kill bacteria that may be on it. Bring 1 cup of the milk to a boil (unless it is raw milk[8]) in a saucepan over medium heat and boil it for one minute. Let it cool to 95°F, using the digital thermometer to monitor the temperature as it cools. Stir the culture into the warm milk and put the milk in a yogurt maker container or glass jar. Incubate the milk overnight in a yogurt maker or proofing box. See pages 62 to 63 for information about proofing boxes. You may use a yogurt maker if you have or can get an older model that does not get too hot, such as the Yogourmet™ yogurt maker. See page 62 for more about yogurt makers. It will take about 12 to 24 hours of incubation for it to thicken with the length of time depending on the culture used.

Second Day

The next day, when the 1 cup of acidophilus milk has thickened, bring the remaining milk to a boil (unless it is raw milk[8]) over medium heat and boil it for one minute. Immerse the metal tip of a digital thermometer in boiling water while the milk is heating. Cool the milk to 95°F, using the digital thermometer to monitor the temperature as it cools. If you are in a hurry, you can speed this process by putting the pan in a sink of cold water. Stir a little of the warm milk into of the previous day's 1-cup batch of acidophilus milk; then stir this mixture into the rest of the milk in the saucepan.

---

8 If you are using raw milk in this recipe, you have hopefully made sure the dairy from which you purchase it uses "clean" practices. Do not boil this milk; do not destroy enzymes such as phytase which will help you deal with phytic acid. High temperature will also make the calcium less easily absorbable. Using the digital thermometer to monitor progress, gently heat the milk to 95°F before adding the culture.

Pour the milk into yogurt maker container(s) or glass jar(s) to go into your proofing box. Incubate it for 24 hours. A 24-hour acidophilus milk will contain almost no lactose and the protein will be partially digested, which makes it easier to tolerate.

After 24 hours, when the large batch of acidophilus milk has thickened, save some of the acidophilus milk in a clean container in the refrigerator to use to make your next batch. Reserve ¼ to ⅓ cup of acidophilus milk for each quart of it you plan to make next time. Use what you reserve to start at the "second day" point in this recipe when making the next batch of acidophilus milk. Serve the rest of the acidophilus milk immediately or refrigerate it for up to one week. Serve it plain or in a smoothie. (See the smoothie recipe on the next page). Makes about 1 quart of acidophilus milk

NOTE: Acidophilus milk does not get very thick. However, if does not thicken at all or has an off odor, do not eat it. Begin again with fresh starter. If the acidophilus milk is thinner than usual and it has been 3 to 4 weeks since you started with a fresh culture, start over with fresh probiotic starter next time. If you have made several batches since you used fresh starter and the quality of the acidophilus milk has begun to deteriorate, begin with fresh starter the next time.

Yogurt

Yogurt has been called "the milk of life" and is indeed a great health-promoting food. It is made by fermenting milk with the organisms <u>Lactobacillus bulgaricus</u> and <u>Streptococcus thermophilus</u>. Although these organisms do not permanently colonize the human intestine, they assist colonization by <u>Lactobacillus acidophilus</u> and <u>Bifidobacterium bifidum</u>.

> 1 quart whole goat, sheep, cow or other animal milk
> ¼ to ⅓ cup of plain yogurt containing live cultures OR ½ teaspoon of yogurt culture such as dairy-free GI Pro Start™ Yogurt Starter
> (See "Sources," page 261 to order from GI Pro Start™)

While heating the milk, immerse the metal tip of a digital thermometer in boiling water to kill bacteria that may be on it. Bring the milk to a boil (unless it is raw milk[9]) in a saucepan over medium heat and boil it for one minute. Let it cool to 95°F, using the digital thermometer to monitor the temperature as it cools. If you are in a hurry, you can speed this process by putting the pan in a sink of cold water. Stir a little of the warm milk into your fresh yogurt starter or powdered culture; then stir this mixture into the rest of the milk in the saucepan.

---

9 If you are using raw milk in this recipe, you have hopefully made sure the dairy from which you purchase it uses "clean" practices. Do not boil this milk; do not destroy enzymes such as phytase which will help you deal with phytic acid. High temperature will also make the calcium less easily absorbable. Using the digital thermometer to monitor progress, gently heat the milk to 95°F before adding the culture.

Pour the milk into yogurt maker container(s) or glass jar(s) to go into your yogurt maker or proofing box. You may use a yogurt maker if you have or can get an older model that incubates at about 95ºF, such as the Yogourmet™ yogurt maker. See page 62 for more about yogurt makers.

Incubate the yogurt until it thickens (5 to 10 hours) or for up to 24 hours. Yogurt that is incubated for 24 hours will contain almost no lactose and the protein will be partially digested, which makes it easier to tolerate. The only dairy products allowed on the specific carbohydrate and GAP diets are 24-hour fermented yogurt and acidophilus milk, which are essentially lactose-free.

Save some of the yogurt in a clean container in the refrigerator to use to make the next batch of yogurt. Reserve ¼ to ⅓ cup of yogurt for each quart of yogurt you plan to make the next time. Serve the rest of the yogurt immediately or you can refrigerate it for up to one week. Serve it plain, with fresh fruit with or without stevia or a low-GI sweetener, or as a smoothie (recipe below), if desired. Makes about 1 quart of yogurt.

NOTE: If the yogurt does not thicken or has an off odor, do not eat it. Begin again with fresh starter. If it has been 3 to 4 weeks since you started with a fresh culture, start over with fresh starter next time. If you have made several batches since you used fresh starter and the quality of the yogurt has begun to deteriorate, begin with fresh starter next time.

Yogurt or Acidophilus Milk Smoothie

1 cup of yogurt or acidophilus milk
Sweetener of your choice:
    Enzyme-treated white stevia powder – 1 pinch or to taste (optional)
    1 to 2 teaspoons agave or to taste
Flavoring of your choice:
    ½ teaspoon natural flavoring such as Frontier™ brand which is
        corn- and alcohol-free
    Fresh or frozen fruit, mashed or pureed to yield about ¼ cup

Stir the yogurt or acidophilus milk until it is smooth. Add agave or a pinch of white stevia powder, if desired, and stir it in. Add natural flavoring or ¼ cup pureed frozen or fresh fruit. Stir thoroughly and enjoy. Makes one serving

Yogurt "Sour Cream" or Yo-Cheese

One batch of thick yogurt made with high-fat and/or high-protein milk,
    page 123, or one quart of commercially made yogurt which does not
    contain thickeners

To make this easily, use naturally thick yogurt, meaning that it is made from a high-fat or high-protein milk such as sheep or cow yogurt. Line a colander with two double layers of cheesecloth or use a yogurt strainer purchased from a cooking store or catalogue or online. Place a pan or bowl beneath the colander or strainer, allowing plenty of room for the liquid to drain without touching the bottom of the colander or strainer. Place the yogurt in the colander or strainer and refrigerate it for 4 to 6 hours, overnight, or for up to 24 hours. The length of time you must drain your yogurt to obtain the consistency you desire will depend on how thick the yogurt was to begin with; very thick sheep yogurt will achieve a "sour cream" or soft cheese consistency sooner than thin yogurt will.

Serve immediately or refrigerate for up to a week. Yogurt sour cream is delicious on baked potatoes. Yo-cheese is great as a spread or in recipes such as lasagne. Makes about 1½ to 2½ cups of yogurt sour cream or yo-cheese.

Coleslaw Dressing

½ cup tahini or light colored smooth nut butter such as blanched almond or
    macadamia butter
3 to 4 teaspoons unbuffered vitamin C powder, to your taste, (see "Sources,
    page 259) or ⅓ cup lemon juice or rhubarb concentrate (recipe on page 190)
½ to ¾ teaspoon salt
⅛ teaspoon enzyme-treated white stevia powder or 2 teaspoons agave
Water – ⅔ cup if using the vitamin C, ⅓ cup with the lemon juice or rhubarb
    concentrate
1 cup olive, canola, walnut or other healthy oil
1 teaspoon caraway or celery seeds (optional)

Combine the tahini or nut butter, vitamin C (see "Sources," page 259), lemon juice or rhubarb concentrate, salt, sweetener and water in the bowl of a food processor or blender or the container for a hand blender. Blend until smooth. With the blender running, drizzle in the oil in a slow stream. Stir in the seeds. Serve soon or refrigerate any leftover sauce. Makes about 2¼ cups of dressing. Toss with shredded cabbage or jicama to make coleslaw.

Herbed Yogurt Dressing

1 cup of yogurt or acidophilus milk

2 tablespoons lemon juice or 4 tablespoons rhubarb concentrate (recipe on
page 190) or ¼ teaspoon tart-tasting unbuffered vitamin C powder
(See "Sources," page 259).

⅛ to ¼ teaspoon black pepper, to taste

¼ teaspoon salt

1 tablespoon fresh chopped oregano or sweet basil or 1 teaspoon dry oregano
or sweet basil or 1 teaspoon mixture such as Penzeys™ Italian herb mix[10]

If you are using the vitamin C powder, stir it into a few tablespoons of the yogurt
or acidophilus milk until it is completely dissolved. Add the rest of the ingredients and
stir. Serve the dressing immediately or refrigerate leftover dressing. Makes about 1 cup
of dressing.

Sweet Yogurt Dressing

1 cup thick yogurt such as sheep or full fat cow yogurt

2 tablespoons lemon juice or 3 tablespoons rhubarb concentrate (recipe on
page 190), or ¼ teaspoon tart-tasting unbuffered vitamin C powder
(See "Sources," page 259).

¼ cup apple juice concentrate, thawed

¼ teaspoon salt

1 teaspoon celery or poppy seeds (optional)

If you are using the vitamin C powder, stir it into the fruit juice concentrate until
it is completely dissolved. Add the rest of the ingredients and stir. Serve the dressing
immediately or refrigerate leftover dressing. Makes about 1⅓ cups of dressing.

Health Dressing

*Make this dressing with flax oil to provide omega-3 fatty acids. The yogurt and herbs will
mask the taste of the flax oil.*

½ cup yogurt

¼ cup oil, preferably flax oil

⅛ to ¼ teaspoon salt, or to taste

Dash of pepper (optional)

1 to 3 teaspoons fresh oregano or sweet basil or ½ to 1 teaspoon dry oregano
or sweet basil or 1 teaspoon mixture such as Penzeys™ Italian herb mix[10]

---

10 Visit https://www.penzeys.com/ to purchase this mixture or to find a Penzeys store near you.

Stir together all of the recipe ingredients. Serve the dressing immediately or refrigerate any that is left over. Makes ¾ cup of dressing.

Oil and Vinegar Salad Dressing

Because they are not heated, salad dressings are a great place to add fragile oils which are high in essential fatty acids to your diet. Canola and walnut oil are good sources of omega-3 fatty acids which most of our diets lack in sufficient quantities.

> ½ cup oil, preferably walnut or canola because they are high in essential
>   fatty acids
> ½ teaspoon dried oregano, sweet basil or 1 teaspoon mixture such as Penzeys™
>   Italian herb mix (optional)[10]
> ½ teaspoon salt
> Dash of pepper
> ⅓ cup wine vinegar, apple cider vinegar, or lemon juice or 1 to 1½
>   teaspoons unbuffered vitamin C powder plus 1 tablespoons water
>   (See "Sources," page 259 for the vitamin C).

Combine all of the ingredients in a jar and shake. The dressing may be refrigerated at this point. Shake the dressing again to thoroughly mix it right before pouring it on your salad. Makes about ¾ cup of dressing. Refrigerate leftover dressing.

For more recipes for cultured dairy products see *Nourishing Traditions*[11], pages 82 to 87. **For where to purchase cultured dairy products** including sheep and goat yogurt already made, see "Sources," page 256.

---

11 Fallon, Sally with Mary Enig, PhD. *Nourishing Traditions.*, (Brandywine, MD, NewTrends Publishing, 2001), 82-87.

Bone Broth

Homemade bone broth contains an abundance of easily absorbed nutrients which are extracted from bones by long simmering. Nutrients are also extracted from any meat and vegetables simmered with the bones. Another benefit of bone broth is that it is very satisfying and delicious. It is real broth as it has been made for centuries, unlike the products labeled "broth" in grocery stores that contain chemicals that simulate the flavor of meat, high fructose corn syrup, monosodium glutamate (MSG), and other artificial ingredients. Good hand-made bone broth is the basis of many of the delicious sauces used in gourmet cooking.

Homemade chicken soup, also known as Jewish penicillin, really does help recovery from colds. Dr. Stephen Renard demonstrated this in a study on colds using a family recipe handed down from his wife's Lithuanian grandmother.[1] This soup, made by starting with a chicken, shares with other bone broth the ability to boost the immune system. Bone broth also promotes digestive and joint health and aids detoxification.[2]

A crockpot is ideal for making bone broth. Although the broth cooks for up to twenty four hours, it does not require much tending when made in a crock pot. Longer cooking times extract more nutrients from the bones and other ingredients, but also extract more natural glutamates. Therefore, individuals allergic to MSG may do better with broth that is only cooked for six to eight hours. To extract minerals, an acidic ingredient is added to the water and bones before beginning to cook them, and then the broth ingredients are allowed to "rest" for an hour before heating them.

This chapter contains recipes for bone broth made from game meat and less common fowl; options for making bone broth with chicken and beef also are provided. See the end of this chapter for where to find recipes made with more additional ingredients or for fish stock recipes. Enjoy the satisfaction of this delicious broth and the improved health it can bring.

Turkey Bone Broth

Small batch of broth cooked in a small to medium size crockpot
> One small roasted turkey weighing up to about 10 pounds before roasting
> About 2 quarts of purified water
> 1½ teaspoons unbuffered vitamin C powder or 3 tablespoons lemon juice or vinegar (if tolerated – Use the vitamin C if you have citrus or yeast allergies)

---

1 Parker-Hope, Tara. "The Science of Chicken Soup." *The New York Times*, October 12, 2007. https://well.blogs.nytimes.com/2007/10/12/the-science-of-chicken-soup/

2 Axe, Josh, DMN. "Bone Broth Benefits for Digestion, Arthritis and Cellulite." https://draxe.com/the-healing-power-of-bone-broth-for-digestion-arthritis-and-cellulite/

1 to 1½ pounds of vegetables of your choice such as carrots, celery, onions or
    other tolerated non-cabbage family vegetables (optional)
1½ teaspoons whole black peppercorns (optional)

Large batch of broth cooked in a large crock pot holding at least six quarts
    One roasted turkey weighing up to 20 pounds before roasting
    About 4 quarts of purified water
    1 tablespoon unbuffered vitamin C powder or ½ cup vinegar or lemon juice
        (if tolerated – Use the vitamin C if you have citrus or yeast allergies)
    2 to 2½ pounds of vegetables of your choice such as carrots, celery, onions or
        other tolerated non-cabbage family vegetables (optional)
    1 tablespoon whole black peppercorns (optional)

Choose one set of ingredients above, depending on the size of your turkey. You may be able to use a 3-quart crock pot for a small batch if you can pack the bones into it efficiently. It is also fine to use a large crock pot for a small batch of broth. Use a large 6-quart crock pot for a large batch. If you roast a turkey larger than 20 pounds, divide the turkey carcass between two crock pots. Use the amounts of water, acidic ingredient, and vegetables in the ingredient list above for the size of each crockpot.

Roast the turkey, saving the neck and any skin you cut off. (See the "Roasted Poultry" recipe on page 132 for more about to do this). When the turkey is cool enough to handle or the day after a turkey dinner, remove any remaining breast, leg, and thigh meat and reserve it to put in turkey soup or for future meals. Break apart the carcass and place it in the crockpot(s). Add the uncooked neck and skin. Add enough water to cover all the bones in the pot(s). Stir in the vitamin C, lemon juice or vinegar and allow the pot(s) to rest for about one hour. Then turn the crockpot(s) on to "high."

When the broth is near a simmer, reduce the heat and cook it on "low" for 6 to 24 hours. If necessary, set the lid ajar to keep the broth at a low simmer rather than allowing it to boil. You want a bare simmer, steaming with a few bubbles only. Skim and discard any scum that comes to the top after it simmers.

Peel the carrots. Keep the vegetables whole or halve them because larger pieces are easier to retrieve after the cooking time than small pieces. When the broth produces no more scum, add the vegetables and peppercorns to the pot(s).

If you are new to bone broth and are sensitive to glutamates, stop the cooking at six hours of simmering time. As your health improves, you may be able to cook the broth longer which will extract more of the healing nutrients. Twenty four hours of simmering results in almost complete dissolution of the cartilage.

When the broth has simmered for the correct length of time for your personal needs, remove the bones and pieces of meat with tongs and place in a bowl. Remove the vegetables and set them aside to cut up for soup. Strain the broth from the pot and from the bottom of the bowl. Put the broth in jars and refrigerate or freeze. The fat layer that will congeal at the top of the jars helps keep the broth fresh. For intestinal healing this fat should be consumed with the broth. Pick off and save the useable meat from the bones. Serve the broth plain, salted, or made into soup by adding pieces of meat picked from the bones or left from the roasted turkey, vegetables cut into pieces and sea salt. Makes 2 quarts (small batch) to 4½ quarts (large batch) of broth. If you use two crockpots for a very large turkey, this recipe will yield 7 to 8 quarts of broth.

Guinea Hen Bone Broth

2 large or 3 small guinea hens, roasted (See "Sources," page 265).
3 to 4 quarts of purified water
1½ teaspoons unbuffered vitamin C powder or 3 tablespoons lemon juice or vinegar (if tolerated – use vitamin C if you have citrus or yeast allergies)
1 to 1½ pounds of vegetables of your choice such as carrots, celery, onions or other tolerated non-cabbage family vegetables (optional)
1½ teaspoons whole black peppercorns (optional)

Roast the guinea hens, saving the necks and any skin you cut off. (See the "Roasted Poultry" recipe on page 132 for more about to do this). When the birds are cool enough to handle after your meal, remove any remaining breast, leg, and thigh meat and reserve it to put in the soup or for future meals. Break apart the carcasses and place them in a 6-quart crockpot. Add the uncooked necks and skin. (If you are cooking the birds at different times, each carcass and its neck and skin can be frozen until you are ready to make broth). Add enough water to cover all the bones in the pot. Stir in the vitamin C, lemon juice or vinegar and allow the pot to rest for about one hour. Then turn the crock pot on to "high."

When the broth is near a simmer, reduce the heat and cook it on "low" for 6 to 24 hours. If necessary, set the lid ajar to keep the broth at a low simmer rather than allowing it to boil. You want a bare simmer, steaming with a few bubbles only. Skim and discard any scum that comes to the top after it simmers.

Peel the carrots. Keep the vegetables whole or halve them because larger pieces are easier to retrieve after the cooking time than small pieces. When the broth produces no more scum, add the vegetables and peppercorns to the pot.

If you are new to bone broth and are sensitive to glutamates, stop the cooking at six hours of simmering time. As your health improves, you may be able to cook the broth longer which will extract more of the healing nutrients. Twenty four hours of simmering results in almost complete dissolution of the cartilage.

When the broth has simmered for the correct length of time for your personal needs, remove the bones and pieces of meat with tongs and place in a bowl. Remove the vegetables and set them aside to cut up for soup. Strain the broth from the pot and from the bottom of the bowl. Put the broth in jars and refrigerate or freeze. The fat layer that will congeal at the top of the jars helps keep the broth fresh. For intestinal healing this fat should be consumed with the broth. Pick off and save the useable meat from the bones. Serve the broth plain, salted, or made into soup by adding pieces of meat picked from the bones or left from the roasted birds, vegetables cut into pieces and sea salt. Makes 3 to 4 quarts of broth.

Chicken Bone Broth

Substitute two free-range chickens for the guinea hens in the recipe above.

Duck Bone Broth

2 ducks, roasted
3 to 3½ quarts of purified water
1½ teaspoons unbuffered vitamin C powder or 3 tablespoons lemon juice or vinegar (if tolerated – Use vitamin C if you have citrus or yeast allergies)
1 to 1½ pounds of vegetables of your choice such as carrots, celery, onions or other tolerated non-cabbage family vegetables (optional)
1½ teaspoons whole black peppercorns (optional)

Roast the ducks, saving the necks and any skin you cut off. (See the "Roasted Poultry" recipe on page 132 for more about to do this). When the birds are cool enough to handle after your meal, remove any remaining breast, leg, and thigh meat and reserve it to put in the soup or for future meals. Break apart the carcasses and place them in a 6-quart crockpot. Add the uncooked necks and skin. (If you are cooking the birds at different times, each carcass and its neck and skin can be frozen until you are ready to make broth). Add enough water to cover all the bones in the pot. Stir in the vitamin C, lemon juice or vinegar and allow the pot to rest for about one hour. Then turn the crock pot on to "high."

When the broth is near a simmer, reduce the heat and cook it on "low" for 6 to 24 hours. If necessary, set the lid ajar to keep the broth at a low simmer rather than allowing it to boil. You want a bare simmer, steaming with a few bubbles only. Skim and discard any scum that comes to the top after it simmers.

Peel the carrots. Keep the vegetables whole or halve them because larger pieces are easier to retrieve after the cooking time than small pieces. When the broth produces no more scum, add the vegetables and peppercorns to the pot.

If you are new to bone broth and are sensitive to glutamates, stop the cooking at six hours of simmering time. As your health improves, you may be able to cook the broth longer which will extract more of the healing nutrients. Twenty four hours of simmering results in almost complete dissolution of the cartilage.

When the broth has simmered for the correct length of time for your personal needs, remove the bones and pieces of meat with tongs and place in a bowl. Remove the vegetables and set them aside to cut up for soup. Strain the broth from the pot and from the bottom of the bowl. Put the broth in jars and refrigerate or freeze. The fat layer that will congeal at the top of the jars helps keep the broth fresh. For intestinal healing this fat should be consumed with the broth. Pick off and save the useable meat from the bones. Serve the broth plain, salted, or made into soup by adding pieces of meat picked from the bones or left from the roasted ducks, vegetables cut into pieces and sea salt. Makes 3 to 4 quarts of broth.

Roasted Poultry

> One turkey, duck, goose, guinea hen, chicken, or any other type of poultry
> Unrefined salt

If you are using frozen poultry, be sure to purchase it far enough in advance to thaw it. The easiest way to thaw poultry is by putting it in the refrigerator. However, a large turkey can take several days to thaw in the refrigerator, so you can thaw it, still in its wrapping, by placing it in a sink filled with cool water to cover. Begin thawing the turkey one day or more before it will be roasted. Change the water in the sink every half-hour to hour. When the breast feels spongy, remove the turkey from the sink and return it to the refrigerator until it is almost cooking time.

Calculate how many hours the poultry should be roasted using the roasting time information below. Count back from dinner time that number of hours to know when to put the bird in the oven. Shortly before that time, cut the wrapping open and remove the bird. Remove and discard the giblets which are usually in a bag in the neck cavity. Use your fingers to scrape out any excess tissue in the body cavity. Rinse out the neck cavity and body cavity with cool water. Cut off excess skin and fat including the "tail" at the lower end of the body cavity. Rub the body cavity with salt or stuff the bird with quinoa poultry stuffing, page 142. Do not cover smaller birds. Do not cover turkey initially. About one third of the way into the cooking time, when the turkey's breast is nicely browned, cover the breast only with a piece of aluminum foil to keep it from getting too brown before the rest of the turkey is ready.

For a turkey, preheat your oven to 450°F. Place it breast up on a rack in the roasting pan. Put the it in the oven and immediately lower the heat to 350°F. After the turkey is getting brown, cover it with a piece of aluminum foil trimmed to cover the breast only.

For other birds, a rack is not necessary nor is pre-heating the oven. Place smaller birds in a glass casserole dish or baking dish. Turn the oven on to 350°F when you put the bird in the oven.

The approximate roasting times for unstuffed birds are:

Turkey: 20 minutes per pound for birds up to 6 pounds; 15 minutes per pound for larger birds

Duck or goose: 2½ to 3½ hours, or about 20 minutes per pound

Guinea hen or chicken: 1½ to 2½ hours.

Grouse, squab, or Cornish hen: about 1 hour or until nicely browned.

Stuffed birds will take 5 minutes per pound longer to roast.

Baste all birds with the pan drippings occasionally during the roasting time. Watch them and when they are nicely browned, use a digital meat thermometer to check the temperature in the deepest part of the breast. The temperature in the deepest part of the breast should reach 185°F. If the bird is almost up to the correct temperature and you let it rest before carving, the temperature will rise a few degrees during the rest. Smaller birds such as ducks, geese, guinea hens or chickens are less likely than turkey to dry out, so don't worry about overcooking them. If you lack a meat thermometer, just cook the smaller birds until they are nicely browned and the leg joints are quite loose.

There is sometimes concern about food safety when cooking a turkey. As long as you thaw the bird completely in the refrigerator or sink before cooking it and check the temperature with a thermometer to make sure it is high enough before removing it from the oven, you need not fear. The procedure for roasting a turkey and the recommendations above are from my very old *Joy of Cooking* and have kept my family safe from food poisoning for over forty years. This temperature is higher than what the USDA[3] recommends at the time of this writing, and actually *The Joy of Cooking* says to cook until the internal temperature is 190°F. If you remove your turkey from the oven when its temperature is 180-185°F, it will be very tender and juicy if you have basted it about once an hour and covered the breast with foil. Three caveats are: (1) Do not thaw the bird at room temperature or in a microwave, (2) The turkey really must be totally thawed all the way through before you cook it, and (3) For food safety reasons, it is much better to overcook than undercook a turkey!

When the bird has finished roasting, remove it from the pan and put it on a cutting board. Let a large bird such as turkey stand for 10 to 15 minutes before carving it. Smaller birds can be cut apart into breasts, legs, and wings immediately if you wish.

A final piece of advice is to buy a turkey that is going to be good tasting, meaning that it has not been injected with MSG or other chemicals. Free-range turkeys taste great! Years ago, one of my sons asked why turkey cooked by a family member did not taste as good as turkey at home. I told him it had nothing to do with the skill of the cook, but was because the turkey was an inexpensive grocery store special injected with chemicals and unpronounceable man-made ingredients.

---

3 Let's Talk Turkey: A Consumer Guide to Safely Roasting a Turkey. USDA Food Safety and Inspection Service.
https://www.fsis.usda.gov/wps/portal/fsis/topics/food-safety-education/get-answers/food-safety-fact-sheets/poultry-preparation/lets-talk-turkey/CT_Index

Elk Bone Broth

4 to 5 pounds of elk soup bones, knuckle bones if possible, or neck bones if
    you are getting the elk meat from Elk USA[4]
About 3 to 4 pounds of meaty elk bones such as ribs and osso bucco
Purified water, about 3 to 4 quarts
1½ to 2½ teaspoons unbuffered vitamin C powder or ¼ cup lemon juice or
    vinegar (if tolerated – Use vitamin C if you have citrus or yeast allergies)
1 to 2 pounds of vegetables of your choice such as carrots, celery, onions or
    other tolerated non-cabbage family vegetables (optional)
1 to 2 teaspoons whole black peppercorns (optional)

The meat and bones used in this recipe are available from Elk USA. See "Sources," page 265, for more information.

Browning some of the bones adds flavor and color to your broth but it can be skipped if time is lacking. It may be convenient to brown bones the day before you start the broth or it can be done the same day. Place the meaty bones (all except the knuckle bones) in a stainless steel or glass roasting pan. Roast them in a 350°F oven for 20 minutes. Turn the bones and then brown them for another 20 minutes on the second side. Cool until they are easy to handle. Use a narrow knife to remove the marrow from the bones. (I use a Rada tomato knife). Scrape up any drippings in the pan and put them and the marrow in a glass jar. Heat 1 to 1½ cups of purified water to boiling and pour about half of it into the baking pan. Scrape any dried brown bits into the water and add it to the jar. Repeat with some or all of the remaining hot water to capture as much of the flavorful meat and drippings as possible. Refrigerate the jar overnight or until you start making the broth.

On the day you are making the broth, use a narrow knife to ream out the marrow from the osso bucco and any knuckle bones if not already done. Put the knuckle or neck bones, meaty bones, marrow, and reserved liquid with brown bits (if you browned the bones) in a 6 quart crock pot. Add enough water to cover all the ingredients in the pot. Stir in the vitamin C, lemon juice or vinegar and allow to stand for about one hour. Then turn the pot on to "high" and bring the broth to a bare simmer.

When the broth is near a simmer, reduce the heat and cook it on "low" for 6 to 24 hours. If necessary, set the lid ajar to keep the broth at a low simmer rather than allowing it to boil. You want a bare simmer, steaming with a few bubbles only. Skim and discard any scum that comes to the top after it simmers.

---

4 Knuckle bones from Elk USA come with a 22 inch long femur bone, which will be useable in a crock pot only if you cut the bone into small pieces with a band saw. If this broth is made with neck bones, the broth gels lightly, not firmly. You may wish to search online for small knuckle bones, which I have not been able to find at the time of this writing.

Peel the carrots. Keep the vegetables whole or halve them because larger pieces are easier to retrieve after the cooking time than small pieces. When the broth produces no more scum, add the vegetables and peppercorns to the pot.

If you are new to bone broth and are sensitive to glutamates, stop the cooking at six hours of simmering time. As your health improves, you may be able to cook the broth longer which will extract more of the healing nutrients. Twenty four hours of simmering results in almost complete dissolution of the cartilage.

When the broth has simmered for the correct length of time for your personal needs, remove the bones and pieces of meat with tongs and place in a bowl. Remove the vegetables and set them aside to cut up for soup. Strain the broth from the pot and from the bottom of the bowl. Put the broth in jars and refrigerate or freeze. The fat layer that will congeal at the top of the jars helps keep the broth fresh. For intestinal healing this fat should be consumed with the broth. Pick off and save the useable meat from the bones. Serve the broth plain, salted, or made into soup with pieces of the meat from the meaty bones, vegetables cut into small pieces and sea salt. Makes 3 to 4 quarts of broth.

Venison Bone Broth

5 to 6 pounds of venison knuckle bones
About 4 pounds of meaty venison bones, including osso bucco
Purified water, about 3 to 4 quarts
2 teaspoons unbuffered vitamin C powder or ¼ cup lemon juice or
    vinegar (if tolerated – Use vitamin C if you have citrus or yeast allergies)
1 to 2 pounds of vegetables of your choice such as carrots, celery, onions, or
    other tolerated non-cabbage family vegetables (optional)
2 teaspoons whole black peppercorns (optional)

The meat and bones used in this recipe are available from Broken Arrow Ranch. See "Sources," page 265, for more information.

Browning some of the bones adds flavor and color to your broth but it can be skipped if time is lacking. It may be convenient to brown bones the day before you start the broth or it can be done the same day. Place the meaty bones (all except the knuckle bones) in a stainless steel or glass roasting pan. Roast them in a 350°F oven for 20 minutes. Turn the bones and then brown them for another 20 minutes on the second side. Cool until they are easy to handle. Use a narrow knife to remove the marrow from the bones. (I use a Rada tomato knife). Scrape up any drippings in the pan and put them and the marrow in a glass jar. Heat 1 to 1½ cups of purified water to boiling and pour about half of it into the baking pan. Scrape any dried brown bits into the water and add it to the jar. Repeat with some or all of the remaining hot water to capture as much of the flavorful meat and drippings as possible. Refrigerate the jar overnight or until you start making the broth.

On the day you are making the broth, use a narrow knife to ream out the marrow from the osso bucco and any knuckle bones if not already done. Put the knuckle or neck bones, meaty bones, marrow, and reserved liquid with brown bits (if you browned the bones) in a 6 quart crock pot. Add enough water to cover all the ingredients in the pot. Stir in the vitamin C, lemon juice or vinegar and allow to stand for about one hour. Then turn the pot on to "high" and bring the broth to a bare simmer.

When the broth is near a simmer, reduce the heat and cook it on "low" for 6 to 24 hours. If necessary, set the lid ajar to keep the broth at a low simmer rather than allowing it to boil. You want a bare simmer, steaming with a few bubbles only. Skim and discard any scum that comes to the top after it simmers.

Peel the carrots. Keep the vegetables whole or halve them because larger pieces are easier to retrieve after the cooking time than small pieces. When the broth produces no more scum, add the vegetables and peppercorns to the pot.

If you are new to bone broth and are sensitive to glutamates, stop the cooking at six hours of simmering time. As your health improves, you may be able to cook the broth longer which will extract more of the healing nutrients. Twenty four hours of simmering results in almost complete dissolution of the cartilage.

When the broth has simmered for the correct length of time for your personal needs, remove the bones and pieces of meat with tongs and place in a bowl. Remove the vegetables and set them aside to cut up for soup. Strain the broth from the pot and from the bottom of the bowl. Put the broth in jars and refrigerate or freeze. The fat layer that will congeal at the top of the jars helps keep the broth fresh. For intestinal healing this fat should be consumed with the broth. Pick off and save the useable meat from the bones. Serve the broth plain, salted, or made into soup with pieces of the meat from the meaty bones, vegetables cut into small pieces and sea salt. Makes 3 to 4 quarts of broth.

Buffalo (Bison) Bone Broth

About 4 to 5 pounds of buffalo knuckle bones
About 2 to 3 pounds of buffalo ribs
Purified water, about 3 to 3½ quarts
2 to 3 teaspoons unbuffered vitamin C powder or ¼ cup lemon juice or
    vinegar (if tolerated – Use vitamin C if you have citrus or yeast allergies)
1 to 2 pounds of vegetables of your choice such as carrots, celery, onions or
    other tolerated non-cabbage family vegetables (optional)
2 teaspoons whole black peppercorns (optional)

The meat and bones used in this recipe are available from North American Bison. See "Sources," page 264, for more information.

Browning some of the bones adds flavor and color to your broth but it can be skipped if time is lacking. It may be convenient to brown bones the day before you start the broth or it can be done the same day. Place the ribs in a stainless steel or glass roasting pan. Roast them in a 350°F oven for 20 minutes. Turn the bones and then brown them for another 20 minutes on the second side. Cool until they are easy to handle. Scrape up any drippings in the pan and put them and the marrow in a glass jar. Heat 1 to 1½ cups of purified water to boiling and pour about half of it into the baking pan. Scrape any dried brown bits into the water and add it to the jar. Repeat with some or all of the remaining hot water to capture as much of the flavorful meat and drippings as possible. Refrigerate the jar overnight or until you start making the broth.

On the day you are making the broth, use a narrow knife to ream out the marrow from the knuckle bones. Put the knuckle bones, ribs, marrow and reserved liquid with brown bits in a 6 quart crock pot. Add enough water to cover all the ingredients in the pot. Stir in the vitamin C, lemon juice or vinegar and allow to stand for about one hour. Then turn the pot on to "high" and bring the broth to a bare simmer.

When the broth is near a simmer, reduce the heat and cook it on "low" for 6 to 24 hours. If necessary, set the lid ajar to keep the broth at a low simmer rather than allowing it to boil. You want a bare simmer, steaming with a few bubbles only. Skim and discard any scum that comes to the top after it simmers.

Peel the carrots. Keep the vegetables whole or halve them because larger pieces are easier to retrieve after the cooking time than small pieces. When the broth produces no more scum, add the vegetables and peppercorns to the pot.

If you are new to bone broth and are sensitive to glutamates, stop the cooking at six hours of simmering time. As your health improves, you may be able to cook the broth longer which will extract more of the healing nutrients. Twenty four hours of simmering results in almost complete dissolution of the cartilage.

When the broth has simmered for the correct length of time for your personal needs, remove the bones and pieces of meat with tongs and place in a bowl. Remove the vegetables and set them aside to cut up for soup. Strain the broth from the pot and from the bottom of the bowl. Put the broth in jars and refrigerate or freeze. The fat layer that will congeal at the top of the jars helps keep the broth fresh. For intestinal healing this fat should be consumed with the broth. Pick off and save the useable meat from the bones. Serve the broth plain, salted, or made into soup with pieces of the meat from the meaty bones, vegetables cut into small pieces and sea salt. Makes 3 to 3½ quarts of broth.

Beef Bone Broth

Substitute beef knuckle bones and ribs for the buffalo bones in the recipe above.

Alpaca Bone Broth

3 to 4 pounds of alpaca knuckle bones
About 4 pounds of meaty bones alpaca such as ribs and osso bucco
Purified water, about 3 quarts
1½ teaspoons unbuffered vitamin C powder or ¼ cup lemon juice or
      vinegar (if tolerated – Use vitamin C if you have citrus or yeast allergies)
1 to 2 pounds of vegetables of your choice such as carrots, celery, onions or
      other tolerated non-cabbage family vegetables (optional)
1½ teaspoons whole black peppercorns (optional)

The meat and bones used in this recipe are available from Many Pastures Alpaca. See "Sources," page 265, for more information.

Browning some of the bones adds flavor and color to your broth but it can be skipped if time is lacking. It may be convenient to brown bones the day before you start the broth or it can be done the same day. Place the meaty bones (all except the knuckle bones) in a stainless steel or glass roasting pan. Roast them in a 350°F oven for 20 minutes. Turn the bones and then brown them for another 20 minutes on the second side. Cool until they are easy to handle. Use a narrow knife to remove the marrow from the bones. (I use a Rada tomato knife). Scrape up any drippings in the pan and put them and the marrow in a glass jar. Heat 1 to 1½ cups of purified water to boiling and pour about half of it into the baking pan. Scrape any dried brown bits into the water and add it to the jar. Repeat with some or all of the remaining hot water to capture as much of the flavorful meat and drippings as possible. Refrigerate the jar overnight or until you start making the broth.

On the day you are making the broth, use a narrow knife to ream out the marrow from the osso bucco and any knuckle bones if not already done. Put the knuckle or neck bones, meaty bones, marrow, and reserved liquid with brown bits (if you browned the bones) in a 6 quart crock pot. Add enough water to cover all the ingredients in the pot. Stir in the vitamin C, lemon juice or vinegar and allow to stand for about one hour. Then turn the pot on to "high" and bring the broth to a bare simmer.

When the broth is near a simmer, reduce the heat and cook it on "low" for 6 to 24 hours. If necessary, set the lid ajar to keep the broth at a low simmer rather than allowing it to boil. You want a bare simmer, steaming with a few bubbles only. Skim and discard any scum that comes to the top after it simmers.

Peel the carrots. Keep the vegetables whole or halve them because larger pieces are easier to retrieve after the cooking time than small pieces. When the broth produces no more scum, add the vegetables and peppercorns to the pot.

If you are new to bone broth and are sensitive to glutamates, stop the cooking at six hours of simmering time. As your health improves, you may be able to cook the broth longer which will extract more of the healing nutrients. Twenty four hours of simmering results in almost complete dissolution of the cartilage.

When the broth has simmered for the correct length of time for your personal needs, remove the bones and pieces of meat with tongs and place in a bowl. Remove the vegetables and set them aside to cut up for soup. Strain the broth from the pot and from the bottom of the bowl. Put the broth in jars and refrigerate or freeze. The fat layer that will congeal at the top of the jars helps keep the broth fresh. For intestinal healing this fat should be consumed with the broth. Pick off and save the useable meat from the bones. Serve the broth plain, salted, or made into soup with pieces of the meat from the meaty bones, vegetables cut into small pieces and sea salt. Makes 3 to 3½ quarts of broth.

Antelope Bone Broth

> 5 to 6 pounds of antelope bones including ribs if that is all you can find
> Purified water, about 3 to 3½ quarts
> 2 teaspoons unbuffered vitamin C powder or ¼ cup lemon juice or vinegar
>   (if tolerated – Use vitamin C if you have citrus or yeast allergies)
> 1 to 2 pounds of vegetables of your choice such as carrots, celery, onions or
>   other tolerated non-cabbage family vegetables (optional)
> 2 teaspoons whole black peppercorns (optional)

The meat and bones used in this recipe are available from Broken Arrow Ranch. See "Sources," page 265, for more information.

Browning some of the bones adds flavor and color to your broth but it can be skipped if time is lacking. It may be convenient to brown bones the day before you start the broth or it can be done the same day. Place the bones in a stainless steel or glass roasting pan. Roast them in a 350°F oven for 20 minutes. Turn the bones and then brown them for another 20 minutes on the second side. Cool until they are easy to handle and remove the bones from the pan. Scrape up any drippings in the pan and put them in a glass jar. Heat 1 to 1½ cups of purified water to boiling and pour about half of it into the baking pan. Scrape any dried brown bits into the water and add it to the jar. Repeat with some or all of the remaining hot water to capture as much of the flavorful meat and drippings as possible. Refrigerate the jar overnight or until you start making the broth.

On the day you are making the broth, use a narrow knife to ream out the marrow from any osso bucco or knuckle bones if not already done. Put the bones, marrow and reserved liquid with brown bits (if you browned the bones) in a 6 quart crock pot. Add enough water to cover all the ingredients in the pot. Stir in the vitamin C, lemon juice or vinegar and allow to stand for about one hour. Then turn the pot on to "high" and bring the broth to a bare simmer.

When the broth is near a simmer, reduce the heat and cook it on "low" for 6 to 24 hours. If necessary, set the lid ajar to keep the broth at a low simmer rather than allowing it to boil. You want a bare simmer, steaming with a few bubbles only. Skim and discard any scum that comes to the top after it simmers.

Peel the carrots. Keep the vegetables whole or halve them because larger pieces are easier to retrieve after the cooking time than small pieces. When the broth produces no more scum, add the vegetables and peppercorns to the pot.

If you are new to bone broth and are sensitive to glutamates, stop the cooking at six hours of simmering time. As your health improves, you may be able to cook the broth longer which will extract more of the healing nutrients. Twenty four hours of simmering results in almost complete dissolution of the cartilage.

When the broth has simmered for the correct length of time for your personal needs, remove the bones and pieces of meat with tongs and place in a bowl. Remove the vegetables and set them aside to cut up for soup. Strain the broth from the pot and from the bottom of the bowl. Put the broth in jars and refrigerate or freeze. There will be very little fat from this broth. Pick off and save the meat from the bones if you wish to add it to the broth. If you like to chew meat from ribs, save the meat on the bones. Serve the broth plain, salted, or made into soup with pieces of the meat from the bones, vegetables cut into small pieces and sea salt. Makes 3 to 3½ quarts of broth.

For more bone broth recipes, see *Nourishing Traditions*,[5] pages 119 to 124. For fish stocks see pages 119-121.

For where to purchase bone broth already made, see "Sources," page 254. For sources of game meat, game bones, as well as more common animal bones, see "Sources," page 264 to 265.

---

5 Fallon, Sally with Mary Enig, PhD. *Nourishing Traditions*., (Brandywine, MD, NewTrends Publishing, 2001), 119-124.

Grains

Bread made from grains has been called the staff of life. Because grains keep well in storage longer than many other foods, they have made up a large part of our food supply since human beings began growing grain. This chapter discusses both members of the grain family and alternative grains such as quinoa, amaranth, and buckwheat. These can be treated like grain family members in cooking except for the notable difference in quinoa. It is coated with a soap-like substance which protects the seeds from being eaten by insects, etc. Therefore, it must be thoroughly rinsed before cooking or it will taste like soap.

Both grain-family whole grains and alternative grains are highly nutritious. They are concentrated sources of carbohydrates, high in fiber for good digestion, and contain some protein, although the level is low compared to legumes or animal foods. Most grains contain incomplete protein, meaning that they do not contain all the amino acids that our bodies are unable to synthesize. Quinoa is an exception to this; it is one of the few plant sources of complete protein, albeit a low level. Vegetarians eat beans and grains or alternative grains together to get complete protein nutrition, with each food making up for the amino acid deficit of the other. Grains and grain alternatives are also high in B vitamins and a wide variety of minerals including manganese and selenium.

Like nuts and legumes, grains are the seeds of the plants that produce them. Thus, they contain substances to protect them from being digested by soil bacteria before they can germinate. These enzyme inhibitors and phytic acid also make it less easy for us to digest and absorb nutrients from grains. Phytic acid interferes with the absorption of minerals including calcium, zinc, magnesium, iron and copper. A diet high in vitamin C, vitamins A and D from animal sources and absorbable calcium will help avert the effects of consuming phytic acid. In addition, good intestinal flora can break the phytic acid down, but proper preparation and cooking of grains is still essential.[1]

To gain the best nutrition from grains, they should be soaked for twelve to twenty four hours with an acidic ingredient or fermented before cooking to neutralize the phytic acid and enzyme inhibitors. Lemon juice, vinegar, and fermented milk products are often used as the acidic ingredient for soaking, but, unfortunately, are allergenic foods. Therefore, this chapter contains recipes for whole grains soaked with unbuffered vitamin C, lemon juice or rhubarb concentrate, muffin recipes made from flours soaked with vitamin C and/or acidic fruit juice, and pancakes and breads fermented using yeast and/ or *lactobacilli*. Enjoy these grain-based foods made more digestible and nutritious.

---

1 Nagle, Ramiel. "Living with Phytic Acid." The Weston A. Price Foundation. https://www.westonaprice. org/health-topics/vegetarianism-and-plant-foods/living-with-phytic-acid/

Quinoa Pilaf or Poultry Stuffing

1 cup quinoa, thoroughly washed
1 tablespoon of lemon juice or rhubarb concentrate (recipe on page 190)
    or ¼ teaspoon unbuffered vitamin C powder or crystals
2 cups sliced celery
¼ small onion, chopped (optional)
4 tablespoons oil
2 cups purified water plus additional water for soaking
½ to 1 teaspoon unrefined salt, or to taste
¼ teaspoon pepper
3 tablespoons finely chopped fresh parsley or 1 tablespoon dried parsley
1 tablespoon finely chopped fresh sweet basil or 1 teaspoon dried sweet basil
1 teaspoon finely chopped fresh rosemary or ¼ teaspoon ground dried
    rosemary (optional)

Place the quinoa in a strainer and run water over it until the water is no longer sudsy. This removes the soap-like coating on the quinoa. Place the quinoa in a bowl and add the lemon juice, rhubarb concentrate, or vitamin C. Add warm water to cover by an inch or two. Allow the quinoa to soak for 12 to 24 hours. Then drain and replace the water two or three times to rinse it thoroughly. Drain off all of the water.

Using a saucepan, sauté the celery and onion in the oil until they just begin to brown. Add the quinoa and purified water, bring the mixture to a boil, and simmer it for 15 to 20 minutes, or until the quinoa is translucent. Stir in the seasonings thoroughly and allow the quinoa to stand for a few minutes so that the flavors can blend. Serve it as a side dish or stuff it into a large chicken and then roast the chicken. To use this stuffing for a turkey, double the recipe for a 12-pound turkey or triple it for a 24-pound turkey. The cooking time should be increased 5 minutes per pound if you stuff a bird. Makes 4 to 6 side-dish servings.

Stovetop Grains

Soaking whole grains overnight before cooking them (as in the next two recipes) makes them tender and creamy plus easier to digest.

RYE
1 cup rye
1 tablespoon of lemon juice or rhubarb concentrate (recipe on page 190)
    or ¼ teaspoon unbuffered vitamin C powder or crystals
4 cups purified water plus additional water for soaking
¼ teaspoon unrefined salt
Cooking time: 1½ to 2 hours

TEFF

1 cup teff

1 tablespoon of lemon juice or rhubarb concentrate (recipe on page 190)
   or ¼ teaspoon unbuffered vitamin C powder or crystals

3 cups purified water plus additional water for soaking

¼ teaspoon unrefined salt

Cooking time: 15 to 20 minutes

KAMUT

1 cup kamut

1 tablespoon of lemon juice or rhubarb concentrate (recipe on page 190)
   or ¼ teaspoon unbuffered vitamin C powder or crystals

3 cups purified water plus additional water for soaking

¼ teaspoon unrefined salt

Cooking time: 2 hours

BARLEY

1 cup barley, whole or pearled

1 tablespoon of lemon juice or rhubarb concentrate (recipe on page 190)
   or ¼ teaspoon unbuffered vitamin C powder or crystals

3 cups purified water plus additional water for soaking

¼ teaspoon unrefined salt

Cooking time: 1½ to 1¾ hours for whole barley or 45 to 55 minutes for pearled barley

AMARANTH

1 cup amaranth

1 tablespoon of lemon juice or rhubarb concentrate (recipe on page 190)
   or ¼ teaspoon unbuffered vitamin C powder or crystals

2½ cups purified water plus additional water for soaking

¼ teaspoon unrefined salt

Cooking time: 30 to 35 minutes

SORGHUM

1 cup sorghum

1 tablespoon of lemon juice or rhubarb concentrate (recipe on page 190)
   or ¼ teaspoon unbuffered vitamin C powder or crystals

3½ cups purified water plus additional water for soaking

¼ teaspoon unrefined salt

Cooking time: 1 to 1¼ hours

OAT GROATS

    1 cup oat groats

    1 tablespoon of lemon juice or rhubarb concentrate (recipe on page 190)
        or ¼ teaspoon unbuffered vitamin C powder or crystals

    3 cups purified water plus additional water for soaking

    ¼ teaspoon unrefined salt

Cooking time: 2 to 2½ hours

BROWN RICE

    1 cup brown rice

    1 tablespoon of lemon juice or rhubarb concentrate (recipe on page 190)
        or ¼ teaspoon unbuffered vitamin C powder or crystals

    2½ cups purified water plus additional water for soaking

    ¼ teaspoon unrefined salt

Cooking time: 45 to 50 minutes

WILD RICE

    1 cup wild rice

    1 tablespoon of lemon juice or rhubarb concentrate (recipe on page 190)
        or ¼ teaspoon unbuffered vitamin C powder or crystals

    4 cups purified water plus additional water for soaking

    ¼ teaspoon unrefined salt

Cooking time: 60 minutes

SPELT

    1 cup spelt

    1 tablespoon of lemon juice or rhubarb concentrate (recipe on page 190)
        or ¼ teaspoon unbuffered vitamin C powder or crystals

    3 cups purified water plus additional water for soaking

    ¼ teaspoon unrefined salt

Cooking time: 1½ to 2½ hours

MILLET

    1 cup millet

    1 tablespoon of lemon juice or rhubarb concentrate (recipe on page 190)
        or ¼ teaspoon unbuffered vitamin C powder or crystals

    3 cups purified water plus additional water for soaking

    ¼ teaspoon unrefined salt

Cooking time: 25 to 35 minutes

QUINOA
  1 cup quinoa, thoroughly washed
  1 tablespoon of lemon juice or rhubarb concentrate (recipe on page 190)
      or ¼ teaspoon unbuffered vitamin C powder or crystals
  2 cups purified water plus additional water for soaking
  ¼ teaspoon unrefined salt
Cooking time: 20 minutes

BUCKWHEAT, white or raw
  1 cup buckwheat
  1 tablespoon of lemon juice or rhubarb concentrate (recipe on page 190)
      or ¼ teaspoon unbuffered vitamin C powder or crystals
  3 cups purified water plus additional water for soaking
  ½ teaspoon unrefined salt
Cooking time: 20 to 25 minutes

BUCKWHEAT, roasted
  1 cup buckwheat
  1 tablespoon of lemon juice or rhubarb concentrate (recipe on page 190)
      or ¼ teaspoon unbuffered vitamin C powder or crystals
  2½ cups purified water plus additional water for soaking
  ½ teaspoon unrefined salt
Cooking time: 20 to 30 minutes

Choose one set of ingredients from above or from the previous three pages. If you are using quinoa, place it in a strainer and run water over it until the water is no longer sudsy. This removes the soap-like coating on the quinoa. If you wish, you can rinse other whole grains also. The advice given to not rinse grains before cooking applies *only* to *refined* grains such as white rice. Refined grains are required by law to be enriched with vitamins which are water soluble and are removed by rinsing. Whole grains have not had the vitamins removed. Therefore, they do not need to be enriched and there are no water soluble vitamins to wash away.

In a saucepan, combine the grain, lemon juice, rhubarb concentrate, or vitamin C, and warm water to cover the grain by an inch or two. Place the lid on the pan and allow it to soak for 12 to 24 hours. Then drain and replace the water two or three times to rinse it thoroughly. Drain off all of the water.

Add the salt to the pan. Also add the amount of purified water for cooking given in the ingredient list for the grain you are using. Bring the pan to a boil, then lower the heat and simmer for the time specified above. Check the pan during the cooking time and add more purified water if the grain seems to be drying out. If the water is not absorbed at the end of the cooking time, cook it longer. Remove the pan from the heat. Fluff the grain. Season with butter or oil if desired and serve. Makes 4 to 6 servings.

Oven Grains

If the oven is already on to cook a main dish, this recipe invites cooking a grain side dish at the same time.

SPELT
> 1 cup spelt
> 1 tablespoon of lemon juice or rhubarb concentrate (recipe on page 190)
>> or ¼ teaspoon unbuffered vitamin C powder or crystals
> 3½ cups purified water plus additional water for soaking
> 1 tablespoon oil
> ½ teaspoon unrefined salt

Cooking time: 2 to 2½ hours

MILLET
> 1 cup millet
> 1 tablespoon of lemon juice or rhubarb concentrate (recipe on page 190)
>> or ¼ teaspoon unbuffered vitamin C powder or crystals
> 3½ cups purified water plus additional water for soaking
> 1 tablespoon oil
> ½ teaspoon unrefined salt

Cooking time: 30 to 45 minutes

TEFF
> 1 cup teff
> 1 tablespoon of lemon juice or rhubarb concentrate (recipe on page 190)
>> or ¼ teaspoon unbuffered vitamin C powder or crystals
> 3 cups purified water plus additional water for soaking
> 1 tablespoon oil
> ½ teaspoon unrefined salt

Cooking time: 1 to 1½ hours

BUCKWHEAT
> 1 cup buckwheat, white or roasted
> 1 tablespoon of lemon juice or rhubarb concentrate (recipe on page 190)
>> or ¼ teaspoon unbuffered vitamin C powder or crystals
> 3½ cups purified water plus additional water for soaking
> 1 tablespoon oil
> ½ teaspoon unrefined salt

Cooking time: 1 to 1½ hours

KAMUT

    1 cup kamut

    1 tablespoon of lemon juice or rhubarb concentrate (recipe on page 190)
        or ¼ teaspoon unbuffered vitamin C powder or crystals

    3½ cups purified water plus additional water for soaking

    1 tablespoon oil

    ½ teaspoon unrefined salt

Cooking time: 1¾ to 2 hours

BARLEY

    1 cup pearled or hulless barley

    1 tablespoon of lemon juice or rhubarb concentrate (recipe on page 190)
        or ¼ teaspoon unbuffered vitamin C powder or crystals

    3½ cups purified water plus additional water for soaking

    1 tablespoon oil

    ½ teaspoon unrefined salt

Cooking time: 1 to 1½ hours for hulless barley, 2 to 2½ hours for pearled barley

SORGHUM

    1 cup sorghum

    1 tablespoon of lemon juice or rhubarb concentrate (recipe on page 190)
        or ¼ teaspoon unbuffered vitamin C powder or crystals

    3½ cups purified water plus additional water for soaking

    1 tablespoon oil

    ½ teaspoon unrefined salt

Cooking time: 2½ to 3 hours

RYE

    1 cup rye

    1 tablespoon of lemon juice or rhubarb concentrate (recipe on page 190)
        or ¼ teaspoon unbuffered vitamin C powder or crystals

    3¾ cups purified water plus additional water for soaking

    1 tablespoon oil

    ½ teaspoon unrefined salt

Cooking time: 2 hours

QUINOA

1 cup quinoa
1 tablespoon of lemon juice or rhubarb concentrate (recipe on page 190)
      or ¼ teaspoon unbuffered vitamin C powder or crystals
2½ cups purified water plus additional water for soaking
1 tablespoon oil
½ teaspoon unrefined salt
Cooking time: 1 hour

BROWN RICE

1 cup brown rice
1 tablespoon of lemon juice or rhubarb concentrate (recipe on page 190)
      or ¼ teaspoon unbuffered vitamin C powder or crystals
2½ cups purified water plus additional water for soaking
1 tablespoon oil
½ teaspoon unrefined salt
Cooking time: 1 to 1½ hours

WILD RICE

1 cup wild rice
1 tablespoon of lemon juice or rhubarb concentrate (recipe on page 190)
      or ¼ teaspoon unbuffered vitamin C powder or crystals
4 cups purified water plus additional water for soaking
1 tablespoon oil
½ teaspoon unrefined salt
Cooking time: 1½ to 2 hours

OAT GROATS

1 cup oat groats
1 tablespoon of lemon juice or rhubarb concentrate (recipe on page 190)
      or ¼ teaspoon unbuffered vitamin C powder or crystals
2¾ cups purified water plus additional water for soaking
1 tablespoon oil
½ teaspoon unrefined salt
Cooking time: 2 hours

Choose one set of ingredients from above or from the previous two pages. If you are using quinoa, place it in a strainer and run water over it until the water is no longer sudsy. This removes the soap-like coating on the quinoa. If you wish, you can rinse other whole grains also. We are told to not rinse *refined* grains before cooking only because they are enriched with vitamins which are washed away by rinsing. This is not an issue with the unrefined whole grains used in this recipe.

In a 2- to 3-quart casserole dish, combine the grain, lemon juice, rhubarb concentrate, or vitamin C, and warm water to cover the grain by an inch or two. Place the lid on the casserole and allow it to soak for 12 to 24 hours. Then drain and replace the water two or three times to rinse it thoroughly. Drain off all of the water.

Add the oil and salt to the casserole. Also add the amount of purified water for cooking given in the ingredient list for the grain you are using. Put the lid on the casserole. Bake at 350°F until the grain is tender and all the water is absorbed. Approximate baking times are given with the ingredient list for each grain.

The first time you make this recipe with each grain, or if you are using a different oven temperature to cook a main dish with the grain, check the grain during baking and add more purified water if it is beginning to dry out. Fluff the grain and serve. Makes 4 to 6 servings

NON-YEAST BAKED GOODS

Nourishing Muffins

Soaking flour before baking with it makes it more digestible, but it makes leavening tricky especially with gluten-free flours. It's a new baking experience, but worth the effort.

QUINOA

 2 cups quinoa flour
 ⅝ cup tapioca flour
 ¼ teaspoon unrefined salt
 ¼ teaspoon unbuffered vitamin C powder or crystals
 1½ teaspoons cinnamon
 1 cup unsweetened applesauce
 ⅜ cup apple juice concentrate, thawed
 2 tablespoons oil
 1 teaspoon baking soda

BUCKWHEAT

 2¼ cups buckwheat flour
 ¼ teaspoon unrefined salt
 ¼ teaspoon unbuffered vitamin C powder or crystals
 1½ teaspoons cinnamon or caraway seeds (optional)
 ¾ cup pureed soft fruit such as pear or peach
 ¾ cup white or purple grape juice concentrate, thawed
 3 tablespoons oil
 1 teaspoon baking soda

SORGHUM

>   2½ cups sorghum flour
>   ¼ teaspoon unrefined salt
>   ⅔ cup fresh pineapple with juice to cover[2]
>   ½ cup pineapple juice concentrate, thawed
>   2 tablespoons oil
>   1 teaspoon baking soda

SPELT

>   3¼ cups whole spelt flour
>   ¼ teaspoon unrefined salt
>   ¼ teaspoon unbuffered vitamin C powder or crystals
>   1½ teaspoons cinnamon (optional)
>   ¾ cup unsweetened applesauce
>   ⅜ cup apple juice concentrate, thawed
>   2 tablespoons oil
>   1 teaspoon baking soda

Choose one set of ingredients above.

The day or evening before you plan to bake these muffins, stir together the flour(s), salt, vitamin C (if using) and cinnamon or caraway seeds (if using) in a bowl.

For the sorghum muffins, use a hand blender, blender or food processor to puree the pineapple with its juice. Add the pineapple juice concentrate and mix.

For the buckwheat muffins, if you don't have fruit ripe enough to be soft, cook the fruit. You will need 2 to 3 peaches or pears for this recipe. Puree the ripe or cooked fruit with a hand blender or blender. Add the grape juice concentrate to the puree and stir.

For the quinoa and spelt muffins, mix together the applesauce and apple juice concentrate.

Thoroughly stir the liquid ingredients into the dry ingredients. Cover the bowl and allow the mixture to stand at room temperature for 12 to 24 hours. The mixture will not be like soft batter, but rather like cookie dough. The quinoa is like soft drop cookie dough, spelt and buckwheat are intermediate, and the sorghum is like rolled cookie dough.

The next day, preheat your oven to 375ºF and line the wells of a muffin tin with paper liners. Check the consistency of the muffin dough. If it crumbles when you stir it (most likely to happen with the sorghum dough), add one tablespoon of water to the dough and stir it in thoroughly. If it is still crumbly after adding one tablespoon of water, add more water, one teaspoon at a time. The dough should still be stiff but should stick together.

---

2 Unsweetened canned pineapple in its own juice can also be used in this recipe. However, cancer patients should avoid canned foods because of the plastic lining in the cans.

If the dough holds together in a solid mass when stirred (common with the buckwheat dough), you may to need to use your hands to mix in the oil and baking soda below.

Thoroughly stir together the oil and baking soda in a small bowl or glass. Add the oil mixture to the flour mixture and quickly but thoroughly mix it into the dough with a large spoon until just mixed and the dough is just starting to develop the leavening gas. If the oil mixture does not incorporate into the dough with stirring, use your hands to mix it in. (This is normal with the buckwheat muffins). Work quickly and DO NOT OVERMIX or the leavening gasses will dissipate in the bowl rather than causing the muffins to rise in the oven.

Quickly spoon the batter into the muffin tin, filling the cups to the top. Bake for 17 to 22 minutes or until the muffins are golden brown and a toothpick inserted in the center of the largest muffin comes out dry. Cool the muffins for about 5 minutes in the pan and then remove them to finish cooling on a rack. Makes about 10 to 11 sorghum or quinoa muffins or 12 to 13 buckwheat or spelt muffins.

Sourdough Pancakes

WHOLE SPELT
   Sourdough starter:
      2⅜ cups whole spelt flour
      1¼ cups purified water at 85 to 90°F
      ¼ teaspoon Fermapan™ French-style freeze dried sourdough starter
   Pancakes:
      1 cup of sourdough starter
      2 tablespoons apple juice concentrate, thawed
      1 tablespoon oil
      ⅛ teaspoon unrefined salt
      ⅛ teaspoon baking soda

WHITE SPELT
   Sourdough starter:
      2 cups white spelt flour
      1 cup purified water at 85 to 90°F
      ¼ teaspoon Fermapan™ French-style freeze dried sourdough starter
   Pancakes:
      1 cup of sourdough starter
      2 tablespoons apple juice concentrate, thawed
      1 tablespoon oil
      ⅛ teaspoon unrefined salt
      ⅛ teaspoon baking soda

SORGHUM

Sourdough starter:

   2¼ cups Bob's Red Mill™ white sorghum flour

   1⅛ cups purified water at 85 to 90°F, with an additional tablespoon or two if
      needed to get a batter-like consistency

   ¼ teaspoon Fermapan™ French-style freeze dried sourdough starter

This starter may thicken overnight. In the morning, mix in about ⅛ to ¼ cup of
water when you stir it up before measuring out one cup of starter and adding the other
ingredients below.

Pancakes:

   1 cup of sourdough starter

   1 tablespoon oil

   ⅛ teaspoon unrefined salt

   Additional water to bring it to a "pancake batter" consistency, 2 tablespoons or
      more if needed

   ⅛ teaspoon baking soda

TEFF

Sourdough starter:

   2 cups Bob's Red Mill™ teff flour

   1 cup purified water at 85 to 90°F, with an additional tablespoon if needed to
      get a batter-like consistency

   ¼ teaspoon Fermapan™ French-style freeze dried sourdough starter

This starter may thicken overnight. In the morning, mix in about 1 to 2
tablespoons of water when you stir it up before measuring out one cup of starter and
adding the other ingredients below.

Pancakes:

   1 cup of sourdough starter

   1 tablespoon oil

   ⅛ teaspoon unrefined salt

   Additional water to bring it to a "pancake batter" consistency, 2 tablespoons
      or more if needed

   ⅛ teaspoon baking soda

Chose one set of ingredients above. Mix the ingredients in the "starter" ingredient
list in a glass bowl or programmable bread machine. (See "Sources," page 262, to get the
Fermapan™ sourdough starter). Set the bowl in a cozy spot or put the bread machine
pan in the machine and start a sourdough cycle consisting of a 10 to 15 minute mix followed by up to 24 hours of rising time. Let the flour mixture rise for 18 to 24 hours. If
the starter thickens overnight, add more water (suggested amount in the ingredient list)
to return the batter to its original consistency.

The next day stir the starter, adding more water if the dough is crumbly (likely with the spelt flour) to return it to its original consistency. Oil and heat the griddle. (Electric griddles are ideal because they have a pancake setting with an indicator light to show when they are hot enough). If the batter is too thick, add water to bring it to a pancake-batter consistency.

Measure out one cup of starter to use. Put the remaining starter in a glass jar with a lid and store it in the refrigerator for up to a week to use for more pancakes. Stir together the ingredients in the "pancakes" part of the ingredient list, except **reserve the baking soda.**

When the griddle is hot enough, stir the soda into the batter thoroughly immediately before cooking the pancakes. Scoop up three to four tablespoons of batter for each pancake. A one-fourth cup measuring cup (part of a set of measuring cups for dry ingredients) is ideal for scooping the batter. Pour the batter on the griddle and cook each pancake until it has holes and is beginning to dry on the edges. It should be light brown on the bottom. Then turn and cook the second side until light brown. If you are cooking some of these to freeze rather than eat immediately, cool them on a wire cooling rack. Otherwise, serve them immediately.

Refrigerate the remaining starter for a few days to a week. Then use it to make pancakes on other mornings. However, if your family is large or hungry, make a double batch of pancakes the day after making the starter.

If the pancakes are fragile, difficult to turn, or stick to the griddle, re-oil the griddle with a paper towel between cooking successive batches. Pancake batter tends to thicken as it stands. You may need to add an additional one to three tablespoons of water to the batter as you cook successive batches to keep the consistency of the batter right. If the pancake batter becomes too thick, the pancakes will be thick and may not cook well in the middle.

Each batch of pancakes made with one cup of starter makes 7 to 8 pancakes 3 to 4 inches in diameter.

YEAST BREAD

The easiest way to make yeast bread is to use an appliance such as a heavy duty mixer or a bread machine. In fact, you must use a mixer or bread machine for developing the structure of the bread when making gluten-free bread. All of the yeast bread recipes here give a choice of appliances for making them. Instructions for making bread totally by hand are available online and in many general cookbooks, so they are not included here. For the allergy and gluten-free version of hand-made yeast bread technique, see *Allergy Cooking With Ease* or *The Ultimate Food Allergy Cookbook and Survival Guide* as described on the last pages of this book. Information that will help with the decision of whether to purchase a bread machine and how to choose the machine that is best for your special diet is on pages 242 to 245.

If you already have a bread machine, you may be able to use it for special breads. Almost any machine can be used on the dough cycle to perform the initial mixing and kneading and the first rise for your bread. Then restart the cycle and allow the dough to knead for another 3 to 5 minutes. Remove the dough from the machine and put it in a prepared loaf pan. Proceed with the second rise and baking as in the recipes below.

Most gluten-free breads are made with a combination of grains plus multiple stabilizers. This seems to produce bread with a more conventional texture in most cases. However, as you have read on previous pages, this book takes a different approach to combining several grains and stabilizers in each recipe both to save time on measuring and, more importantly, to prevent the development of allergies to foods that are eaten every day. Therefore, the recipes in this book are made with a single grain/grain alternative or a single grain/grain alternative plus a starch which acts as a binder. My two favorite single-grain gluten-free bread recipes are included on the next few pages of this chapter. For more bread recipes made by hand, mixer, or bread machine, see the books mentioned at the end of this chapter.

Quinoa Raisin Bread

Try this tasty bread toasted for breakfast.

  ¼ cup purified water
  ⅓ cup apple juice concentrate
  About 4 large or 3 extra large eggs[3] (enough to measure ¾ cup in volume) at
        room temperature
  2 tablespoons oil
  ¾ teaspoon unrefined salt
  1 teaspoon cinnamon
  4 teaspoons guar or xanthan gum[4]
  2½ cups quinoa flour
  ¾ cup tapioca starch
  2¼ teaspoons (1 packet) active dry yeast
  ½ cup raisins

---

3 If you are allergic to eggs, use ¾ cup warm purified water in their place. If you do not take the eggs out of the refrigerator early enough for them to come to room temperature before you are ready to bake, put them in a bowl of warm water for 5 or 10 minutes before using them in this recipe.

4 On guar or xanthan gum: When making the dough for this bread in a bread machine, mix together the guar or xanthan gum and flour before adding them to the machine. If you just add the ingredients to the machine in the order listed, during the time before mixing begins, the water and gum can form lumps that routine mixing may not completely eliminate.

If you wish to use a non-programmable bread machine to mix this bread, use the method described in the first paragraph on the previous page. After the first rise, start the cycle again and re-mix the dough for a few minutes. Add the raisins and mix for a minute or two more until they are evenly distributed in the dough. Proceed with this recipe as in the fourth paragraph of these directions.

If you have a programmable bread machine, set the knead time to 20 minutes, the first rise(s) to the lowest time possible, last rise to 40 to 60[5] minutes, and bake to 50 minutes. Add the raisins 5 minutes before the end of the kneading time.

To make this bread with a mixer (which need not be a heavy-duty mixer), heat the water and apple juice concentrate to about 115°F. Beat the eggs slightly and add them to the other liquids. Stir together the dry ingredients in the large mixer bowl. With the mixer running at low speed, gradually add the liquid mixture and oil. Beat the dough for three minutes at medium speed. Scrape the dough from the beaters and the sides of the bowl into the bottom of the bowl. Oil the top of the dough and the sides of the bowl, and cover the bowl with a towel. Put the bowl in a warm (85°F to 90°F) place and let the dough rise for 1 to 1½ hours. Beat the dough again for three minutes at medium speed. Stir in the raisins by hand.

Oil and flour an 8 by 4 inch loaf pan. Put the dough in the pan and let it rise in a warm place for about 20 to 30 minutes or until it barely doubles. Preheat the oven to 375°F. Bake the loaf for about 50 to 70 minutes, loosely covering it with foil after the first 15 minutes to prevent excessive browning. Remove the loaf from the pan and cool it completely on a cooling rack. Makes one loaf.

Spelt Bread

When made with white spelt, this bread is so "normal" in taste and texture that guests may be surprised that they are not eating wheat. It can be made using the basic bread cycle of any bread machine that does not knead much too vigorously. Always use Purity Foods™ flour to make spelt yeast bread. See page 89 to read why.

    1 cup purified water
    ¼ cup apple juice concentrate, thawed
    1½ tablespoons oil
    1 teaspoon unrefined salt
    About 3¼ to 3¾ cups whole spelt flour or 4½ to 5¼ cups white spelt flour
    2¼ teaspoons (1 packet) active dry yeast

---

5 When making this bread the first time, begin with the lowest last rise time of 40 minutes. Then increase the time by five minutes each time you make the bread. If it over rises and falls, return to previous length of time and record that as the correct rising time for your conditions.

To make this recipe with a bread machine[6], add the ingredients to the pan in the order listed using the smaller amount of the flour. Chose the basic cycle and a loaf size of 1½ pounds for whole spelt bread or 2 pounds for white spelt bread. Start the machine. After a few minutes of mixing, look in the machine. If the dough is very soft, begin adding more flour about 2 tablespoons at a time until it reaches a consistency that is tacky but not sticky. After about 10 minutes of mixing, re-check the consistency of the dough and add flour if needed. It should be tacky but not sticky and be starting to become elastic and not too soft. Re-check the dough near the end of the kneading time, such as when the "add raisins" timer sounds, because it can soften with kneading and may need more flour. Then allow the rest of the cycle to run.

To make this recipe with a mixer, put one-half to two-thirds of the flour, the yeast, and the salt in the mixer bowl. Mix on low speed for about 30 seconds. Warm the liquid ingredients to 115 to 120°F. With the mixer running on low speed, add the liquids to the dry ingredients in a slow stream. Continue mixing until the dry and liquid ingredients are thoroughly mixed. If your mixer is not a heavy-duty mixer, at this point beat the dough for 5 to 10 minutes. You will be able to tell that the gluten is developing because the dough will begin to climb up the beaters. Then knead the rest of the flour in by hand, kneading for about 10 minutes, or until the dough is very smooth and elastic.

If your mixer is a heavy-duty mixer, after the liquids are thoroughly mixed in, with the mixer still running, begin adding the rest of the flour around the edges of the bowl ½ cup at a time. Mix well after each addition before adding more flour until the dough forms a ball and cleans the sides of the bowl. Knead the dough on the speed directed in your mixer manual for 5 to 10 minutes, or until the dough is very elastic and smooth. Turn the dough out onto a floured board and knead it briefly to check the consistency of the dough, kneading in a little more flour if necessary.

Put the dough into an oiled bowl and turn it once so that the top of the ball is also oiled. Cover it with a towel and let it rise in a warm (85°F to 90°F) place until it has doubled in volume, about 45 minutes to 1 hour.

While the dough is rising, prepare your baking pan. Spelt flour is different than any other flour in that it can be very difficult to remove the bread from the pan. To solve this problem, rub the inside of an 8 by 4 inch or 9 by 5 inch loaf pan with oil. Cut a piece of parchment or waxed paper the length of the pan and put it in the pan so the bottom and sides are covered with the paper. Oil the paper also.

When the dough has doubled in volume, punch it down and shape it into a loaf. Put the loaf into the prepared loaf pan. Let the dough rise until double again. Bake bread at 375°F for 45 minutes to an hour or until it is nicely browned. Check it midway through the baking time, and if it is already getting brown, cover it with a piece of foil to prevent

---

6 Note on spelt in bread machine recipes: Even if you use Purity Foods™ flour, spelt flour is more variable from batch to batch on how much it takes to make the right consistency of dough. In this recipe, you will probably have to check the dough several times throughout the kneading time and add more flour.

over-browning. At the end of the baking time, remove the loaf from the pan. You may need to run a knife along any parts of the ends of the pan that are not lined with paper in order to loosen the loaf. When the bread has been baked long enough it will sound hollow when tapped on the bottom with your knuckles. Cool it completely on a cooling rack before slicing it. If you can't wait to eat it, slice it carefully with a serrated knife. Makes one loaf or about 14 slices.

Buckwheat "Rye" Bread

The caraway seeds and rye flavor powder give this bread a delicious rye-like taste. If you do not like rye, this bread is also delicious without the rye flavor.

½ cup purified water
¼ cup apple juice concentrate
About 4 large or 3 extra large eggs[7], or enough to measure ¾ cup in volume,
    at room temperature
3 tablespoons oil
1¼ teaspoon unrefined salt
1 tablespoon caraway seed (optional)
¾ teaspoon rye flavor powder, to taste (optional - See "Sources," page 259).
1 tablespoon guar or xanthan gum[8]
2 cups buckwheat flour
1¼ cup tapioca starch
2¼ teaspoons (1 packet) active dry yeast

If you wish to use a non-programmable bread machine to mix this bread, use the method described in the first paragraph on page 154. After the first rise, re-start the cycle and re-mix the dough for a few minutes. Then proceed with this recipe as in the fourth paragraph of these directions.

If you have a programmable bread machine, set the knead to 25 minutes, first rise(s) to the lowest time possible, last rise to 25 to 35[9] minutes, and bake to 55 to 60 minutes.

---

7 If you are allergic to eggs, use ¾ cup warm purified water in their place. If you do not take the eggs out of the refrigerator early enough for them to come to room temperature before you are ready to bake, put them in a bowl of warm water for 5 or 10 minutes before using them in this recipe.

8 On guar or xanthan gum: When making the dough for this bread in a bread machine, mix together the guar or xanthan gum and flour before adding them to the machine. If you just add the ingredients to the machine in the order listed, during the time before mixing begins, the water and gum can form lumps that routine mixing may not completely eliminate.

9 When making this bread the first time, begin with the lowest last rise time of 25 minutes. Then increase the time by five minutes each time you make the bread. If it over rises and falls, return to previous length of time and record that as the correct rising time for your conditions.

To make this bread using a mixer, (which need not be a heavy-duty mixer) heat the purified water and apple juice concentrate to about 115°F. Beat the eggs slightly and add them to the other liquids. Stir together the dry ingredients in a large electric mixer bowl. With the mixer running at low speed, gradually add the liquid mixture and oil. Beat the dough for three minutes at medium speed. Scrape the dough from the beaters and the sides of the bowl into the bottom of the bowl. It will be very sticky. Oil the top of the dough and the sides of the bowl, and cover the bowl with a towel. Put the bowl in a warm (85°F to 90°F) place and let the dough rise for 1 to 1½ hours. Beat the dough again for three minutes at medium speed.

Oil and flour an 8 by 4 inch loaf pan. Put the dough in the pan and let it rise in a warm place for about 20 to 35 minutes, or until it barely doubles. Preheat the oven to 375°F. Bake the loaf for about 50 to 65 minutes, loosely covering it with foil after the first 30 to 45 minutes if it is getting excessively brown. Remove the loaf from the pan and cool it completely on a cooling rack. Makes one loaf.

Bread Machine 100% Stone Ground Whole Wheat Bread

This whole wheat bread is delicious and nearly effortless to make with almost any bread machine. However, due to its high fiber content, the middle of the loaf may fall a little. If you are fussy about how the loaf looks, try the recipe for oven-baked bread on the next page.

> 1⅛ cups warm purified water
> 1 tablespoon agave or Fruit Sweet™
> 1½ tablespoons oil or 1 tablespoon oil plus ½ tablespoon lecithin
> 1 teaspoon unrefined salt
> 3 cups stone ground whole wheat flour such as Guisto's™ or Bob's Red Mill™ brand
> 3 tablespoons vital gluten such as Bob's Red Mill™ brand
> 2¼ teaspoons (1 packet) active dry yeast

Stir the gluten into part of the flour. Then add the ingredients to the pan in the order listed in your bread machine's instruction manual. (For most machines this will be the order given above). Chose a loaf size of 1½ pounds and start the basic cycle or a quick wheat cycle if your machine has one. (Do not use a "regular" non-quick whole wheat cycle with a long rising time. A programmable cycle is given below to use if you have a Zojirushi machine). Start the machine.

After 5 to 10 minutes of mixing, touch the dough. If it is sticky, add one tablespoon of flour. After a few more minutes of mixing, re-check the consistency of the dough; if it is still sticky, add another tablespoon of flour. If it is just tacky, you have added enough flour. If you live in a humid climate and your flour absorbs moisture from the air, you may need to add a total of one to four additional tablespoons of flour to the dough to achieve the right consistency – tacky but not sticky. In a dry climate during a dry season, you may need to add one to three teaspoons of water, one at a time, to make the dough supple.

Let the cycle run to completion. Remove the bread from the machine and let the loaf completely cool on a wire rack before slicing it. Makes one 1½ pound loaf, or about 14 slices.

Note on the cycle to use with this bread recipe: Because this bread has a high fiber content, it may fall a little. If this happens with the first cycle you try on your bread machine, the next time you make this bread, change to another cycle that has a shorter last rise time. Another option is if you have a programmable machine, try using a cycle similar to this: Knead – 20 minutes; Rise 1 and 2 – Off; Rise 3 (or the last rise) – 30 minutes; Bake – 60 minutes. Be prepared to tweak this cycle to fit your machine and baking conditions such as climate and elevation. If the loaf over-rises and falls, decrease the time of the last rise. If the loaf is dense, increase the last rise progressively – such as 5 minutes each time you make the bread – until it falls a little in the middle of the loaf. Then decrease it to the previous setting. Another possible help with the problem of over-rising and then falling is to add an extra ½ tablespoon of gluten. Experiment with the various cycles on your machine, especially any that have a short (30 minute or less) last rise. The whole wheat cycle on most machines includes a lot of rising time, which is the opposite of the shorter rise needed when your bread over-rises and falls. The basic cycle for white bread is more likely to work well.

Oven-Baked 100% Stone Ground Whole Wheat Bread

My husband likes his bread tall and with a perfectly domed top because if the bread isn't tall enough, he ends up with a skimpy sandwich. Since I could not always get the perfect shape and height in a bread machine, I used this recipe until we discovered his favorite low-GI bread, "San Francisco Sourdough." See the recipe on page 164.

> 1⅛ cups warm purified water
> 1 tablespoon agave or Fruit Sweet™
> 1½ tablespoons oil or 1 tablespoon oil plus ½ tablespoon lecithin
> 1 teaspoon unrefined salt
> 3 cups stone ground whole wheat flour such as Guisto's™ or Bob's Red Mill™ brand
> 3 tablespoons vital gluten such as Bob's Red Mill™ brand
> 2¼ teaspoons (1 packet) active dry yeast

Stir the gluten into part of the flour. Then prepare this dough by the mixer method as described in the second and third paragraphs of the spelt bread recipe on pages 156 or with the dough cycle of a bread machine. When using a bread machine, add the ingredients to the pan in the order listed in your bread machine's instruction manual. (For most machines this will be the order given above). Start the dough cycle. After 5 to 10 minutes of vigorous mixing, touch the dough. If it is sticky, add one tablespoon of flour. After a few more minutes of mixing, re-check the consistency of the dough. If it is still sticky, add another 1 tablespoon of flour. If it is just tacky, you have added enough flour. If you live in a humid climate and your flour absorbs moisture from the air, you may need to add a total of one to three additional tablespoons of flour to the dough to achieve the right consistency – tacky but not sticky. In a dry climate during a dry season, you may need to add one to three teaspoons of water (one at a time) to make the dough supple. Allow the dough cycle to run to completion.

While the cycle is running or your mixer-made dough is rising, oil an 8 by 4-inch loaf pan. Line it with waxed or parchment paper and oil the paper. When the cycle is finished or the mixer-made dough has doubled in size, remove the dough from the machine or rising place, knead it, and form it into a loaf. Place it in the prepared pan. Let it rise in a cozy spot for 30 to 45 minutes or until it is a little more than doubled.* Preheat oven to 350°F. Put the loaf in the oven and bake it for 45 minutes, covering after the first 30 minutes with foil to prevent excessive browning. Remove the loaf from the pan. When the loaf has been baked long enough it will sound hollow when tapped on the bottom with your knuckles. After it has cooled for a few minutes, peel the wax or parchment paper from the loaf and let the loaf completely cool on a wire rack before slicing it. Makes one 1½ pound loaf, or about 14 slices.

Note on the second rise: When I let this loaf rise in the bread pan, my goal is to produce the tallest loaf I can without letting it rise for so long that it will fall. For my pans, I let the loaf rise until it is about ¾ inch above the top of the pan; the time that this takes varies. This is probably nearly triple the volume of the original tightly wrapped, totally deflated roll of dough I put in the pan. You may want to experiment to see how much you can let your loaf rise before it falls in the oven.

SOURDOUGH BREAD

Sourdough is yeast bread that is leavened by a sourdough starter or culture. Traditional cultures contain wild yeast, which produces gas and causes the bread to rise, and bacteria of the genus *Lactobacillus* which give the bread a sour flavor. There are many different sourdough cultures, each with a special flavor of its own and unique rising characteristics.

The use of traditional sourdough cultures may be too time-consuming for many with major health problems. However, some people who are allergic to commercial baker's yeast and the bread made with it seem to tolerate sourdough bread. Sourdough bread is not yeast-free; perhaps these people are not allergic to the wild yeast but are allergic to baker's yeast much as one may be allergic to lettuce but not to endive. If you are allergic to yeast, you may want to ask your doctor about trying sourdough bread. See *Easy Breadmaking for Special Diets*, 3rd Edition, if you wish to bake with traditional sourdough cultures. For more about *Easy Breadmaking* see the last pages of this book.

Another dietary reason to make sourdough bread is because it has a lower glycemic index (GI) score than bread made with the same grain but leavened with yeast only. The acid produced in bread by *lactobacilli* decreases the bread's impact on blood sugar and insulin levels and thus makes sourdough bread good for cancer patients and for the glycemic control weight loss program on pages 27 to 30 of this book.

A final reason to make your own sourdough bread is for the flavor of the bread itself. If you have eaten at Fisherman's Wharf in San Francisco and are a fan of the sourdough bread there, you may consider the time spent making sourdough worthwhile (especially if the process is made easier by using a freeze-dried starter) when you taste how delicious really fresh sourdough bread can be.

MAKING BREAD WITH A FREEZE-DRIED SOURDOUGH STARTER

In the last several years, new products have become available which enable us to make sourdough bread easily and without keeping and maintaining a traditional sourdough starter. The most work-saving of these products is the Florapan™ freeze-dried sourdough starter which is called French-style sourdough starter in the King Arthur Flour Baker's Catalogue. In addition, bread machines have become more sophisticated than in the past, and with the programmable Zojirushi™ machines we can make this next generation sourdough bread totally in the machine. Both the bread machine (Zojirushi™ Home Bakery Supreme, model BBCEC20) and sourdough starter are available from King Arthur Flour™. See "Sources," page 262.

The Florapan™ freeze-dried starter makes assertively sour bread which my husband says is "just like real San Francisco sourdough." This starter is gluten-free and wheat-free (but may contain traces of beef) so it makes truly wheat and gluten-free sourdough bread. Unlike breads made with traditional starters, bread made with this starter rises predictably from batch to batch, which allows us to use a programmable bread machine for the whole sourdough process.

The **procedure for making sourdough bread using a freeze-dried starter** is as follows: the morning or early afternoon of the day before you plan to serve sourdough bread for dinner, mix the ingredients above the line in the recipe you are using – usually flour, purified (chlorine-free) water and the Florapan™ starter – using a wooden or plastic spoon in a glass or ceramic mixing bowl or using a bread machine's dough cycle or this programmable cycle:

Knead 1 – 10 minutes; Rise 1 – 23½ hours, Rise 2 and 3 – off, Bake – off.
Allow this sponge to rise in a cozy spot (70° to 85° F) or in the machine on the programmed cycle above for 18 to 20 hours.

The next morning, add the ingredients listed below the line in the recipe you are using. If you are making **wheat containing bread**, allow the dough to mix in the machine, assisting with a narrow spatula, for just a minute or two until a shaggy mass forms. Then turn off the machine. If you are making this by hand, mix briefly to just make a shaggy mass of dough. Allow the dough to rest for 20 to 30 minutes. This part of the process is called autolyse and enables the gluten in the flour to absorb water before you start kneading. If you are making bread which does not contain a gluten-containing flour such as wheat, rye or spelt, a rest at this point is not needed. Proceed as in the second paragraph on the next page.

If you are using a programmable bread machine and wish to bake your wheat or spelt bread in the machine, after the autolyse, start the second day cycle given in the recipe you are using. If the bread is less than totally perfect, the next time you make this you may adjust rising and baking times slightly (start with 5 minute changes) for your baking conditions. If the dough over-rises and falls, decrease the rising time; if it is too dense, increase the rising time; if it over browns, decrease the baking time. When you achieve the best loaf possible, record the times you used for future use.

If you would like a **traditional crisp, cracking sourdough crust** on your wheat or spelt bread, do not bake the bread in a bread machine. Use the dough cycle or the programmable cycle above to knead the bread after the autolyse, or knead it by hand to produce elastic but not sticky dough. To make spelt bread, after the kneading is finished, hand-shape the dough into a loaf and put it into a loaf pan that has been oiled and floured. Let it rise and bake it as described below and on the next page.

To make wheat bread, allow the dough to rise for about 3 hours in a warm place or in the machine on the programmable cycle above. Deflate the dough at hourly intervals during this time. Then gently divide the dough, form it into a ball or balls and place it on a lightly oiled surface. Oil the top of the ball(s) and cover them with plastic wrap and a towel. Let them rest for 20 to 30 minutes. Oil and flour a loaf pan or baking sheet. Gently, without deflating them too much, form the ball(s) into the desired shapes – either a roll to go in a loaf pan or two round or long loaves to be baked on a baking sheet. Put the dough on the baking sheet or in the loaf pan.

Allow both wheat and spelt loaves to rise in a warm place for 3 to 5 hours or until they are doubled (or for wheat more than doubled, depending on how light and holey you prefer your bread). Near the end of the rising time, put a small broiler pan and a baking stone (if you have one) in the oven and preheat the oven to 375°F for 20 to 30 minutes. (I place the broiler pan on the bottom rack underneath and on the opposite side of where I will put the baking stone and bread). Slash the top of the loaf with a sharp serrated knife or lamé. Put the bread in the oven. Pour a cup of boiling water into the broiler pan. Bake until it is golden brown and sounds hollow when tapped on the bottom. If the top is getting too brown before the bottom browns, cover the loaf with foil part way through baking. Remove it from the pan and cool it on a cooling rack before cutting it.

If you are making **gluten-containing wheat-free breads** such as rye and spelt **without a programmable machine**, on the second day, add the ingredients below the line in the recipe to the starter mixture that has been incubating overnight. Knead the dough, adding enough flour to make supple but not sticky dough. Oil a loaf pan; for spelt bread also line the pan with parchment paper. Place the dough in the prepared pan and let it rise in a cozy place for two to three hours until doubled. Then bake it in a preheated 375°F oven. If the top is getting too brown before the bottom browns, cover the loaf with foil part way through baking. Remove it from the pan and cool it on a cooling rack before cutting it.

For gluten-free breads, on the second day, add the ingredients below the line in the recipe to the bread machine pan. Start the programmable cycle given in the recipe for the second day. No resting time for an autolyse is needed because there is no gluten. Use a narrow spatula to assist the kneading process and spread the dough evenly in the pan at the end of the kneading time. You will see fibrous strands of guar or xanthan gum developing in the thick batter as the kneading progresses.

To make gluten-free sourdough bread without a bread machine, on the second day, add the ingredients below the line in the recipe. Mix the ingredients with an electric mixer to "develop" the guar or xanthan gum. Let the dough rise in a warm place for about an hour. Oil and flour a loaf pan. Gently scrape the dough into the prepared pan. Let it rise in a warm place until it is just doubled or barely doubled. Preheat your oven to 375°F and bake the loaf until it is brown on the bottom. If the top is browning quickly, cover it with foil part way through the baking time to give the bottom of the loaf time to brown without burning the top of the loaf. Remove it from the pan and cool it on a cooling rack before cutting it.

"San Francisco" Sourdough Bread

Ingredients:	2 hand-shaped loaves	1 bread machine loaf
King Arthur™ bread flour	1¼ cups	1¼ cups
King Arthur™ white whole wheat or whole wheat flour	¼ cup	¼ cup
Unbuffered vitamin C crystals (divided, reserve about ⅔ of this to add on day 2)	⅛ teaspoon	⅛ teaspoon
Fermapan™ starter	⅛ teaspoon	⅛ teaspoon
Purified water, 85°F	¾ cup	¾ cup
Additional bread flour	2 to 2¾ cups	2 to 2½ cups
Unrefined sea salt	1¼ teaspoons	1¼ teaspoons
Vitamin C reserved from above	Reserved amount	Reserved amount
SAF™ instant yeast	⅜ teaspoon	⅜ teaspoon
Purified water, 85°F	⅝ cup	½ cup plus 1 tbsp.

Cycle for day 1 and for hand shaped loaves on day 2: Dough cycle or this programmable cycle: Knead 1 – 10 minutes; Rise 1 – 23½ hours, Rise 2 and 3 – off, Bake – off.

Cycle for day 2 for bread machine baked loaf: Knead 1 – 10 minutes, Rise 1 – 3½ hours, Rise 2 and 3 – off, Bake – 1 hour, 10 minutes.

In the morning or early afternoon of the day before you want to serve this bread, follow the procedure on page 161 for making the sponge from the ingredients above the line in the ingredient list. Let it rise in the bread machine or in a cozy place (70° to 85°F) for 18 to 20 hours overnight.

The next morning, follow the procedure on page 162 for adding the ingredients below the line and making the dough. After mixing the dough briefly to form a shaggy mass, let it rest (autolyse) for 20 to 30 minutes. Then start the day 2 cycle above for a bread machine-baked loaf. For oven-baked bread with a crisp crust, knead the dough (in the machine or by hand) and continue the process on page 162. After the dough has risen 3 hours, hand shape the dough into two free-form loaves on a oiled baking sheet or one sandwich loaf in an oiled loaf pan. Let the bread rise in a cozy place for an additional 3½ to 4½ hours or until doubled. Prepare your oven as on page 162 and preheat it to 450°F for 20 to 30 minutes. Slash the loaves and bake the hand-shaped loaves for 35 minutes, or the sandwich loaf for 50 minutes. Cover the loaves with foil after the first 20 minutes of baking.

Whole Wheat Sourdough Bread

Ingredients:	2 hand-shaped loaves	1 bread machine loaf
Whole wheat bread flour such	1 cup	¾ cup
as Guisto's™ high protein stone ground whole wheat flour		
King Arthur™ bread flour	1 cup	1 cup
Unbuffered vitamin C crystals	⅛ teaspoon	⅛ teaspoon
(divided, reserve about ⅔ of this to add on day 2)		
Fermapan™ starter	¼ teaspoon	$3/_{16}$ teaspoon
Purified water, 85°F	1¼ cups	1¼ cups
Additional whole wheat flour	1 cup	1¼ cups
Additional bread flour	1⅝ cups	1½ cups
Unrefined sea salt	1½ teaspoons	1¼ teaspoons
Vitamin C reserved from above	Reserved amount	Reserved amount
SAF™ instant yeast	½ teaspoon	⅜ teaspoon
Purified water, 85°F	½ cup	½ cup

Cycle for day 1 and for hand shaped loaves on day 2: Dough cycle or this programmable cycle: Knead 1 – 10 minutes; Rise 1 – 23½ hours, Rise 2 and 3 – off, Bake – off.

Cycle for day 2 for bread machine baked loaf: Knead 1 – 10 minutes, Rise 1 – 4½ hours, Rise 2 and 3 – off, Bake – 1 hour, 10 minutes.

    In the morning or early afternoon of the day before you want to serve this bread, follow the procedure on page 161 for making the sponge from the ingredients above the line in the ingredient list. Let it rise in the bread machine or in a cozy place (70° to 85° F) for 18 to 20 hours overnight.

    The next morning, follow the procedure on page 162 for adding the remaining ingredients and making the dough. After mixing the dough briefly to form a shaggy mass, allow it to rest for 20 to 30 minutes. Then start the day 2 cycle above for a bread machine-baked loaf. For oven-baked bread, knead the dough (in the machine or by hand) and continue the process on page 162. Allow the dough to rise for 2 to 3 hours. Oil and flour a baking sheet or loaf pan. After the dough has risen 2 to 3 hours. Hand shape the dough into two free-form loaves and place them on the baking sheet or put all of the dough in a loaf pan. Let the bread rise for additional 3½ to 4½ hours or until doubled. Prepare your oven as on page 162; preheat it to 450°F for 20 to 30 minutes. Slash the loaves. Bake the hand-shaped loaves 35 minutes, the sandwich loaf 50 minutes.

Whole Spelt Sourdough Bread

Ingredients: **1 hand-shaped or bread machine loaf**

Whole spelt flour	2½ cups
Unbuffered vitamin C crystals	Generous ⅛ teaspoon
(divided, reserve about ⅔ of this to add on day 2)	
Fermapan™ starter	¼ teaspoon
Purified water at 85° F to 90°F	1½ cups
Additional whole spelt flour	3¾ cups + more after autolyse
Unrefined sea salt	2 teaspoons
Vitamin C reserved from above	Reserved amount
SAF™ instant yeast	¾ teaspoon
Purified water at 85° F to 90°F	1¼ cups

Cycle for day 1: Dough cycle or this programmable cycle: Knead 1 – 10 minutes; Rise 1 – 23½ hours, Rise 2 and 3 – off, Bake – off.

Cycle for day 2 for bread machine baked loaf: Knead 1 – 10 minutes (Spread the dough evenly in the pan at the end of the kneading time), Rise 1 – 3 hours, Rise 2 and 3 – off, Bake – 1 hour.

In the morning or early afternoon of the day before you want to serve this bread, follow the procedure on page 161 for making the sponge from the ingredients above the line in the ingredient list. Let it rise in the bread machine or in a cozy place (70° to 85° F) for 18 to 20 hours overnight.

The next morning, follow the procedure on page 162 for adding the ingredients below the line (start with the smaller amount of flour) and making the dough. After mixing the dough briefly to form a shaggy mass, let it rest (autolyse) for 20 to 30 minutes. Then start the day 2 cycle above for a bread machine- baked loaf, or knead the dough in the machine or by hand for 10 minutes. **Add more flour as needed (½ cup or more) to make a firm dough.** For oven baked bread, oil and flour a loaf pan with spelt flour and, for sticking problems, also line the pan with parchment paper. After kneading, shape the dough into a roll and put it in the prepared pan. Let the bread rise for 3 to 3 ½ hours until just doubled. Place a baking stone (if you have one) and a small broiler pan in the oven. Preheat your oven to 450°F for 20 to 30 minutes. Slash the loaf. Pour 1 cup of boiling water in to the boiler pan. Bake for 40 minutes, covering the top of the loaf with foil after the first 20 minutes. Cool the bread completely on a wire rack before slicing.

White Spelt Sourdough Bread

Ingredients: **1 hand-shaped or bread machine loaf**

White spelt flour	2¼ cups
Unbuffered vitamin C crystals	Generous ⅛ teaspoon
(divided, reserve about ⅔ of this to add on day 2)	
Fermapan™ starter	¼ teaspoon
Purified water at 85° F to 90°F	1 cup
Additional white spelt flour	3¾ cups + more after autolyse
Unrefined sea salt	1½ teaspoons
Vitamin C reserved from above	Reserved amount
SAF™ instant yeast	¼ teaspoon
Purified water at 85° F to 90°F	¾ cup

Cycle for day 1: Dough cycle or this programmable cycle: Knead 1 – 10 minutes; Rise 1 – 23½ hours, Rise 2 and 3 – off, Bake – off.

Cycle for day 2 for bread machine baked loaf: Knead 1 – 10 minutes (Spread the dough evenly in the pan after kneading), Rise 1 – 4 hours, Rise 2 and 3 – off, Bake – 1 hour 10 minutes.

In the morning or early afternoon of the day before you want to serve this bread, follow the procedure on page 161 for making the sponge from the ingredients above the line in the ingredient list. Let it rise in the bread machine or in a cozy place (70° to 85° F) for 18 to 20 hours overnight.

The next morning, follow the procedure on page 162 for adding the ingredients below the line and making the dough. After mixing the dough briefly to form a shaggy mass, allow it to rest (autolyse) for 20 to 30 minutes. Then start the day 2 cycle above for a bread machine-baked loaf, or knead the dough in the machine or by hand for 10 minutes. **Add more flour as needed (½ cup or more) to make a firm dough.** For oven baked bread, oil and flour a loaf pan with spelt flour and, for sticking problems, also line the pan with parchment paper. After kneading, shape the dough into a roll and put it in the prepared pan. Let the bread rise for about 4 hours until just doubled. Place a baking stone (if you have one) and a small broiler pan in the oven. Preheat your oven to 450°F for 20 to 30 minutes. Slash the loaf. Pour 1 cup of boiling water in to the boiler pan. Bake for 40 minutes, covering the top of the loaf with foil after the first 20 minutes. Cool the bread completely on a wire rack before slicing.

Volkorn 100% Rye Sourdough Bread

Ingredients: **1 hand-shaped or bread machine loaf**

Rye flour such as King Arthur™ medium rye (See "Sources," page 260).	2 cups
Fermapan™ starter	$3/16$ teaspoon
Purified water at 85° F to 90°F	¼ cup
Additional rye flour	2½ cups
Unrefined sea salt	2¼ teaspoons
Caraway seed (optional)	1 to 1½ tablespoons
SAF™ instant yeast	¾ teaspoon
Purified water at 85° F to 90°F	½ cup + 1 tablespoon

Cycle for day 1: Dough cycle or this programmable cycle: Knead 1 – 10 minutes; Rise 1 – 23½ hours, Rise 2 and 3 – off, Bake – off.

Cycle for day 2 for bread machine baked loaf: Knead 1 – 10 minutes (Spread the dough evenly in the pan after kneading), Rise 1 – 4 hours, Rise 2 and 3 – off, Bake – 1 hour 10 minutes.

In the morning or early afternoon of the day before you want to serve this bread, follow the procedure on page 161 for making the sponge from the ingredients above the line in the ingredient list. Let it rise in the bread machine or in a cozy place (70° to 85° F) for 18 to 20 hours overnight.

The next morning, follow the procedure on page 162 for adding the ingredients below the line and making the dough. After mixing the dough briefly to form a shaggy mass, allow it to rest (autolyse) for 20 to 30 minutes. Then start the day 2 cycle above for a bread machine-baked loaf. For oven-baked bread, knead the dough in the machine or by hand for 10 minutes. The dough will be sticky. Let it rise in a cozy place for 2 hours. Oil and flour a loaf pan with rye flour. Scrape the dough into the pan without deflating it too much, and let it rise for another 2 to 3 hours until doubled. Place a baking stone (if you have one) and a small broiler pan in the oven. Preheat your oven to 375°F for 20 to 30 minutes. Pour 1 cup of boiling water in to the boiler pan. Bake for 1 hour, covering the top of the loaf with foil after the first 20 minutes if needed. Cool the bread completely on a wire rack before slicing.

Light Rye Sourdough Bread

Ingredients: **2 hand-shaped or 1 bread machine loaf**

Whole rye flour such as King Arthur™ medium rye (See "Sources," page 260).	1 cup
Fermapan™ starter	¼ teaspoon
Purified water at 85° F to 90°F	1 cup
Bread flour, preferably King Arthur™ flour	2⅞ to 3⅛ cups
Unrefined sea salt	1 teaspoon
Caraway seed (optional)	1 tablespoon
SAF™ instant yeast	½ teaspoon
Apple juice concentrate, thawed and warmed	⅛ cup
Purified water at 85° F to 90°F	⅜ cup

Cycle for day 1: Dough cycle or this programmable cycle: Knead 1 – 10 minutes; Rise 1 – 23½ hours, Rise 2 and 3 – off, Bake – off.

Cycle for day 2 for bread machine baked loaf: Knead 1 – 10 minutes (Spread the dough evenly in the pan after kneading), Rise 1 – 4 hours, Rise 2 and 3 – off, Bake – 1 hour 10 minutes.

In the morning or early afternoon of the day before you want to serve this bread, follow the procedure on page 161 for making the sponge from the ingredients above the line in the ingredient list. Let it rise in the bread machine or in a cozy place (70° to 85° F) for 18 to 20 hours overnight.

The next morning, follow the procedure on page 162 for adding the ingredients below the line and making the dough. After mixing the dough briefly to form a shaggy mass, allow it to rest (autolyse) for 20 to 30 minutes. Then start the day 2 cycle above for a bread machine-baked loaf. For oven-baked bread, knead the dough in the machine or by hand for 10 minutes. Let it rise in a cozy place for 2 hours. Divide the dough into two balls and let it rest for 30 minutes. Oil and flour a baking sheet. Shape two loaves, put them on the baking sheet and let them rise for about 3 hours until doubled. Place a baking stone (if you have one) and a small broiler pan in the oven. Preheat your oven to 450°F for 20 to 30 minutes. Pour 1 cup of boiling water in to the boiler pan. Bake for 35 to 45 minutes, covering the top of the loaf with foil after the first 20 minutes if needed. Cool the bread before slicing.

Buckwheat Sourdough Bread

Ingredients: **1 hand-shaped or bread machine loaf**

Buckwheat flour	1½ cups
Fermapan™ starter	⅛ teaspoon
Purified water at 85° F to 90°F	¾ to ⅞ cup[10]
Additional buckwheat flour	½ cup
Tapioca starch/flour	1⅜ cups
Guar or xanthan gum	1 tablespoon
Unrefined sea salt	1¼ teaspoons
Caraway seeds (optional)	1 tablespoon
Oil	3 tablespoons
SAF™ instant yeast	½ teaspoon
Combined liquids: 3 eggs at room temperature +	¾ cup total volume
1 tablespoon apple juice concentrate + purified water at 85° F to 90°F	

Cycle for day 1: Dough cycle or this programmable cycle: Knead 1 – 10 minutes; Rise 1 – 23½ hours, Rise 2 and 3 – off, Bake – off.

Cycle for day 2 for bread machine baked loaf: Knead 1 – 10 minutes (Spread the dough evenly in the pan after kneading), Rise 1 – 2 hours, 30 minutes, Rise 2 and 3 – off, Bake – 1 hour.

In the morning or early afternoon of the day before you want to serve this bread, follow the procedure on page 161 for making the sponge from the ingredients above the line in the ingredient list. Let it rise in the bread machine or in a cozy place (70° to 85° F) for 18 to 20 hours overnight.

The next morning, mix the guar or xanthan gum into some of the flour. Then follow the procedure on page 162 for adding the ingredients below the line and making the dough. Use the day 2 cycle above for a bread machine-baked loaf. For oven-baked bread, mix the dough using the dough cycle of the bread machine or with a mixer for 10 minutes to develop the guar or xanthan gum fibers. Oil and flour a loaf pan with buckwheat flour. Scrape the dough into the pan and let it rise for about 2½ hours until barely doubled. Place a baking stone (if you have one) in the oven. Preheat your oven to 375°F for 20 minutes. Bake the bread on the stone for 50 to 65 minutes, covering the top of the loaf with foil after the first 30 minutes if needed. Cool the bread completely on a wire rack before slicing.

---

10 When making the sponge on the first day, initially use the smaller amount of water. If it is not the consistency of a thick batter after a few minutes of mixing, add the additional ⅛ cup of water or slightly more. The extra water may be needed due to variation in the buckwheat flour.

Rice Sourdough Bread

Ingredients: **1 hand-shaped or bread machine loaf**

Brown rice flour	3 cups
Fermapan™ starter	¼ teaspoon
Purified water at 85° F to 90°F	1½ cups
Additional brown rice flour	2 cups
Tapioca starch/flour	1 cup
Guar or xanthan gum	2 tablespoons + 2 teaspoons
Unrefined sea salt	2 teaspoons
SAF™ instant yeast	½ teaspoon
Combined liquids: 4 large eggs at room temperature + purified water at 85° F to 90°F (about ⅝ cup water)	1½ cups total volume

Cycle for day 1: Dough cycle or this programmable cycle: Knead 1 – 10 minutes; Rise 1 – 23½ hours, Rise 2 and 3 – off, Bake – off.

Cycle for day 2 for bread machine baked loaf: Knead 1 – 10 minutes (Spread dough evenly in the pan after kneading), Rise 1 – 2½ to 3 hours, Rise 2 and 3 – off, Bake – 1 hour, 10 minutes.

In the morning or early afternoon of the day before you want to serve this bread, follow the procedure on page 161 for making the sponge from the ingredients above the line in the ingredient list. Let it rise in the bread machine or in a cozy place (70° to 85° F) for 18 to 20 hours overnight.

The next morning, mix the guar or xanthan gum into some of the flour. Then follow the procedure on page 162 for adding the ingredients below the line and making the dough. Use the day 2 cycle above for a bread machine-baked loaf. For oven-baked bread, mix the dough using the dough cycle of the bread machine or with a mixer for 10 minutes to develop the guar or xanthan gum fibers. Oil and flour a loaf pan with rice flour. Scrape the dough into the pan and let it rise for about 2½ hours until barely doubled. Place a baking stone (if you have one) in the oven. Preheat your oven to 375°F for 20 minutes. Bake the bread on the stone for about 1 hour, covering the top of the loaf with foil after the first 30 minutes, if needed. Cool the bread completely on a wire rack before slicing.

Quinoa Sourdough Bread

Ingredients: **1 hand-shaped or bread machine loaf**

Quinoa flour	1 cup
Unbuffered vitamin C crystals	⅛ teaspoon
(divided, reserve about ⅔ of this to add on day 2)	
Fermapan™ starter	⅛ teaspoon
Purified water at 85° F to 90°F	½ cup
Additional quinoa flour	2⅛ cups
Tapioca starch/flour	1 cup
Vitamin C reserved from above	Reserved amount
Guar or xanthan gum	1 tablespoon + 1 teaspoon
Unrefined sea salt	¾ teaspoon
SAF™ instant yeast	¾ teaspoon
Combined liquids: 4 eggs at room temperature	1¼ cups total volume
+ 1 tablespoon apple juice concentrate + purified water at 85° F to 90°F	

Cycle for day 1: Dough cycle or this programmable cycle: Knead 1 – 10 minutes; Rise 1 – 23½ hours, Rise 2 and 3 – off, Bake – off.

Cycle for day 2 for bread machine baked loaf: Knead 1 – 10 minutes (Spread the dough evenly in the pan after kneading), Rise 1 – 2 hours, 30 minutes, Rise 2 and 3 – off, Bake – 1 hour.

In the morning or early afternoon of the day before you want to serve this bread, follow the procedure on page 161 for making the sponge from the ingredients above the line in the ingredient list. Let it rise in the bread machine or in a cozy place (70° to 85° F) for 18 to 20 hours overnight.

The next morning, mix the guar or xanthan gum into some of the flour. Then follow the procedure on page 162 for adding the ingredients below the line and making the dough. Use the day 2 cycle above for a bread machine-baked loaf. For oven-baked bread, mix the dough using the dough cycle of the bread machine or with a mixer for 10 minutes to develop the guar or xanthan gum fibers. Oil and flour a loaf pan with quinoa flour. Scrape the dough into the pan and let it rise for about 2½ hours until barely doubled. Place a baking stone (if you have one) in the oven. Preheat your oven to 375°F for 20 minutes. Bake the bread on the stone for about 1 hour, covering the top of the loaf with foil after the first 30 minutes if needed. Cool the bread completely on a wire rack before slicing.

For more recipes for cooked grains and breads see *Nourishing Traditions,* pages 452 to 494.[11] For more allergy non-yeast bread recipes see *The Ultimate Food Allergy Cookbook and Survival Guide,* pages 150 to 179. See allergy and gluten-free yeast bread recipes on pages 180 to 220 of *The Ultimate Food Allergy Cookbook and Survival Guide,* which is described on the last pages of this book.[12]

For more special-diet yeast bread or sourdough bread recipes made by hand, mixer, or bread machine see *Easy Breadmaking for Special Diets, 3rd Edition* as described on the last pages of his book.[13]

To purchase bread, English muffins, pocket bread, cereal and other grain products made from sprouted grains, including gluten-free grains, see "Sources," page 252 to 253.

11 Fallon, Sally with Mary Enig, PhD. *Nourishing Traditions.*, (Brandywine, MD, NewTrends Publishing, 2001), 452-594.

12 Dumke, Nicolette. *The Ultimate Food Allergy Cookbook and Survival Guide.* (Louisville, CO, Allergy Adapt Inc., 2006) 150-220.

13 Dumke, Nicolette. *Easy Breadmaking for Special Diets, 3rd Edition.* (Louisville, CO, Allergy Adapt Inc., 2012).

Legumes

Legumes not only are delicious but are very nutritious additions to our diet. Since they are high in protein, they may be used in place of meat in vegetarian and money-saving meals. Because the protein in legumes is not "complete" (does not contain all of the amino acids we are unable to synthesize), they should be eaten with grains or alternative grains. The beans compensate for the amino acid deficit in the grains and vice versa so that a complete complement of amino acids is consumed.

Legumes also contain B vitamins, minerals including iron, zinc, calcium and magnesium, and plenty of fiber. The fiber promotes both satiety and good digestion.

A common reason for avoiding eating legumes is "gas." This problem is due to carbohydrates in legumes which we cannot digest and absorb but our intestinal bacteria can digest, thus producing gas in the process. This problem can be reduced by soaking the beans at least overnight and rinsing them in three changes of water in the morning before cooking them. In addition, consuming beans in small quantities and gradually increasing the quantity will increase our digestive systems' ability to handle larger quantities of beans.

Dried beans must be soaked before cooking to rehydrate them and to neutralize the phytates and enzyme inhibitors they contain. In the recipes in *Nourishing Traditions*, Sally Fallon recommends soaking some legumes with an acidic ingredient such as vinegar or whey. True confessions: I do not use an acidic ingredient to soak beans. Because vinegar and whey are allergenic, I tried soaking beans in water containing unbuffered vitamin C. When cooked, the beans took forever to begin to soften and never softened sufficiently. I then tried vitamin C in the soaking water for lentils which some cooking experts say do not need to be soaked for rehydration because they are small and thin-skinned. (However, all legumes should be soaked to remove indigestible carbohydrates and neutralize phytic acid and enzyme inhibitors). The lentils did not soften when cooked all day and overnight that night in a crockpot. I learned that, at least for vitamin C, the advice which applies to cooking legumes also applies to soaking them. That advice is not to add salt or acidic ingredients to legumes until after they have cooked long enough to soften as much as you prefer.

Crockpot cooking is well suited for dry legumes. Using a crockpot to cook dry beans makes it possible for cancer patients and individuals with limited time or low energy to avoid chemicals from plastic linings in cans of beans by cooking their beans from scratch without the effort of tending the pot. While a crockpot saves the work of tending a pan while cooking a large batch of beans, an additional benefit is leftovers to freeze for future use. See the recipe for crockpot cooked legumes on page 176.

Beans may be combined with vegetables in the crockpot to produce delicious soups for hearty and economical meals. I sometimes peel and cut the vegetables the evening before I plan to serve soup. The next morning, I rinse the beans, add the other vegetables to the crock pot, and the soup can cook all day while I am away. I hope you will enjoy the bean soup recipes at the end of this chapter.

Stovetop Cooked Legumes

LENTILS OR SPLIT PEAS
    1 cup of dry lentils or split peas
    2 cups purified water
    ¼ teaspoon unrefined salt

ADZUKI, BLACK, SOY, OR GREAT NORTHERN BEANS
    1 cup of dry beans
    3 cups purified water
    ¼ teaspoon unrefined salt

ANASAZI, CRANBERRY, CANNELLINI, GARBANZO, KIDNEY, LIMA, NAVY, PINTO, OR RED BEANS OR BLACK-EYED PEAS
    1 cup of dry beans
    4 cups purified water
    ¼ teaspoon unrefined salt

Choose one set of ingredients above. Wash the dry legumes by placing them in a strainer and running water through them. Check the water that is coming out of the bottom of the strainer for dirt and continue rinsing until all traces of dirt are gone. Discard any shriveled or bad looking beans.

Put the legumes in a saucepan and cover them with three times their volume of water. Soak them for 12 to 24 hours or at least overnight. The next morning thoroughly drain the water from the beans, holding the lid over the top of the pan with just a crack open to let water escape. Replace the water with fresh water and pour it off the beans again. Repeat this rinsing three times. This removes gas-causing carbohydrates.

Add the amount of water specified in the ingredient list above to the drained legumes. Place the pan on the stove and bring it to a boil. Reduce the heat and simmer the legumes until they are tender to soft. (Beans are more easily digested if they are soaked for a long time and cooked until they are soft rather than just tender). Check them during cooking and add more water if necessary. Add the salt during the last ten minutes of cooking. Approximate cooking times are:
    Adzuki beans: 2 to 2½ hours
    Anasazi beans: 2 to 2½ hours
    Black beans: 2 to 2½ hours

Cannellini beans: 1½ to 2 hours
Cranberry beans: 1½ to 2 hours
Garbanzo beans: 3 to 3½ hours
Great northern beans: 2 to 2½ hours
Kidney beans: 2½ to 3 hours
Lentils: 1 to 2 hours
Lima beans: 1 to 1½ hours
Navy (small white) beans: 3 to 3½ hours
Pinto beans: 2 to 2½ hours
Red beans: 2 to 2½ hours
Soybeans: 3½ to 4½ hours
Split peas: 1 to 2 hours

Makes 2 to 2½ cups of cooked legumes, or 4 to 5 servings

Crockpot Cooked Legumes

The easiest way to cook dried legumes is using a crockpot. An additional benefit is that there are usually leftover beans which freeze well for future meals. If you want to stock your freezer, use a six-quart crockpot and double this recipe.

1 pound of any kind of dry legume
4 to 5 cups of purified water
1 teaspoon unrefined salt

The morning of the day before you plan to serve the dry legumes for dinner, wash the legumes, removing any shriveled or bad looking beans. Place them in a strainer and rinse them until all traces of dirt have disappeared from the rinse water. Put the legumes in a 3-quart crockpot and fill the pot almost to the top with water. The volume of the water should be two to three times the volume of the legumes. Soak the beans for 12 to 24 hours.

The next morning pour the water off the beans and replace it with fresh water three times. This removes gas-causing carbohydrates. Drain off all of the water after the last rinse. Add 4 cups of purified water to the pot and put the cover on. Cook the legumes on low for 8 to 10 hours or on high for 4 to 6 hours. Check them during cooking and add more purified water if necessary. Record how much water was used for each type of beans (possible in the margin of this page) and the next time you cook that type, you can add that much initially. Stir the salt into the legumes during the last fifteen minutes of the cooking time. Makes 8 to 10 servings

Crockpot Baked Beans

1 pound small white or small navy beans
Purified water
One sweetening option of your choice:

> ¾ cup apple juice concentrate
> ¾ cup white grape juice concentrate
> ¾ cup pineapple juice concentrate
> ¾ cup purified water plus ⅓ cup or coconut or date sugar
> ¾ cup purified water plus $1/16$ to ⅛ teaspoon white stevia powder,
>   or to taste

1½ teaspoons unrefined salt
¼ teaspoon pepper (optional)
1 tablespoon finely chopped onion or 1 teaspoon dried onion flakes (optional)
1 tablespoon finely chopped fresh sweet basil or 1 teaspoon dried sweet basil
1½ teaspoons paprika or 6 ounces of tomato paste (optional)

The day or evening before you plan to serve baked beans for dinner, wash the beans by placing them in a strainer and running water through them. Check the water that is coming out of the bottom of the strainer for dirt. Then continue rinsing until all traces of dirt are gone. Discard any shriveled or bad looking beans. Put the beans in a 3-quart crockpot and fill the pot almost to the top with water. (The volume of the water should be two to three times the volume of the beans). Soak the beans for 12 to 24 hours.

The next morning pour the water off the beans and replace it with fresh water three times. This removes gas-causing carbohydrates. Drain off all of the water after the last rinse. Add 4 cups of purified water to the pot and cover the pot. Cook the beans on high for 4 to 5 hours or until they are tender. Check them during cooking and add more purified water if necessary.

Add the fruit juice concentrate or ¾ cup purified water plus the coconut sugar, date sugar or stevia, onion and seasonings to the crock pot. Stir them into the beans thoroughly. Cover the pot and cook the beans on high another 2 to 2½ hours. If you are using the optional tomato paste, wait to add it a half hour before serving. Also a half hour before serving, stir the salt into the crock pot thoroughly. Then cook the beans for the last half hour.

If you like a thick sauce, smash a few beans against the side of the pot an hour or so before they finish cooking. Check the beans during cooking and add more purified water if necessary. Makes 6 to 8 servings

Bean Soups

NAVY BEAN SOUP

1 pound dry navy beans

Purified water

2 carrots, peeled and sliced

3 stalks of celery, sliced

2 teaspoons unrefined salt

½ teaspoon pepper (optional)

3 tablespoons fresh chopped parsley or 1 tablespoon dry parsley

1 tablespoon fresh chopped sweet basil or 1 teaspoon dry sweet basil

1 potato, peeled and grated (optional)

LIMA BEAN SOUP

1 pound dry baby lima beans

Purified water

1 large or 2 small carrots, peeled and sliced

3 to 4 stalks of celery, sliced

2 teaspoons unrefined salt

½ teaspoon pepper (optional)

1 bay leaf

3 tablespoons fresh chopped parsley or 1 tablespoon dry parsley

1 tablespoon fresh chopped sweet basil or 1 teaspoon dry sweet basil

BLACK BEAN SOUP

1 pound dry black beans

Purified water

2 bell peppers, preferably one green and one red, seeded and diced

1 small onion, diced (optional)

1 pound tomatoes, chopped (optional)

1 teaspoon ground cumin (optional)

2 teaspoons unrefined salt

2 tablespoons fresh chopped oregano or 2 teaspoons dry oregano

½ teaspoon black pepper or a 2 inch chili pepper, seeded and crumbled

WHITE BEAN AND ESCAROLE SOUP

1 pound white beans

Purified water

½ small head of cabbage, chopped (about ¾ pound)

2 teaspoons unrefined salt

¼ teaspoon pepper (optional)

1 tablespoon fresh chopped sweet basil or 1 teaspoon dry sweet basil

1 head of escarole or endive, washed and chopped (about ¾ pound)
2 medium potatoes, peeled and diced

LENTIL SOUP

1 pound lentils
Purified water
3 to 5 carrots, peeled and sliced
3 stalks of celery, sliced
2 teaspoons unrefined salt
¼ teaspoon pepper (optional)

SPLIT PEA SOUP

1 pound split peas
Purified water
3 to 4 carrots, peeled and sliced
3 stalks of celery, sliced
2 teaspoons unrefined salt
¼ teaspoon pepper (optional)
1 bay leaf (optional)

MULTI-BEAN SOUP

1 pound of Bob's Red Mill 13-bean mix OR a total of 1 pound dried beans
composed of as many of the varieties below as you can find and tolerate
Lentils
Yellow split peas
Green split peas
Black beans
Small navy beans
Medium or large lima beans
Blackeyed peas
Small red beans
Kidney beans
Pinto beans
Purified water
3 carrots, about ½ pound, peeled and sliced
3 stalks of celery, sliced
2 teaspoons unrefined salt
¼ teaspoon pepper (optional)

Choose one set of ingredients from above or the previous page. The morning of day before you plan to serve the soup for dinner, wash the dry legumes by placing them in a strainer and running water through them. Check the water that is coming out of the bottom of the strainer for dirt and continue rinsing until all traces of dirt are gone. Discard any shriveled or bad looking beans. Put the legumes in a 3-quart crockpot and cover them with two to three times their volume of water. Soak them for 12 to 24 hours overnight.

The next morning, pour the water off the beans and replace it with fresh water three times. This removes gas-causing carbohydrates. Drain off all of the water after the last rinse. Add purified water to the beans in the pot in the following amounts:

Navy bean soup: 6 cups
Lima bean soup: 6 cups
Black bean soup: 3 cups if you are using the tomatoes, or 4 cups if you are not
    using the tomatoes
White bean and escarole soup: 5½ cups
Lentil soup: 5 cups
Split pea soup: 5 cups
Multi-bean soup: 6 cups

Add the rest of the ingredients to the pot EXCEPT for the salt, the tomatoes in the black bean soup, or the potatoes and escarole in the navy bean and white bean and escarole soups. Cover the crockpot with the lid and cook the soup on high for 5 to 6 hours or on low for 8 to 10 hours.

Add the potatoes and escarole, if you are using them, about two hours before the end of the cooking time. Add the salt to all of the soups about a half hour before the end of the cooking time. Add the tomatoes to the black bean soup about a half hour before the end of the cooking time. Check the soup near the end of the cooking time and add a little boiling purified water if you like your soup thinner. Makes 6 to 8 servings or about 2½ quarts of soup.

For more recipes for legumes see *Nourishing Traditions*[14], pages 495 to 510.

Jovial Foods™ prepares **cooked beans in glass jars**, which are helpful for cancer patients who may be unable to cook but should not consume foods in cans due to the chemicals in the can linings. To purchase cooked beans packed in glass, see "Sources," page 253.

---

14 Fallon, Sally with Mary Enig, PhD. *Nourishing Traditions*., (Brandywine, MD, NewTrends Publishing, 2001), 533-582.

Nuts

Nuts are nutritional giants and posses many positive health effects. Eating one small handful of nuts a day four or five days a week improves outcomes with medical conditions such as heart health and diabetes.[1] In the area of cardiovascular health, eating nuts regularly reduces the incidence of cardiovascular events such as heart attacks and strokes by 30% to 50%. Eating nuts also reduces the incidence of diabetes by 50% and the incidence of metabolic syndrome, a precursor of diabetes, by 26%.

Nuts contain protein, healthy fats including omega-3 fatty acids, fiber, B vitamins including folic acid, minerals such as calcium, magnesium, potassium, iron and zinc, antioxidant minerals such as selenium, manganese and copper, and phytonutrients such as flavonoids and resveratrol.[1] Seeds offer a strong nutritional profile similar to nuts, with some of them being very high in omega-3 fats. Amazingly, chia seeds are a better source of omega-3 fats than salmon. Seeds are helpful for blood sugar control and weight loss as well as lowering the risk of some types of cancer and obesity.[2]

Like grains and legumes, seeds and nuts are the seeds of the plants that produce them. Thus they contain enzyme inhibitors and variable amounts of phytic acid to protect them from digestion by soil bacteria during germination. These substances may also make seeds and nuts difficult for us to digest. Soaking them in salted[3] water for twelve to twenty four hours neutralizes the enzyme inhibitors and phytic acid. Salt is essential for neutralizing these substances in nuts and seeds. However, if you prefer nuts not to have the slightest taste of salt, rinse them after soaking them. See pages 67 to 69 for why whole (unrefined) salt is good for our health.

Nuts and seeds are easily portable non-perishable snacks that are high in protein so they help maintain stable blood sugar levels. Their nutrients are easily absorbed if the seeds or nuts are soaked in salted water for twelve to twenty four hours and then dried. Recipes for preparing nuts and seeds by soaking and drying are on the next page. For nut or seed milk, puree the nuts or seeds after soaking. These milk recipes are in the "Beverages" chapter on pages 187 to 189. Soaked and dried nuts are also used instead of flour in several of the dessert recipes in this book. See these recipes on pages 193 to 196.

---

1 "Nuts and Health," Nutrition Australia. http://www.nutritionaustralia.org/national/frequently-asked-questions/general-nutrition/nuts-and-health

2 Goesch, Heather A. "9 Super Seeds are Small but Mighty." Food & Nutrition. http://www.foodandnutrition.org/July-August-2016/Super-Seeds/

3 Cottis, Halle. "Is Soaking Nuts Necessary & How To Properly Soak Your Organic Raw Nuts!" https://wholelifestylenutrition.com/recipes/appetizers-snacks/is-soaking-nuts-necessary-how-to-properly-soak-your-organic-raw-nuts/

Nourishing Nuts

About 1 pound of raw nuts
1 to 2 tablespoons unrefined sea salt
Purified water

Put the nuts in a bowl or two quart glass canning jars, filling jars to about one inch from the top. Add the salt to the bowl or jars. Fill the bowl to cover the nuts or fill the jars to the top with purified water and stir or invert a few times to dissolve the salt. Soak the nuts for up to 24 hours. This long soak makes nuts easier to digest, although some online recipes say to soak them only 7 to 12 hours or overnight. I soak pecans, walnuts, almonds, macadamia nuts, filberts, pine nuts, and Brazil nuts for 24 hours. Cashews only require a 6 hour soak because they are not actually raw nuts. The GAPS diet instructs that nuts be soaked for 24 hours.

Drain the water from the nuts. Spread the nuts in a single layer on dehydrator trays or baking sheets. Place them in a food dehydrator set at 145°F or oven rigged with the door open to maintain a temperature of up to 150°F to dry. Dry until the nuts are dry and crisp. (Let them cool a bit before judging crispness). I dry most nuts for 24 hours. When drying whole macadamias, some of the nuts may remain soft after 24 hours, so I have dried them up to 34 hours. The solution to this problem is to use macadamia pieces which are smaller. See "Sources," page 266, for where to get macadamia pieces.

Store the dried nuts in glass jars with the lids a little loose or in cellophane bags.

Nourishing Seeds

About 1 pound of raw seeds such as sunflower or pumpkin seeds
2 tablespoons unrefined sea salt
Purified water

Put the raw seeds in a bowl or two quart glass canning jars, filling jars to about one inch from the top. Add the salt to the bowl or jars. Fill the bowl to cover the seeds or the jars to the top with purified water and stir or invert is a few times to dissolve the salt. Soak the seeds for 8 to 14 hours. Being smaller, seeds take less time to soak than nuts and also dry more quickly.

Drain the water from the seeds. Spread the seeds in a single layer on dehydrator trays or baking sheets. Place them in a food dehydrator set at 145°F or oven rigged with the door open to maintain a temperature of up to 150°F to dry. Dry until the seeds are dry and crisp. Pumpkin seeds may begin to brown when they are ready. Smaller pumpkin seeds may be dry in 6 to 8 hours. Sunflower and larger pumpkin seeds and sunflower seeds take 12 to 15 hours.

Store the dried seeds in glass jars with the lids a little loose or in cellophane bags.

Nourishing Nut Pesto

Although "pesto alla Genovese" is traditionally made with sweet basil, pine nuts and olive oil, the combinations below are all delicious and will give you pesto sauce to use on any day if you are on a rotation diet. If you are not on a rotation diet, feel free to use olive oil for any of the varieties of pesto. Because this sauce freezes well, I make it in large batches to freeze for future use.

TRADITIONAL PESTO
½ pound (about 7 cups) sweet basil
1 to 2 cup soaked and dried pine nuts or nuts of your choice
1 to 3 cloves of garlic, optional
1 cup olive oil
1 to 1½ teaspoons unrefined sea salt
¼ teaspoon pepper, optional

PARSLEY PESTO
½ pound (about 7 cups) Italian flat-leaf parsley
1 to 2 cup soaked and dried walnuts or nuts of your choice
1 to 3 cloves of garlic (optional)
1 cup walnut oil
1 to 1½ teaspoons unrefined sea salt
¼ teaspoon pepper, optional

ARUGULA PESTO
½ pound (about 7 cups) arugula
1 to 2 cup soaked and dried cashews or nuts of your choice
1 to 3 cloves of garlic, optional
1 cup canola oil
1 to 1½ teaspoons unrefined sea salt
¼ teaspoon pepper, optional

SPINACH PESTO
½ pound (about 7 cups) spinach
1 to 2 cup soaked and dried almonds or nuts of your choice
1 to 3 cloves of garlic, optional
1 cup almond oil
1 to 1½ teaspoons unrefined sea salt
¼ teaspoon pepper, optional

Remove the stems from the vegetables and wash the leaves in several changes of water. Spread them out on a dishcloth or paper towel. Blot them to remove most of the water. If you are using the garlic, chop it in a blender or a food processor with the metal blade using a pulsing action. Add the vegetable leaves to the processor or blender and use a pulsing action to chop the leaves. Add the nuts to the processor or blender and process continually until they are ground. With the machine running, add the oil in a thin stream. Add the seasonings and process briefly. Serve the sauce over pasta or use it as a condiment or for a spread on bread, crackers, or other baked goods. Makes about 2¼ cups of sauce, or enough for 2 to 4 pounds of pasta.

For other recipes in this book that use nuts and seeds that have been soaked or soaked and dried to make them digestible, see the dessert recipes on pages 192 to 196 and the nut and seed milk recipes on pages 187 to 189.

For more recipes for nourishing nut snacks, see *Nourishing Traditions*[4], pages 513 to 517.

Nuts prepared this way can be found in parts of the world other than the United States under the description of "activated nuts." **Wise Choice Market sells nut butters made from soaked nuts.** See "Sources," page 266, for more information about ordering these nut butters.

---

4 Fallon, Sally with Mary Enig, PhD. *Nourishing Traditions.*, (Brandywine, MD, NewTrends Publishing, 2001), 513-517.

Beverages

Sodas are possibly the most dangerous "food" Americans consume. When we are hot and thirsty and have sodas, it very easy to ingest a large amount of quickly-absorbed carbohydrate. Sodas contain inorganic phosphates which deplete calcium and can stimulate lung cancer. (See pages 12 to 13 for more about inorganic phosphates and other problems with sodas). Diet soda contains ever changing artificial sweeteners, none of which have been adequately tested for safety. However, we do enjoy fizzy drinks. This chapter will give you the experience of a soda without high fructose corn syrup, sugar, or chemicals.

The thirst quenching beverages here are sweetened with stevia, agave, or fruit sweeteners. If you are controlling carbohydrates strictly for weight loss or are on a low yeast diet for *Candida,* try the stevia sweetened lemonade, cranberry soda, or ginger ale. The stevia-containing recipes give a range for the amount of stevia to be used. The reason is that the amount that tastes right varies from person to person and between various brands and kinds of stevia, especially in beverages. Furthermore, as people grow more accustomed to using stevia, some may prefer more of it. For pure sweetness and the least licorice-like taste, I recommend enzyme-treated stevia from Berlin Seeds. To order it, see "Sources," page 267.

The nut and seed milks and smoothies provide protein, omega-3 fats, fiber for satiety, and many vitamins and minerals. With protein from the seeds and nuts to balance the carbohydrate, the nutritive sweeteners in the recipes give quick energy without a slump later. The sweetener choices for the nut and seed milk include agave, dates, fruit sweeteners and stevia. The energizing smoothie recipes in this chapter are made with nut or seed milks.

Finally, this chapter includes tea recipes. Ginger tea is great for quelling inflammation. Cranberry tea is good for urinary tract problems. Rhubarb tea is like hibiscus and is allowed on the LDA diet. It also is handy to have rhubarb concentrate as another option in acid ingredients for leavening and for soaking grains.

Give these easy recipes a try and enjoy healthy beverages.

Lemonade

⅔ cup lemon juice squeezed from two to three lemons
¼ to 1 teaspoon enzyme-treated white stevia powder, or to taste
3 to 4 cups cold purified water or chilled carbonated water
Ice

Stir the juice and the smallest amount of stevia together until the stevia is completely dissolved. Add three cups of water, stir and taste. If it's too strong, add more of the water. If it's not sweet enough, add more stevia and taste after each small addition. When you achieve "just right," record the amounts of water and stevia used, possibly in the margin of this page, for next time. Serve with ice. Makes about 4 servings.

Cranberry Soda

¾ cup pure unsweetened cranberry juice, such as Knudsen™ "Just Cranberry" juice OR ⅓ cup cranberry juice concentrate, such as Knudsen™ cranberry juice concentrate
½ to 1 teaspoon enzyme-treated white stevia powder
3 to 4 cups chilled carbonated water
Ice

Stir the juice and smallest amount of stevia together until the stevia is completely dissolved. Add three cups water, stir, and taste. If it's too strong or too sour, add the additional cup of water. If it's not sweet enough, add more stevia and taste after each small addition. When you achieve "just right," record the amounts of water and stevia used, possibly in the margin of this page, for next time. Serve with ice. Makes about 4 servings.

Cherry Soda

⅓ cup black cherry juice concentrate such as Bernard Jensen's™ or Knudsen™ black cherry juice concentrate, or more to taste
4 cups chilled carbonated water
Ice

Stir the cherry juice concentrate and water together. Serve the drink with ice if desired. Makes about 4 servings.

Fruit Sodas

¼ cup sugar-free frozen fruit juice concentrate such as apple, grape, pineapple or orange
¾ cup carbonated water or more to taste
Ice

Several hours or the night before you want to make this, remove the frozen fruit juice from the freezer and allow it to thaw in the refrigerator. After using a can for the first time, I transfer the remaining juice concentrate to a glass jar to keep in the refrigerator or freezer for future use.

Just before serving, pour the fruit juice concentrate into a glass. Add about half of the carbonated water and stir. Add ice cubes and fill the glass with carbonated water. Give a quick stir if needed and serve. Makes one serving.

Ginger Ale

2 to 4 tablespoons ginger concentrate on page 191, or to taste
Sweetener of your choice -
    $1/16$ teaspoon enzyme-treated white stevia powder, or to taste
    2 to 3 teaspoons agave, or to taste
1 cup carbonated water
Ice

Measure 2 tablespoons of the ginger concentrate and the smaller amount of the sweetener into a glass and stir them together thoroughly. Add the carbonated water and stir. Taste the ginger ale and add more ginger concentrate or sweetener if desired. Record how much ginger and sweetener make it taste "just right" to you, perhaps in the margin of this page, for next time. Add ice and serve. Makes 1 serving.

Nut Milk

1½ cups walnuts, almonds, cashews or other nuts
1 teaspoon unrefined salt
Purified water for soaking plus an additional 3 to 4 cups to make the milk
½ teaspoon cinnamon or ½ to 1 teaspoon vanilla extract, optional
Optional sweetener of your choice–
    2 to 3 tablespoons apple juice concentrate, thawed
    1 to 2 tablespoons agave or Fruit Sweet™
    2 to 4 soft small pitted dates
    $1/16$ to ⅛ teaspoon enzyme-treated white stevia powder, or to taste

Combine the nuts and salt in a quart canning jar or bowl. Add enough water to cover the nuts by at least a few inches. Soak for twelve to twenty four hours at room temperature. After soaking, drain the water and rinse the nuts thoroughly. Put the nuts and 3 cups of purified water in a blender. Blend at highest speed for three minutes or until smooth. Add the flavoring and sweetener and blend again briefly for liquid sweeteners and stevia or a minute or two for dates. If the milk seems too thick add more water and blend briefly. Refrigerate and use within a day or two, or divide into four 1 cup portions and freeze any milk you won't use soon for smoothies. Makes about 4 servings of milk, or use it as a base for the smoothies on page 189.

Many recipes for nut milk advise straining the milk with a nut milk bag. I purchased two bags and tried this. Along with being messy, my impression was that fiber, which can stabilize blood sugar levels, and possibly other nutrients were being discarded. Therefore, no straining is included in this recipe. If your blender leaves pieces of nuts, you may want to pour the milk through a wire mesh sieve. If you prefer nut milk that has no texture, try straining your milk with a nut milk bag.

Seed Milk

This milk is a delicious way to get nutrients such as omega-3 fats from super-food seeds. It has texture, thus making it ideal to use in the smoothies on the next two pages. It is also tasty and filling alone.

FLAX MILK
¾ cup flaxseed
3¾ cups purified water
Sweetener of your choice –
    2 to 4 tablespoons **agave** or Fruit Sweet™
    ¼ cup apple juice concentrate, thawed
    4 to 6 soft small pitted dates
    ⅛ to ¼ teaspoon enzyme-treated white stevia powder, or to taste
2 to 3 teaspoons cinnamon or to taste (optional)

SACHA INCHI SEED MILK
1¾ cups sacha inchi seeds (about 8 ounces, or half of a 16-ounce jar of
    Imlak'esh Organics™ sacha inchi seeds)
Purified water for soaking + 2¾ cups purified water
Sweetener of your choice –
    2 to 4 tablespoons agave or **Fruit Sweet™**
    ¼ cup apple juice concentrate, thawed
    6 to 8 soft small pitted dates
    ⅛ teaspoon enzyme-treated white stevia powder, or to taste
2 to 3 teaspoons cinnamon or to taste (optional)

HEMP MILK
1¾ cup hemp seeds
1⅞ cups purified water
Sweetener of your choice –
    ¼ cup **apple or grape juice concentrate**, thawed,
    2 to 4 tablespoons agave or Fruit Sweet™
    4 to 6 soft small pitted dates
    $1/16$ to ¼ teaspoon enzyme-treated white stevia powder, or to taste
2 to 3 teaspoons cinnamon or to taste (optional)

CHIA MILK
½ to ⅔ cup chia seeds (Use ½ cup for thin milk or ⅔ cup to make a thick
    smoothie even without frozen fruit).
3 cups purified water

Sweetener of your choice –
>   2 to 4 tablespoons agave or Fruit Sweet™
>   ¼ cup apple juice concentrate, thawed
>   4 to 6 soft small **pitted dates**
>   ⅛ to ¼ teaspoon enzyme-treated white stevia powder, or to taste
> 2 to 3 teaspoons cinnamon or to taste (optional)

Choose one set of ingredients above. There are four sets to enable this recipe to be used by those on rotation diets. One sweetener is in bold in each ingredient set to help with rotation but feel free to use a different sweetener. Be consistent in which sweetener is used with each kind of seed if you are on a rotation diet.

In a glass bowl or one-quart canning jar, combine the flax, hemp, or chia seeds with the amount of water specified in the ingredient list. Let the seeds soak in the water for two hours to overnight. For the sacha inchi seeds[5], add enough purified water to cover them by a few inches and refrigerate them overnight. In the morning drain and rinse the seeds.

After soaking, pour the flax, hemp or chia seeds and their soaking water into the blender. Combine the drained sacha inchi seeds with 2¾ cups of purified water in the blender. Blend at highest speed for 2 to 3 minutes or until smooth. Add the sweetener and spice and blend again briefly for liquid sweeteners or a minute or two for dates. Refrigerate and use within a day or two, or divide into four 1 cup portions and freeze any milk you won't use soon for smoothies. Makes about 4 cups or 4 servings of milk.

Nut or Seed Milk Smoothie

This is a take-off on Dr. Baker's Rhythmic Shake on the next page for those who are allergic to some of the ingredients in his shake.

>   1 cup of nut or seed milk (recipes above and on the previous two pages)
>   ⅓ to ⅔ cup of blueberries, strawberries, other berries, cherries, or pieces of
>   other fruit to taste, fresh or frozen
>   Other nourishing additions such as green powders or probiotics (optional)

If not just made, thaw or partially thaw the frozen milk overnight in the refrigerator or place it in a sink or pan of warm water in the morning. In a blender or using a hand blender, combine the milk with fruit and additional ingredients. If made with frozen fruit, this is like ice cream. Makes one serving.

---

5 The directions for the sacha inchi seeds are different than for the other seeds because they are very firm so require long soaking and because I had sacha inchi seeds from nuts.com begin a yeast-type fermentation and smell alcoholic when they were soaked overnight at room temperature. Since yeast is something many allergic people must avoid, soak sacha inchi seeds overnight in the refrigerator. For those on rotation diets, sacha inchi is in the spurge family with castor oil, tapioca and cassava.

Dr. Baker's Basic Rhythmic Shake

If you can have cow milk, flaxseed and soy, Dr. Sidney Baker's[6] recipe is easier to make than the smoothies above and also contains anti-cancer nutrients.

3 ounces whole milk
3 ounces regular yogurt
1 tablespoon ground flax seeds
3 tablespoons soy protein isolate
¼ cup blueberries, fresh or frozen, or other berries

Put the yogurt and milk in a blender. With the blender on low speed, add ground flaxseeds, soy protein isolate, and blueberries. Increase the speed until ingredients are well blended. Makes one serving.

Rhubarb Concentrate

Use this to make rhubarb tea (below) or as an acidic ingredient for leavening and for soaking grains.

1 pound rhubarb
2 cups purified water

Clean the rhubarb and cut it into ½ inch slices. Place it in a saucepan with the water. Place the lid on the pan, bring it to a boil, reduce the heat and simmer for one hour. Pour the mixture into a wire mesh strainer or colander and let it stand for about ½ hour to thoroughly strain the liquid from the rhubarb slices. If you are making this to use at the time of LDA treatment, reserve the slices to use in rhubarb jam or as a condiment with meat. If you are not taking LDA, press the slices in the strainer with the back of a spoon to extract more liquid and then compost or discard the pulp. Refrigerate the concentrate to use within a few days or freeze any leftover concentrate for future use. Makes about 2½ to 3 cups of concentrate.

Rhubarb Tea

This is a tangy tea similar to hibiscus tea.

4 to 6 tablespoons of rhubarb concentrate above, to taste
Purified water, boiling

Put the rhubarb concentrate into a 10-ounce mug and fill with boiling water to make rhubarb tea. One batch of rhubarb concentrate makes about 8 cups of tea.

---

6 Recipe used with permission. Baker, Sidney M., MD. *The Circadian Prescription*, (New York, Berkley Publishing Group, a division of Penguin Putnam Inc., 2000), 74.

Ginger Tea by the Cup

This is the way to drink ginger tea if you want great flavor and the full benefit of its anti-inflammatory effects. Skip the ginger tea bags and make your own tea using this recipe or the recipes below and on the next page.

  1 ounce fresh ginger root
  1¼ cups purified water

Wash the ginger root and cut off any damaged or discolored spots. If you are rushed for time, dice it finely. If you have more time and want more potent tea, peel and grate the ginger root. Combine the ginger and water in a saucepan and bring it to a boil. Reduce the heat and simmer it for 10 to 15 minutes. Strain out the ginger and enjoy the tea immediately. Makes one serving. This recipe may be doubled, tripled, etc. if it is for serving more than one person. To save work if drinking ginger tea often, make a large batch of ginger concentrate using the recipe below.

Ginger Concentrate

With a food processor, you can easily make enough ginger concentrate to last for several weeks of ginger tea or ginger ale. Then you can enjoy these beverages easily when time is tight. Use the freshest ginger you can find – heavy and smooth skinned – for this recipe.

  2 to 2¼ pounds fresh ginger root
  10 cups purified water

Scrub the ginger root and cut off any damaged or discolored spots. Cut the ginger into chunks that will fit into the feed tube of your food processor. Grate it with the processor, cleaning the fiber out of the holes in the blade two or three times when you stop during processing. Reserve the fiber to cook with the grated ginger.

Combine the grated ginger with the water in a large stockpot and bring it to a boil over medium heat. Reduce the heat and simmer it for 30 to 40 minutes. Cool the mixture at room temperature until it is lukewarm or cooler. Working with about two cups of the cooked ginger mixture at a time, strain it through a wire mesh strainer, pressing the grated ginger with the back of a spoon to extract all of the liquid. Freeze the concentrate in small jars containing enough concentrate for you to use in two or three days or put it into ice cube trays to freeze. When the ginger concentrate cubes are frozen, transfer them to a canning jar and return them to the freezer. Makes 9 to 10 cups of concentrate, or enough for about 40 cups of tea.

Quick Ginger Tea

With this recipe you can enjoy ginger tea without much time spent on preparation.

Ginger concentrate on the previous page
Purified water

Fill a cup or mug about ⅙ to ¼ full with ginger concentrate or about ⅓ to ½ full of frozen ginger concentrate cubes. Add water to finish filling the cup or mug. Transfer the mixture to a saucepan, bring it to a boil, and then serve. Makes one serving.

Cranberry Tea

Cranberries are not on the anti-inflammatory food list, but they are closely related to blueberries and this tea contains two anti-inflammatory spices. It's also delicious.

3 tablespoons Knudsen™ cranberry concentrate
1 cup purified water
⅛ teaspoon each ground cinnamon, ginger, and cloves
1 tablespoon lemon juice (optional)
¼ cup orange juice (optional)
$1/16$ teaspoon of enzyme treated stevia powder, or to taste (optional, not
     needed with the orange juice)

Bring the cranberry concentrate and water to a low boil; reduce heat to a simmer. Place cinnamon, ginger and nutmeg into a cloth tea bag or fine mesh tea ball; add to the cranberry juice and water. If you prefer the tea spicier, add the spices directly to the liquid. Simmer 15 minutes. Remove the tea ball or bag. Stir in the optional orange and lemon juices and stevia if desired. Return the tea to a boil and pour it into a large mug. Makes one serving. This recipe may be doubled, tripled, etc. if serving more than one person.

For more beverage recipes including some for fermented beverages, see *Nourishing Traditions*[7], pages 584 to 596.

---

7 Fallon, Sally with Mary Enig, PhD. *Nourishing Traditions.*, (Brandywine, MD, NewTrends Publishing, 2001), 584-596.

Treats

Some occasions in life call for a celebration – birthdays, graduations, holidays, new babies, promotions, and more. With the recipes in this chapter no one will feel left out. Everyone who comes to the celebration will be able to enjoy a treat.

Several recipes below are made with nuts rather than flour or starch of any kind. Those on gluten-free diets, blood sugar control protocols, and other special diets will enjoy these treats and the stable blood sugar that follows them. Most of the recipes include an option for sweetening with stevia and many are sweetened with low glycemic index sweeteners such as agave, coconut sugar, or fruit sweeteners. If pressed for time, choose an easy fruit crumble or pudding recipe. If there is more time, see the recipes below for pies, cakes and brownies.

Nourishing Nut Brownies

8 ounces of soaked and dried cashews or nuts of your choice (about 2 cups of cashew splits)
2 large eggs
¼ cup plus 1 tablespoon purified water
1 teaspoon vanilla (optional)
⅛ teaspoon unrefined salt
⅞ teaspoons enzyme-treated white stevia powder (See "Sources," page 267).
¼ cup plus 1 tablespoon cocoa (natural, not Dutch process or alkalinized)
¼ teaspoon baking soda

Preheat your oven to 350°F. Line the bottom and an inch or two up the sides of an 8 or 9 inch square baking pan with parchment paper.

Measure the cocoa into a small bowl. Remove and set aside about ⅛ cup of it. Put the nuts in a food processor bowl with the metal pureeing blade. (Cashews are mild flavored, easy to grind to a fine meal-like consistency and the splits are less expensive than other cashews). Process the nuts for about 30 seconds. Then add the ⅛ cup of cocoa that was set aside and process it with the nuts until the nuts are very finely ground. Scrape the bottom corners of the bowl with a spatula, and process again briefly. Add the eggs, water, vanilla, salt and stevia and blend until well mixed, stopping and scraping the bowl a time or two. Stir the baking soda into the remaining cocoa in the small bowl. Add it to the food processor bowl and very briefly mix it in with a spatula until there is only a little dry powder on the top of the mixture. Process for a few seconds until just blended. Scrape the batter into the prepared pan and bake for 20 minutes. Cool completely before cutting. Makes 12 to 16 brownies.

Stevia-Sweetened Chocolate Layer Cake

1½ pounds soaked and dried almonds, cashews or nuts of your choice (recipe
    on page 182) or 1½ 16-ounce jars of creamy almond butter

6 large eggs (about 1⅛ cup in volume)

1¼ cups purified water

2 to 3 teaspoons vanilla (optional)

¼ teaspoon unrefined salt

1¼ teaspoons enzyme-treated white stevia powder (See "Sources," page 267).

¾ cup cocoa (natural, not Dutch process or alkalinized)

¾ teaspoon baking soda

Preheat your oven to 350°F. Rub the sides of two 8 or 9 inch round baking pans or three 7 inch round pans with fat or oil, preferably with a solid fat like coconut or palm oil or butter. Line the bottom of the pans with parchment paper.

If using the nut butter, blend the nut butter and eggs until smooth in a large bowl with a hand blender or use a food processor. Add the eggs water, vanilla, salt, and stevia and blend until well mixed. Proceed with the recipe as below in the fourth paragraph.

If using the nuts, measure the cocoa into a small bowl. Remove about ⅓ cup of it. Put the nuts in a food processor bowl with the metal pureeing blade and process for about 30 seconds. Then add the ⅓ cup of cocoa and process it with the nuts until the nuts are very finely ground. Scrape the bottom corners of the bowl with a spatula and process again briefly. Add the eggs, water, vanilla, salt and stevia and blend until well mixed, stopping and scraping the bowl a time or two.

Stir the baking soda into the remaining cocoa in the small bowl. Add it to the food processor bowl (or bowl used with a hand blender) and quickly and very briefly mix it in with a spatula until there is not much dry powder on the top of the mixture. Process for a few seconds until just blended. Quickly scrape the batter into the prepared pans and level it with the spatula. Quickly pop the pans into the oven and bake for 20 to 30 minutes. If three pans are used, the cake may bake a little more quickly.

Cool completely before frosting with the frosting below or on the nest page.

Chocolate Cream Cheese Frosting

FROSTING FOR BROWNIES OR A SINGLE LAYER CAKE

    1 8-ounce package cream cheese at room temperature

    ½ cup (1 stick) butter at room temperature

    ⅜ cup cocoa

    ⅝ to ⅞ cup agave or Fruit Sweet™ (to taste) or 1½ to 2 teaspoons enzyme-treated
        stevia (to taste) plus ¼ cup milk (See "Sources," page 267).

    1 teaspoon vanilla extract

FROSTING FOR A MULTI-LAYER CAKE

>   2 8-ounce packages cream cheese at room temperature
>
>   1 cup (2 sticks) butter at room temperature
>
>   ¾ cup cocoa
>
>   1¼ to 1¾ cups agave or Fruit Sweet™ (to taste) or 3 to 4 teaspoons enzyme-treated stevia (to taste) plus ½ cup milk (See "Sources," page 267).
>
>   2 teaspoons vanilla extract

Use an electric mixer, blender, food processor or hand blender to mix together the cream cheese and butter. Beat until fluffy. Mix in the cocoa and vanilla extract. Add the agave or Fruit Sweet™ one tablespoon at a time, tasting it as you add the sweetener until you get it to your preferred level of sweetness. (If you add enough sweetener to make the frosting too thin to spread easily, refrigerate it for 15 minutes or more until it is a good spreading consistency). If you are using the stevia, beat in the milk thoroughly. Then add the stevia starting with 1 teaspoon for a single layer batch or 2 teaspoons for a multi-layer batch, tasting, and adding ¼ teaspoon at a time, mixing and tasting until it tastes right for you. Record how much stevia you used, possibly in the margin of this page, for next time. Frost the cake. This frosting will be soft but it gets firmer when chilled. Store any cake frosted with this frosting in the refrigerator. The single layer batch of frosting makes about 1½ cups of frosting or enough to frost a single layer of the chocolate cake recipe. The multi-layer batch makes about 3 cups of frosting or enough for the multi-layer chocolate cake.

Vanilla Cream Cheese Frosting

FROSTING FOR A SINGLE LAYER CAKE

>   1 8-ounce package cream cheese at room temperature
>
>   ½ cup (1 stick) butter at room temperature
>
>   4 to 6 tablespoons agave or Fruit Sweet™ to taste or 1¼ to 1¾ teaspoons enzyme-treated stevia to taste plus 3 tablespoons milk (See "Sources," page 267).
>
>   1 teaspoon vanilla extract

FROSTING FOR A MULTI-LAYER CAKE

>   2 8-ounce packages cream cheese at room temperature
>
>   1 cup (2 sticks) butter at room temperature
>
>   ½ to ¾ cups agave or Fruit Sweet™ to taste or 2½ to 3½ teaspoons enzyme-treated stevia to taste plus ⅜ cup milk (See "Sources," page 267).
>
>   2 teaspoons vanilla extract

Use an electric mixer, blender, food processor or hand blender to mix together the cream cheese and butter. Beat until fluffy. Mix in the vanilla extract. Add the agave or

Fruit Sweet™ one tablespoon at a time, tasting it as you add the sweetener until you get it to your preferred level of sweetness. (If you add enough sweetener to make the frosting too thin to spread easily, refrigerate it for 15 minutes or more until it is a good spreading consistency). If you are using the stevia, beat in the milk thoroughly. Then add the stevia starting with 1 teaspoon for a single layer batch or 2 teaspoons for a multi-layer batch, tasting, and adding ¼ teaspoon at a time, mixing and tasting until it tastes right for you. Record how much stevia you used, possibly in the margin of this page, for next time. Frost the cake. This frosting will be soft but it gets firmer when chilled. Store any cake frosted with this frosting in the refrigerator. The single layer batch of frosting makes about 1½ cups of frosting or enough to frost a single layer of the carrot or chocolate cake recipe. The multi-layer batch makes about 3 cups of frosting or enough for the multi-layer carrot or chocolate cake.

Carrot Cake

SINGLE LAYER CAKE

 ½ pound soaked and dried nuts, any kind, recipe on page 182 or
  ½ 16-ounce jar of creamy almond butter
 ⅛ cup purified water
 4 large eggs
 1 tablespoon lemon juice
 ½ to ¾ teaspoon cinnamon
 ¾ to 1 teaspoon enzyme-treated white stevia powder (See "Sources," page 267).
 ⅛ cup chardonnay grape seed flour, arrowroot, or tapioca starch.
 1 teaspoon baking soda
 ¾ cups grated carrots plus ¼ cup currants or raisins OR 1 cup grated carrots

MULTI-LAYER CAKE

 1 pound soaked and dried nuts, any kind, recipe on pages 182 or
  1 16-ounce jar of creamy almond butter
 ¼ cup purified water
 8 large eggs
 2 tablespoons lemon juice
 1½ teaspoon cinnamon
 1½ to 2 teaspoons enzyme-treated white stevia powder (See "Sources," page 267).
 ¼ cup chardonnay grape seed flour, arrowroot, or tapioca starch.
 2 teaspoons baking soda
 1½ cups grated carrots plus ½ cup currants or raisins OR 2 cups grated carrots

Grease the sides of and parchment-paper line the bottom of an 8 or 9 inch round cake pan for a one layer cake. Prepare two 8 or 9-inch round pans or three 7 inch round pans for a multi-layer cake. Preheat your oven to 375°F.

If using the nut butter, blend the nut butter and eggs till smooth in a large bowl with a hand blender or use a food processor. Add the water, eggs, lemon juice, cinnamon, and stevia and blend until well mixed. Proceed with the recipe as in the third paragraph below.

If using the nuts, place them in the bowl of a food processor and process on "puree" until they become a thick paste. Cashew, almonds, or a mixture of the two are good if you're not limited in your nut choices. Add the water to the paste and process for a few minutes to get the mixture to come together in a nut butter consistency. Add the eggs, lemon juice, cinnamon and stevia and puree until smooth.

In a small bowl stir together the grapeseed flour or starch and baking soda. Add it to the processor bowl by sprinkling it around the top post of the blade. Puree using the pulse control for a few seconds. Do not over mix. Quickly fold in the carrots and optional raisins or currants. Again, do not over mix or all the leavening will happen in the food processor bowl rather than in the oven. Quickly divide the batter between the prepared pans and pop them into the oven.

Bake for about 20 minutes or until a toothpick comes our dry when tested in the middle of a cake layer. Place the pans on a cooling rack and cool for about 15 minutes. Then remove the cake layers from the pans and return them to the rack to cool completely before frosting the cake with vanilla cream cheese frosting on page 195.

For a weight loss glycemic control diet, make this cake with the grape seed flour and all carrots rather than carrots and raisins

Whipped Cream

This is delicious on the pies, puddings and the fruit crumble on the next page. It's just as good made without the thickener if you are allergic to corn or if you will be making it shortly before serving time.

> 1 pint (2 cups) whipping cream
> ¼ teaspoon enzyme treated stevia or 2 teaspoons to 1 tablespoon agave
> 1 tablespoon Signature Secrets Culinary Thickener™, optional (See "Sources," page 259).

TRADITIONAL METHOD

Beat the cream at high speed until soft peaks form. Add the sweetener and beat it in thoroughly. Add the thickener and blend it on low speed until it seems well mixed into the cream. Then beat on high speed for one to two more minutes until the cream forms stiff shapes. The surface of the cream will look chunky. Refrigerate the whipped cream. It will stay whipped for at least several days if using the thickener. If you are allergic to corn, omit the thickener and whip the cream up to an hour or two before you plan to serve it. Makes about 3¾ to 4 cups of whipped cream

FOOD PROCESSOR METHOD

Put all ingredients in the bowl of the food processor with the metal pureeing blade. Process for about 30 seconds. Scrape down the sides of the processor with a rubber spatula to place the thin liquid into the whipped cream in the bowl. Process for another 30 seconds to one minute or until of the desired consistency. If you are allergic to corn, omit the thickener and whip the cream up to an hour or two before you plan to serve it. Makes about 3¾ to 4 cups of whipped cream

No-Grain Easy Fruit Crumble

1½ to 1¾ pounds of apples, peaches, or dark (Bing) cherries OR 1¼ pounds
 frozen blueberries or pitted dark cherries
¼ cup arrowroot or tapioca starch
½ to ¾ cup date sugar, divided
Up to 4 tablespoons purified water
¼ cup soaked and dried nuts ground to meal consistency in a food processor
 or ¼ cup commercially-ground almond meal/flour or pecan meal/flour
 (See "Sources" page 266 for almond flour and 260 for pecan meal/flour).
⅔ cup grated unsweetened coconut
⅓ cup coarsely chopped soaked and dried nuts or purchased sliced almonds or
 chopped pecans
Cinnamon – 1¼ teaspoon with the apples, ¼ teaspoon with the other fruit
¼ to ⅓ cup oil

Preheat the oven to 375°F. Grind the soaked and dried nuts by pulsing in a food processor to a meal consistency if you are not using commercially ground nut meal or flour.

If you are using fresh fruit, peel, core and slice the apples or peaches or pit the cherries. Measure about 4 cups of the prepared fruit in a measuring cup for liquids. I like to use my 4 cup glass liquid measure for this recipe and fill it a little above the line at the top.

Combine the prepared fresh or frozen fruit, arrowroot or tapioca starch, and ¼ to ½ cup of date sugar (depending on how sweet the fruit is) in a deep 8 or 9 inch square baking dish or 2 to 3-quart casserole dish. Add enough of the water to moisten the starch and date sugar. The starch-liquid mixture should be like a thick paste that sticks to the fruit. How much water you need to add will depend on how juicy the fruit is.

In a bowl, stir together the remaining ¼ cup date sugar, nut meal, coconut, nuts, and cinnamon. Pour ¼ cup of oil over the mixture and stir until it is evenly moistened but not soggy with oil. The larger quantity of oil will be needed if the coconut is very finely grated. Sprinkle the nut mixture over the fruit in the baking dish. Bake for 10 minutes. Then cover it with foil to prevent excessive browning. Bake for another 35 to 45 minutes or until the filling is tender and bubbly throughout. Makes about 6 servings.

Almond Pie Crust

This pie crust is a good low-carbohydrate choice for all the pies in this book. However, if there is no one at your celebration who needs this crust and you'd like to make a traditional two-crust fruit pie, see page 201 for a rolled white spelt crust.

1¾ cups finely ground blanched almond flour
¼ teaspoon unrefined salt
$1/16$ teaspoon enzyme-treated stevia (optional – or omit and substitute 1 tablespoon agave for 1 tablespoon of the water below)
¼ cup oil
1 teaspoon vanilla (optional)
2 tablespoons purified water

Preheat the oven to 350°F. Stir together the almond flour, salt and stevia in a large bowl. Add the oil and stir in thoroughly until it is all taken up by the flour and the dough forms lumps. Add the water or water plus agave and stir until it comes together. Press the dough on to the bottom and sides of a 9-inch glass pie dish. Bake for 9 to 15 minutes or until the crust is golden brown. Cool completely before filling.

If you will be filling this with a "wet" filling such as pumpkin (see page 203), the crust may become soggy if the pie is stored in the refrigerator very long and will need the protection of an egg wash.[1] Therefore, again preheat your oven to 350°F. After the crust has cooled enough to handle the pie dish comfortably, slightly beat an egg and brush it on the bottom and sides of the crust. Wrap a 4-inch wide strip of aluminum foil around the edge of the pie dish and fold it over the edge of the crust to protect it from over-browning. Bake for 6 to 9 minutes until the egg is set and dry. Leave the foil on the edge of the crust. Cool the crust completely before filling.

Coconut Pie Crust

2 cups unsweetened shredded or very finely shredded coconut
Coconut oil – ¼ cup with shredded coconut or ⅜ cup with finely shredded coconut

Preheat your oven to 300°F. Melt about ½ cup coconut oil in a small saucepan over low heat. Measure ¼ cup of the liquid coconut oil.

Measure the coconut into a glass pie dish. Pour the ¼ cup coconut oil over the coconut. Mix the oil and coconut thoroughly using a spoon and your hands. If necessary, add more melted coconut oil to get the coconut to stick together. (More oil will be needed if the coconut is finely shredded). Press the mixture evenly onto the bottom and sides of the dish.

---

1 If you are allergic to eggs, omit the egg wash. A slightly soggy crust is better than an allergic reaction.

Bake the crust for 12 to 15 minutes or until it begins to brown. Cool the crust completely on a wire cooling rack. Fill the crust with any fruit filling, pages 205 to 207, which is partially cooled and thickening but not set. Makes one pie crust.

Flour and Oil Pie Crust

With this recipe, pie crust can be made with a variety of flours and healthy oils. Using a pastry cloth, the white (sifted) spelt crust can be rolled and crimped to make a traditional two-crust pie.

KAMUT

      2¾ cups kamut flour
      ½ teaspoon salt
      ⅔ cup oil
      4 to 5 tablespoons purified water

BARLEY

      3 cups barley flour
      ½ teaspoon salt
      ½ cup oil
      6 to 7 tablespoons purified water

AMARANTH

      1½ cups amaranth flour
      ¾ cup arrowroot
      ½ teaspoon salt
      ½ cup oil
      4 to 5 tablespoons purified water

RYE

      2½ cups rye flour
      ½ teaspoon salt
      ⅔ cup oil
      4 to 5 tablespoons purified water

TEFF

      3 cups teff flour
      ½ teaspoon salt
      ½ cup oil
      5 to 6 tablespoons purified water

BUCKWHEAT

> 3 cups buckwheat flour
> ½ teaspoon salt
> ¾ cup oil
> 6 to 8 tablespoons purified water

SPELT

> 3 cups spelt flour
> ½ teaspoon salt
> ½ cup oil
> 5 to 6 tablespoons purified water

WHITE SPELT

> 2½ cups white spelt flour
> ½ teaspoon salt
> ⅜ cup (¼ cup plus 2 tablespoons) oil
> 4 to 6 tablespoons purified water

QUINOA

> 2 cups quinoa flour
> 1 teaspoon baking soda
> ¼ teaspoon unbuffered vitamin C powder
> ½ teaspoon salt (optional)
> ½ teaspoon cinnamon (optional)
> ½ cup oil
> 4 to 6 tablespoons purified water

OAT

> 3 cups oat flour
> ½ teaspoon salt
> ½ cup oil
> 4 to 5 tablespoons purified water

RICE

> 3 cups brown or white rice flour
> ½ teaspoon salt
> ½ cup oil
> 6 to 8 tablespoons purified water

Choose one set of ingredients from the previous page or above. If you are making a pie for which you bake the crust before filling it, preheat your oven to 350°F for the quinoa crust or to 400°F for any of the other kinds of pie crust. If you will be baking the crust with the filling in it, preheat your oven to the temperature given in the filling recipe.

Stir together the dry ingredients such as the flour(s), salt, baking soda, vitamin C and cinnamon in a large bowl. Add the oil and blend it in thoroughly with a pastry cutter. Add the smallest amount of water listed above and mix the dough until it begins to stick together, adding more water if necessary.

For single crust pies, divide the dough in half and press each half of the dough into a glass pie dish. If you are making a type of pie that directs that the crust be baked before adding the filling to it, gently prick the crusts with a fork. Bake the crusts for the following times or until they begin to brown on the bottom:

> Kamut: 13 to 18 minutes
> Barley: 15 to 18 minutes
> Amaranth: 15 to 18 minutes
> Rye: 15 to 20 minutes
> Teff: 15 to 18 minutes
> Buckwheat: 15 to 18 minutes
> Spelt: 18 to 22 minutes
> White spelt: 13 to 17 minutes
> Quinoa: 20 to 25 minutes
> Oat: 15 to 20 minutes
> Rice: 15 to 18 minutes

Completely cool the crusts on a wire cooling rack before filling them. If you are making only one pie, freeze the second crust.

Although not as likely to become soggy as an almond crust, these crusts should be coated with an egg wash[2] if used for pumpkin and other liquid-filling pies. Bake the crust, shielding the edge with a strip of foil wrapped around the pie dish and folded over the edge of the crust. Cool the crust, brush it with beaten egg, and bake it again until the egg is set. Cool the crust again and add the pumpkin filling and bake as directed in the filling recipe. Remove the foil from the crust's edge for the last ten minutes of baking.

For a double crust pie, divide the dough in half and press one half into a glass pie dish. Preheat your oven to the temperature given in the filling recipe. Prepare the filling and add it to the bottom crust. Crumble the second half of the dough over the filling. Bale as directed in the filling recipe.

White spelt pie crust is sturdy enough to be rolled out on a pastry cloth if you wish. Flour the pastry cloth and cloth-covered rolling pin well. Roll half of the dough to about ⅛ inch thick. Use the pastry cloth to fold the crust in half. Then transfer it to the pie dish and unfold it. Ease the dough down into the pie dish without stretching it much. Trim excess pastry even with the edge of the pie plate. For a double crust pie, pour the warm filling into the bottom crust in the pie dish. Roll the second half of the dough, fold it, and transfer it to the pie as described above. Place the top crust over the filling and cut

---

2 If you are allergic to eggs, omit the egg wash. A slightly soggy crust is better than an allergic reaction.

the edge so it overlaps the bottom crust by about ½ inch. Fold the edge of the top crust under the bottom crust and press the three-layer edge together with a fork. Prick the top crust with the fork to let steam escape. Bake as directed in the filling recipe.

Pumpkin Pie

FILLING
>   1 15-ounce can of thick canned pumpkin such as Kuner's™
>   1 teaspoon cinnamon
>   ½ teaspoon nutmeg
>   ¼ teaspoon allspice
>   1 to 1⅛ teaspoon enzyme-treated stevia or to taste (See "Sources," page 267).
>   3 large eggs
>   ⅞ cup milk

CRUST
>   1 single Almond Pie Crust, page 199, or a Flour and Oil Pie crust, page 200
>   1 egg for brushing the crust.

Make the crust as directed in the recipe. Cover the edges of the crust with foil. Bake as directed in the recipe until it is set and just beginning to brown in a place or two. Remove it from the oven and let it cool a little. Brush it with beaten egg and bake for another 6 to10 minutes or until the egg is set. Cool the crust completely. Leave the foil on the crust edges. Fill and bake as below.

For the filling, whisk or beat the eggs and combine them with the other ingredients in a saucepan. Preheat the oven to 375°F while cooking the filling. Cook the filling over medium heat until steamy. Put the filling into the crust. Bake for 30 to 35 minutes or until the filling is just beginning to set in the middle of the pie. Take the foil off the edges of the crust and bake for another 10 to 15 minutes until the edge is brown and a knife inserted in the filling comes out wet but without filling on it. Makes one pie or six servings.

Pumpkin Pudding

>   1 29-ounce can of thick canned pumpkin such as Kuner's™
>   2 teaspoons cinnamon
>   1 teaspoon nutmeg
>   ½ teaspoon allspice
>   2¼ teaspoons enzyme-treated stevia or to taste (See "Sources," page 267).
>   6 large eggs
>   1¾ cups milk

Whisk or beat the eggs and combine them with the other ingredients in a saucepan. Preheat the oven to 375°F. Cook the pudding over medium heat until steamy. Pour it into one or more casserole dishes, leaving at least an inch of two at the top of the dish for expansion during baking. Bake for 45 minutes or until it is set in the middle and a knife inserted in the middle comes out wet but without pudding on it.

Lemon Chiffon Pie

One baked "Almond Pie Crust," page 199, or "Flour and Oil Pie" crust, page 200
2 tablespoons butter, coconut oil, or palm oil shortening (See "Sources," page 259).
2 tablespoons flour (sorghum, unbleached all-purpose, or flour of your choice)
1 cup milk – whole cow milk, goat milk, nut milk, etc.
⅛ teaspoon unrefined salt
1½ teaspoons enzyme-treated stevia or ¾ cup coconut sugar or to taste
     (See "Sources," page 267, for both sweeteners).
¼ cup lemon juice
2 teaspoons grated lemon zest (yellow part of rind) or ½ teaspoon Boyajian
     Pure Lemon Oil (See "Sources," page 258).
5 eggs, separated, for the filling plus an extra egg to coat the almond crust

Prepare and bake the pie crust as directed in the recipe. If using an almond pie crust, coat the bottom and sides with beaten egg, shield the edge of the crust with foil and bake as directed in the recipe until the egg is set. Cool the crust completely, and leave the foil covering the edge. If you are using a flour and oil crust, cover the edge with foil.

Preheat your oven to 325°F. Melt the butter, coconut oil, or palm oil shortening in a saucepan. Stir in the flour and cook, stirring constantly, over medium heat until it bubbles a little. Continue cooking and stirring for at least one minute. Add the milk gradually, stirring continuously until the mixture is smooth. Add the salt and stevia or coconut sugar and cook the mixture over low heat, stirring continuously, until it thickens and begins to barely boil. Continue cooking and stirring for one additional minute. Stir in the lemon juice and flavoring or zest. Remove the pan from the heat and set it aside to cool for a few minutes.

Separate the eggs into yolks and whites, putting the whites into a mixer bowl and the yolks into another bowl. Whisk the yolks. Add a tablespoon of the milk mixture to the yolks and whisk. Continue adding the milk mixture, 1 to 2 tablespoons at a time, whisking after each addition until you've added about ½ cup of the milk mixture. Then pour the yolk mixture into the milk mixture and whisk thoroughly.

Beat the egg whites until stiff peaks form. Fold in the yolk-milk mixture. Pour the lemon filling into the pie crust and bake for one hour or until it is golden brown and a knife inserted into the center of the pie comes out dry. Makes one pie or six servings.

Lemon Chiffon Pudding

Prepare the recipe on the previous page, omitting the pie crust. Put the filling into a casserole dish or single serving glass ramekins and bake at 325°F for 45 to 55 minutes or until golden brown and a knife inserted into the center comes out dry. Makes six servings.

Apple Pie

6 to 7 apples, peeled, cored and sliced to make about 5 cups of slices
⅞ cup thawed apple juice concentrate, divided, or ¾ cup purified water,
    divided, plus ¼ to ½ teaspoon white enzyme-treated stevia powder (See
    "Sources," page 267).
1 teaspoon cinnamon
2 tablespoons arrowroot or tapioca starch OR 3 tablespoons of quick-cooking
    (Minute™) tapioca
1 baked pie crust, recipes on pages 199 to 202

In a saucepan combine the apple slices, ½ cup water plus ¼ teaspoon enzyme-treated stevia or ⅝ cup apple juice concentrate and cinnamon. Bring them to a boil and reduce the heat to a simmer. Simmer for about 15 to 20 minutes or until the apples are tender. While they are cooking, in a separate cup stir together the additional ¼ cup water or apple juice concentrate with the starch or quick-cooking tapioca. If you are using quick-cooking tapioca, let it stand for 5 minutes in the cup before adding it to the apples. Stir the starch or tapioca mixture into the saucepan at the end of the simmering time for the apples. Continue to simmer until the fruit mixture returns to a boil. Cook and stir it for one minute if you are using the quick-cooking tapioca or until it thickens if you are using the starch. Remove the pan from the heat.

If this is the first time you have made this pie with stevia, taste the filling after 3 minutes of cooling. If it is not sweet enough for you, sprinkle an additional ⅛ teaspoon of enzyme-treated stevia powder over the surface and then stir it in very thoroughly. Taste the filling again. If it is still not sweet enough, add another ⅛ teaspoon of stevia and taste after each small addition. Record how much stevia and the variety of apples you use for next time. Allow the filling to cool, stirring it occasionally, for 15 to 30 minutes or until it is lukewarm or cooler and thickening but not set. Put the filling in the pie crust. Chill the pie in the refrigerator for a few hours before serving.

If you wish to make a traditional two-crust fruit pie, make the white spelt "Flour and Oil" pie crust on page 200. Preheat the oven to 400°F while preparing the filling. Roll and fill the crust as directed on pages 202 to 203. Bake the pie at 400°F for 10 minutes. Then reduce the heat to 350°F and bake for 40 to 50 minutes or until the top and bottom of the crust is golden brown. Makes one pie or six servings.

Blueberry Pie

20 ounces fresh or frozen blueberries (about 5 to 6 cups fresh or 1¼
    1-pound bags frozen blueberries)
1 cup thawed apple juice concentrate OR 1 cup purified water plus
    ⅜ to ⅝ teaspoon enzyme-treated stevia powder or to taste (See "Sources,"
    page 267).
2½ to 3 tablespoons quick-cooking (Minute™) tapioca or 2½ tablespoons
    tapioca starch or arrowroot
1 baked pie crust, recipes on pages 199 to 200

Combine the blueberries, water, thickener, and ⅜ teaspoon of the stevia (if you are using it) in a saucepan. If you are using the apple juice concentrate, combine it with the blueberries and thickener. If you are using the Minute™ tapioca, allow the mixture to stand for 5 minutes. Then cook it over medium heat, stirring occasionally, until it comes to a boil. Cook and stir it for one minute if you are using the quick-cooking tapioca or until it thickens if you are using the starch. Remove the pan from the heat.

If you are using the stevia and this is the first time you have made this pie, taste the filling after 3 minutes of cooling. If it is not sweet enough for you, sprinkle an additional ⅛ teaspoon of stevia powder over the surface and then stir it in very thoroughly. Taste the filling again. If it is still not sweet enough, add another ⅛ teaspoon of stevia. Record how much stevia you use for the next time you make this. Let the filling cool, stirring it occasionally, for 15 to 30 minutes or until it is lukewarm or cooler and thickening but not set. Put the filling in the pie crust. Chill the pie in the refrigerator for a few hours before serving.

If you wish to make a traditional two-crust fruit pie, make the white spelt "Flour and Oil" pie crust on page 200. Preheat the oven to 400°F while preparing the filling. Roll and fill the crust as directed on pages 202 to 203. Bake the pie at 400°F for 10 minutes. Then reduce the heat to 350°F and bake for 40 to 50 minutes or until the top and bottom crusts are golden brown. Makes one pie or six servings.

Cherry Pie

Because pie cherries are fairly tart, this recipe may require quite a bit of stevia to taste sweet enough. I prefer pie a little on the tart side to minimize the stevia taste and so use ¾ teaspoon of stevia powder, but you may prefer it sweeter.

1 pound frozen tart cherries (See "Sources," page 260) or 1¼ pounds pitted fresh
    tart cherries, or if you are not a cancer patient avoiding canned foods,
    2 16-ounce cans water-packed tart pie cherries

¾ cup reserved cherry juice or water plus ¾ teaspoon white enzyme-treated stevia powder (or to taste, See "Sources," page 267) or ¾ cup agave or Fruit Sweet™

3 tablespoons arrowroot or tapioca starch OR ¼ cup quick-cooking ("Minute™") tapioca

1 baked pie crust, recipes on pages 199 to 202

Thoroughly drain the liquid from the canned cherries, if you are using them, and reserve ¾ cup of the liquid. Combine the stevia and thickener with the cherry juice or water (if using fresh or frozen cherries) in a saucepan. If you are using quick-cooking tapioca, let it stand in the liquid for at least five minutes before you begin cooking the filling. Add the cherries and stir. Heat the fruit mixture over low to medium heat, stirring frequently, until it comes to a boil and thickens. Boil it for one minute if you are using the quick-cooking tapioca.

If this is the first time you have made this pie and you are using the stevia, taste the filling after 3 minutes of cooling. If it is not sweet enough for you, sprinkle an additional ⅛ teaspoon of stevia powder over the surface and then stir it in very thoroughly. Taste the filling again and adjust the sweetness to your liking. Record how much stevia you use for the next time you make this.

Allow the filling to cool in the pan, stirring occasionally, for 15 to 30 minutes or until it is lukewarm or cooler and thickening but not set. Put it in the baked cooled pie crust and refrigerate for a few hours before serving.

If you wish to make a traditional two-crust fruit pie, make the white spelt "Flour and Oil" pie crust on page 200. Preheat the oven to 400°F while preparing the filling. Roll and fill the crust as directed on page 202 to 203. Bake the pie at 400°F for 10 minutes. Then reduce the heat to 350°F and bake for 40 to 50 minutes or until the top and bottom crusts are golden brown. Makes one pie or six servings.

For more recipes for desserts made with healthy sweeteners see *Nourishing Traditions*[3], pages 533 to 582. **For sugar-free allergy desserts** including twenty easy all-fruit desserts, see *The Ultimate Food Allergy Cookbook and Survival Guide*, pages 201 to 243.[4]

3 Fallon, Sally with Mary Enig, PhD. *Nourishing Traditions.*, (Brandywine, MD, NewTrends Publishing, 2001), 533-582.

4 Dumke, Nicolette. The *Ultimate Food Allergy Cookbook and Survival Guide.* (Louisville, CO, Allergy Adapt Inc. 2006), 201-243.

Appendix A
Using the Glycemic Index for Weight Loss Without Hunger

The glycemic index (GI) is a system of rating carbohydrate foods according to the effect they have on blood sugar levels of volunteers. The GI score of a food reflects what actually happens to the blood sugar level of real people when they eat that food.

Testing the effect of various carbohydrates on blood sugar levels was first done in the 1980s by Dr. David Jenkins at the University of Toronto in Canada. He tested the effect of a large number of foods on blood sugar levels of many human volunteers, both normal and diabetic. This testing became standardized and led to the development of the glycemic index.

The glycemic index has been clinically proven to be useful in its application to diabetes, weight loss, appetite control, and coronary health.[1] It is used in Australia, Canada, the UK, France, Italy, Sweden, and other countries. Unfortunately, the United States medical establishment remains officially opposed to the glycemic index.[2]

Glycemic index testing results have corrected a common misconception that all starches are "good" complex carbohydrates and sugars are all "bad." Actually, baked Russet potatoes and some types of rice have GI scores that are higher than pure glucose and have a more major effect on our blood sugar level. Corn syrup also has a GI score of over 100, but white sugar falls in the intermediate range with a GI score of 68. This is because each sucrose molecule is made of two single sugars, one glucose and one fructose. The fructose must be processed into glucose by the liver, thus slowing the release of glucose from that half of the sucrose molecule into the bloodstream. The GI score of a food cannot be predicted from whether it contains simple or complex carbohydrates or from the scores of foods in the same food category. For example, fruits have a wide range of GI scores; grains have a similar wide range.

Glycemic index scores for foods are determined using the test results from pure glucose as a reference food and comparing the results from glucose to the results from the test food. For standard glycemic index testing, eight to ten volunteers are given a dose of 50 grams of pure glucose. Their blood is drawn and blood sugar levels are measured periodically over the next two hours. For each volunteer these blood test results

---

1 Brand-Miller, Jennie, PhD, Thomas Wolever, MD, Kay Foster-Powell. MND, and Stephen Colaguiri, MD., *The New Glucose Revolution*, (New York: Marlowe and Company, 2003), 31. Also http://www.montignac.com/en/la_methode_scientifique.php and www.montignac.com/en/la_methode_regime._equilibre.php
2 Brand-Miller, et al., 30.

are plotted on a graph of blood sugar level versus time, and the area under the curve of the graph is calculated. The test is repeated on two or three occasions and the results are averaged. Then, at another time, the volunteer eats a portion of the test food which contains 50 grams of carbohydrate. For example, if bread is the test food, the volunteer eats about 3½ slices of bread. The blood sugar levels are again tested over a two-hour period, plotted on a graph, and the area under the curve of the graph is calculated. This area is divided by that volunteer's average result when glucose was tested and the result of the division is multiplied by 100. The number obtained is the approximate glycemic index score (GI score or GI value) for the test food. This number is averaged with the results obtained for the other volunteers to calculate the GI score for the food tested. These GI tests for various foods have been shown to be reproducible in testing done in many countries around the world. The values obtained are reproduciibly the same for both healthy volunteers and diabetics; however, diabetics have their blood drawn for a three hour period after the test meal rather than for two hours.

To control spikes and dips in blood sugar and weight-depositing insulin spikes or chronically high insulin levels, it is best to choose most carbohydrates in the diet from those that are low on the glycemic index with a GI score of 55 or less. Foods with an intermediate score of 56 to 69 can be eaten in moderation. For best blood sugar and insulin control, high GI foods with scores of 70 or above should be eaten only occasionally. However, there are ways to enjoy favorite high-GI foods more often by preparing them with a healthier recipe that results in a moderate or even low glycemic impact. The development of enzyme-treated stevia, which does not have the potent licorice-like aftertaste that stevia used to have, makes this much easier. It can be heated, unlike some chemically made non-nutritive sweeteners, and is a great way to make sweet treats with a lower glycemic impact.

All high carbohydrate foods should be eaten at the same time as a balancing serving of a protein food. The very sensible, balanced diet in *The Insulin Resistance Diet* by Dr. Cheryle Hart, MD and Mary Kay Grossman, RD links each carbohydrate unit containing 15 grams of carbohydrate with a protein unit containing 7 grams of protein.[3] The various *Zone* diets, which are more restrictive, allow 9 grams of carbohydrate for each 7 grams of protein.[4] The amount of protein required to balance carbohydrate can vary from person to person. It you are having cravings for sweets in spite of balancing carbohydrates with proteins, you may want to limit your carbohydrate intake to one 15-gram unit per meal or snack consumed with at least two units (14 grams) of protein and see if that helps. If you still have cravings for sweets after a few weeks, you may have *Candidiasis*. See page 35 for more about how to eat for this condition.

---

3 Hart, Cheryle R., MD and Mary Kay Grossman, RD, *The Insulin Resistance Diet,* (New York: McGraw-Hill, 2001, 2007), 64.

4 Sears, Barry, PhD, *Mastering the Zone,* (New York, Regan Books, 1997), 30-35, 331.

In addition to the glycemic index score of a meal or food, the quantity eaten also determines the impact the meal or food has on blood sugar and insulin levels. If you eat two cups of cooked pasta, it will have about twice the effect of eating one cup of pasta, or twice the glycemic load.

Using the glycemic index to choose what you eat can help you not to over-stimulate the pancreas which would produce a spike of insulin after any meal or snack. This keeps insulin levels stable and low throughout the course of the day, thus promoting the burning of stored fat rather than the formation and storage of new fat from foods recently eaten. Instead, recently eaten food is used for the immediate energy needs of daily activities. Thus, if your insulin is low and stable, you will use both fat stores and your last meal to produce energy and may notice that you have more energy and are less hungry that you were before you began an eating plan based on glycemic control.

See pages 27 to 30 to read about the glycemic control diet. For more information, go to www.foodallergyandglutenfreeweightloss.com or read *Food Allergy and Gluten-Free Weight Loss* as described on the last pages of this book. You do not have to be on an allergy or gluten-free diet to benefit from the information in these sources. The book contains a chapter of wheat and dairy-containing recipes for normal-diet individuals who will also enjoy the special diet recipes.

Appendix B
Glycemic Index Values for Foods

This table contains glycemic index (GI) values and carbohydrate and protein units for most unprocessed foods. Unfortunately, GI scores for many processed foods are not in this table because they vary from brand to brand and at different times as manufacturers change ingredients or change how the food is processed. In addition, there is a lack of GI data on processed foods because GI scores can be determined only by testing using human volunteers, and very little of this is done in the United States.[5] Without testing specific brands or foods made with specific recipes, it is impossible to accurately know a food's GI score because, for example, two brands of whole wheat bread may be made with different ingredients and different leavening systems or yeast rising times. These differences will then affect the glycemic impact of the bread.

In spite of the lack of GI scores for some foods, the GI values table can guide our food choices. It is possible to work around the lack of data for bread, crackers, and other foods made from grains by using the GI scores of cooked whole grains in this table plus the information in this paragraph to determine trends which help us make wide decisions about what to eat. For example, notice that whole wheat and white bread share very similar GI scores. This is because most flour is very finely milled with metal rollers; thus whole wheat flour is as fine and rapidly digested as white flour. However, the GI score for bread made from stone ground whole wheat flour is lower. Therefore, you might read labels and purchase or bake bread and crackers containing stone ground flour of a variety of kinds, such as Bob's Red Mill™ stone ground quinoa flour. You also might choose baked goods made with grains which have lower on the GI scores from the GI scores of cooked whole grains on page 214. In addition, note the one-carbohydrate unit serving sizes as you decide which grains you wish to eat most often, either as cooked grains or in bread products. When you choose grains with larger one-unit serving sizes, you are allowed to eat more of the grain-containing foods.

In the absence of GI testing on many grain-based foods, the advice given by Dr. Jennie Brand-Miller for choosing a commercially made low GI bread is to use bread that contains a high amount of legume flours (garbanzo or chickpea flour, fava bean flour, soy flour, etc.) and/or that includes high-fiber additions such a psyllium husks, whole grain kernels, nuts or seeds.

In the book *AnitCancer,* Dr. David Servan-Schreiber gives similar advice for the type of bread cancer patients should eat. He recommends eating bread with three or

5 GI scores for Australian brands of bread, etc. are found in the *New Glucose Revolution* series of books. In addition, GI scores from many countries around the world are found on www.mendosa.com/gilists. htm and www.glycemicindex.com .

more grains added such as rye, oat, flaxseeds, etc. or eating sourdough bread, which has a lower GI score than other types of yeast bread due to the acid produced by the *Lactobacillus* fermentation.[6]

Do not permit this table to induce you to weigh your food routinely. If you are uncertain about how large a serving size should be, weigh it once, or only occasionally for rarely-eaten foods, and then judge the portion by appearance the next time you eat that food. The best practice is to eat foods that are as close to nature as possible and only use these tables as a guideline for choosing low GI carbohydrate foods and for linking and balancing your carbohydrate and protein foods. Practice listening to your body rather than becoming legalistic about your food.

The information in this table was derived from several sources.[7] Some values are missing from the data for some foods because either it is not available (i.e. many vegetables have such a low carbohydrate content that they cannot be tested for a GI score) or it does not apply to that food (i.e. GI scores do not apply to foods which contain no carbohydrates such as meat).

6 Servan-Schreiber, David, MD, PhD. *AntiCancer: A New Way of Life.* (New York: Penguin Group, Inc., 2009), 69.

7 Hart, Cheryle R., MD and Mary Kay Grossman, RD, *The Insulin Resistance Diet,* (New York: McGraw-Hill, 2001, 2007), 44-61; Brand-Miller, Jennie, PhD, Kate Marsh , and Phillipa Sandall, *The New Glucose Revolution: Low GI and Gluten-Free Eating Made Easy,* (Cambridge, MA: Da Capo Press, 2008), 224-243; Brand-Miller, Jennie, PhD and Kay Foster-Powell. MND, *The New Glucose Revolution Shoppers Guide to GI Values,* (Cambridge, MA: Da Capo Press, 2009 and 2010); www.montignac.com/en/ig_tableau.php ; www.mendosa.com/gilists.htm ; and *Food Processor for Windows, Version 7.7,* by ESHA Research, Inc., P.O. Box 13028, Salem, OR 97309.

Food	Serving Size	Carb Units	Glycemic Index Score	GI Range

Carbohydrate Foods
Fruits

Food	Serving Size	Carb Units	Glycemic Index Score	GI Range
Apple, raw	1 medium (5 oz.)	1 or 0[8]	36	LOW
Applesauce, unsweetened	½ cup	1	42	LOW
Apples, dried	4 rings (1 oz.)	1	29	X-LOW[9]
Apricots, raw	2 large or 4 small (6 oz.)	1	38[10]	LOW
Apricots, dried	7 halves (1 oz.)	1	30	X-LOW
Banana	½ small (4") or ½ cup slices (2¾ oz.)	1	52	LOW
Blueberries	¾ cup (4 oz.)	1	53	LOW
Cantaloupe	⅓ of a 5" melon (6 oz.)	1	65	MED
Cherries, dark	⅝ cup (3½ oz.)	1	63	MED
Cherries, sour	⅝ cup (3½ oz.)	1	22	X-LOW
Dates, pitted	3 medium (1 oz.)	1	45	LOW
Grapefruit	1 small (3½") or ½ large (6 oz. without peel)	1 or 0[8]	25	X-LOW
Grapes	1 cup (3½ oz.)	1	53	LOW
Kiwi fruit	2 small (4 oz.)	1	53	LOW
Mango	½ medium (3½ oz.)	1	51	LOW
Nectarine	1 medium (5 oz.)	1	43	LOW
Orange	1 3-inch diameter (5 oz.)	1	42	LOW
Papaya	½ large (7 oz.)	1	59	MED
Peach, raw	2 small or 1 large (8 oz.)	1 or 0[8]	42	LOW
Peach, canned in juice	2 small halves (5 oz.)	1	45	LOW
Peach, dried	2 halves (1 oz.)	1	35	LOW

[8] Raw apple, pear, peach, plum, and grapefruit don't have to be balanced with protein in a meal or a snack because they are very high in fiber and the carbohydrate they contain is mostly fructose. Therefore, the impact these fruits have on blood sugar and insulin levels is low and slow. However, if these fruits are cooked, juiced, canned, or otherwise processed, the carbohydrate they contain is absorbed more quickly, so they must be balanced with protein. In that case, the serving size given in this table will count as one carbohydrate unit.

[9] X-LOW indicates that the glycemic index score of this food is extremely low (less than 35). These foods are usually included in the low range. On this chart, LOW means a score of 35 to 55, MED means 56 to 69, and HIGH means 70 or greater.

[10] The GI score of raw apricots on mendosa.com is 34. *The New Glucose Revolution: Low GI and Gluten-Free Eating Made Easy* gives it a score of 38 and *The New Glucose Revolution Shopper's Guide* gives it a score of 57 (medium range).

Food	Serving Size	Carb Units	Glycemic Index Score	GI Range
Pear, raw	1 small (4¼ oz.)	1 or 0[8]	38	LOW
Pear, canned in juice	2 halves (5 oz.)	1	44	LOW
Pear, dried	1½ halves (5 oz.)	1	43	LOW
Pineapple chunks, fresh	¾ cup (4½ oz.)	1	66	MED
Pineapple chunks, canned with juice	⅜ cup (3½ oz.)	1	59	MED
Plum, raw	2 medium (4½ oz.)	1 or 0[8]	39	LOW
Plum, dried (prune)	3 medium (1 oz.)	1	29	LOW
Raisins	2 tbsp. (¾ oz.)	1	64	MED
Strawberries, fresh	15 large, 1½ cups (6 oz.)	1	40	LOW
Strawberries, frozen unsweetened	¾ cup thawed (6 oz.)	1	40	LOW
Watermelon, cubed	1½ cups (8 oz.)	1	76	HIGH

Cooked Whole Grains

Food	Serving Size	Carb Units	Glycemic Index Score	GI Range
Barley, pearled	⅓ cup (2½ oz.)	1	25	X-LOW
Buckwheat	½ cup (3 oz.)	1	54	LOW
Millet	⅓ cup (2½ oz.)	1	71	HIGH
Sorghum (milo)	½ cup (3 oz.)	1	39	LOW
Polenta (cornmeal)	⅓ cup (2¾ oz.)	1	68	MED
Quinoa	½ cup (3½ oz.)	1	53	LOW
Rice, brown (most)	⅓ cup (2¾ oz.)	1	50 to 69	MED-HIGH
Rice, brown basmati	⅓ cup (2¾ oz.)	1	58	MED
Rice, white (most)	⅓ cup (2¾ oz.)	1	76 to 98	HIGH
Rice, white, Uncle Ben's™ converted	⅓ cup (2¾ oz.)	1	45	LOW
Rice, wild	½ cup (3 oz.)	1	57	MED
Wheat, cracked (bulgur)	½ cup (3½ oz.)	1	46	LOW
Whole wheat kernels	½ cup (4 oz.)	1	41	LOW

Food	Serving Size	Carb Units	Glycemic Index Score	GI Range

Grain-based Baked Goods
(Bread, Tortillas, Crackers, etc.)

This section probably lacks the information you most want – the one-carbohydrate unit serving size and GI score for your favorite "normal," allergy or gluten-free bread.[11] Lacking that, use the GI scores of cooked whole grains opposite plus the information below to determine trends that you can use in your food choices. Notice that whole wheat and white bread share very similar GI scores because most flour is very finely milled with metal rollers; thus whole wheat flour is as fine and rapidly digested as white flour. However, the GI score for bread made from stone ground whole wheat flour is lower. Therefore, you might read labels and purchase or bake bread and crackers containing stone ground flour of other kinds, such as Bob's Red Mill™ stone ground quinoa flour. Also, notice that the GI scores for sourdough bread are lower, making sourdough bread made with any grain you tolerate a good choice. In addition, note the one-carbohydrate unit serving sizes as you decide which grains you wish to eat most often in bread products. In the absence of GI testing on many grain-based foods, the advice given by Dr. Jennie Brand-Miller for choosing a commercially made low GI bread is to use bread that contains a high amount of legume flours (garbanzo or chickpea flour, fava bean flour, soy flour, etc.) and/or that includes additions such a psyllium husks, whole grain kernels, nuts or seeds.[12]

Food	Serving Size	Carb Units	Glycemic Index Score	GI Range
Bagel, white wheat	½ of a 4" or ⅓ of a 5"	1	72	HIGH
Barley bread[13]	1 slice (1-1½ oz.)	1	43 to 67	LOW-MED
Buckwheat bread[13]	1 slice (1-1½ oz.)	1	47 to 67	LOW-MED
Chickpea bread[13]	1 slice (1-1½ oz.)	1	55 to 67	MED
Corn tortilla	1 thin 6-inch tortilla	1	46 to 52	LOW
Rice bread[13]	1 slice (1 oz.)	1	72	HIGH

---

[11] Since very little GI testing is done in the United States, American brands are not found in the information that was available for compiling this table. This list of GI scores for breads contains only general information, not information from testing American brands, and scores can vary from brand to brand. The rice bread listed here is of unknown composition so its GI score could easily be higher than 58. Read the label on your bread to insure that your serving contains 15 grams of net carbohydrate (total grams of carbohydrate minus grams of fiber) and thus is the amount of bread to equal one carbohydrate unit. The list of GI scores for cooked whole grains is also woefully incomplete because some very useful gluten-free foods such as amaranth have never been tested.

[12] For more about gluten-free bread see question 19 on the FAQs page from the glycemicindex.com website. http://www.glycemicindex.com/faqsList.php

[13] The GI scores from several alternative grain breads in this section of the table are from these breads made in other countries. The scores came from http://www.mendosa.com/gilists.htm and *The New Glucose Revolution: Low GI and Gluten-Free Eating Made Easy*.

Food	Serving Size	Carb Units	Glycemic Index Score	GI Range
Rice cake, puffed	¾ ounce	1	82	HIGH
Rice crackers	¾ ounce	1	91	HIGH
Rye bread, sourdough	1 slice (1-1½ oz.)	1	42	LOW
Rye bread, whole grain[13, 14]	½ to 1 slice (1-1½ oz.)	1	40 to 72	LOW-HIGH
Rye crispbread	½ ounce	1	63	MED
Sourdough wheat bread[13]	1 slice (1-1½ oz.)	1	54	LOW
Spelt bread[13]	1 slice (1-1½ oz.)	1	54 to 74	LOW -HIGH
White bread (average)	1 slice (1-1½ oz.)	1	75	HIGH
Whole wheat bread (average)	1 slice (1-1½ oz.)	1	74	HIGH
Whole wheat bread, stone ground	1 slice (1-1½ oz.)	1	59 to 66	MED
Whole wheat crackers with sesame seeds	½ ounce	1	54	LOW
Whole wheat tortilla[13]	½ 10-inch tortilla	1	30	LOW

Pasta

Pasta may be a low to medium GI food if it is prepared properly; the scores in this table reflect proper preparation. Pasta should be *al dente,* with resistance to the tooth. If it is over-cooked, it will have a higher GI score and more adverse impact on blood sugar levels.

Food	Serving Size	Carb Units	Glycemic Index Score	GI Range
Corn pasta	½ cup (2 oz.)	1	78	HIGH
Mung bean noodles	⅓ cup (2 oz.)	1	59	MED
Rice pasta	⅓ cup (2 oz.)	1	61	MED
Semolina (durum wheat) pasta	½ cup (2 oz.)	1	35 to 59	LOW-MED
Soba (buckwheat) pasta	⅝ cup (2½ oz.)	1	59	MED

Beverages

Food	Serving Size	Carb Units	Glycemic Index Score	GI Range
Apple juice	½ cup (4 oz.)	1	44	LOW
Beer	12 ounces (1 can)	1	66 to 110	MED-HIGH
Carrot juice, fresh	1 cup (8 oz.)	1	43	LOW
Coffee, unsweetened[15]	8 ounces	0[15]	-	-
Cranberry-apple juice,	½ cup (4 oz.)	1	52	LOW
Grape juice, 100% juice	⅜ cup (3 oz.)	1	53	LOW
Grapefruit juice, 100% jc	⅞ cup (7 oz.)	1	45	LOW

---

[14] The GI scores on http://www.mendosa.com/gilists.htm were as low as 40 for some types of rye bread.

[15] Diet soda and coffee or tea prepared without sugar or nutritive sweeteners contain no carbohydrate. However, caffeinated beverages and diet sodas should be consumed with food to moderate caffeine's impact on blood sugar stability.

Food	Serving Size	Carb Units	Glycemic Index Score	GI Range
Pineapple juice, unsweetened	½ cup (4 oz.)	1	46	LOW
Prune juice	⅓ cup (2⅓ oz.)	1	43	LOW
Rice milk, unsweetened[16]	½ cup (4 oz.)	1	86	HIGH
Soy milk, unsweetened[16]	1 cup (8 ounces)	0[17]	43	LOW
Soda, diet	12 ounces (1 can)	0[15]	-	-
Soda, not diet	4 ounces	1	48 to 58	LOW-MED
Tea. unsweetened[15]	8 ounces	0[15]	-	-
Tomato juice, sugar-free	1½ cups (12 oz.)	1	38	LOW
Wine, dessert type	4 ounces	1	not available	MED-HIGH
Wine, no added sugar	8 ounces	0[18]	-	-

Vegetables

Most vegetables are low in carbohydrate, high in vitamins, phytochemicals and other nutrients, and can be eaten in any quantity you'd like. Therefore, the serving size listed in this section of the table for most vegetables is "to satiety." Many vegetables are so low in carbohydrates that they cannot be tested for a GI score, so the score and GI range data for these vegetables is blank. Vegetables such as potatoes and corn are sources of concentrated carbohydrates, so the portion size must be kept to an amount supplying 30 grams of carbohydrate (2 units) or less and must be balanced with protein. Preparation method matters for potatoes, with GI scores higher if baked than if boiled.[19] Baking increases the GI score of Jersey (white) sweet potaotes from 44 to 94; for Russets from 76 to 111. Of sweet potato varieties, orange potatoes have the highest GI scores. Dried legumes are high in protein and count as protein foods when balancing meals or snacks. The carbohydrate they contain is mostly indigestible so is it all right eat these in a quantity sufficient to satisfy your hunger. If you want a vegetable you do not see here, search for its GI score at http://www.mendosa.com/gilists.htm, or if it is not starchy (such as a tuber), eat as much of it as is needed to satisfy hunger.

---

[16] Check the labels on rice and soy milk for sweeteners. If they are sweetened, use the net carbohydrate content to calculate the correct serving size, which will be smaller than for unsweetened milk. See the dairy product section of this table for more about the protein content of soy milk. Rice milk contains a negligible amount of protein and a large amount of high GI carbohydrate.

[17] The carbohydrate in unsweetened soy milk comes from soybeans and, like all carbohydrates from beans, is mostly fiber so doesn't need to be counted or balanced with protein.

[18] The carbohydrates in the grapes used to make wine are completely changed to alcohol during fermentation. This alcohol may or may not (depending on the expert) affect blood sugar balance. Although the zero number of carbohydrate units implies that you do not need to balance wine with protein foods, it is advisable to drink wine with a protein-containing snack.

[19] Scott-Dixon, Krista and Brian St. Pierre. "Sweet vs. Regular Potatoes: Which Potatoes Are Really Healthier?" https://www.precisionnutrition.com/regular-vs-sweet-potatoes

Food	Serving Size	Units	Glycemic Index Score	GI Range
Artichokes	To satiety	-	-	-
Arugula	To satiety	-	-	-
Asparagus	To satiety	-	-	-
Beans, baked	⅓ cup (3 oz.)	1 prot	47 to 55	LOW- MED
Beans, green, wax, etc.	To satiety	-	-	-
Beans, green baby lima	To satiety	-	32	LOW
Beets	To satiety	-	52	LOW
Broccoli	To satiety	-	-	-
Cauliflower	To satiety	-	-	-
Cabbage, any kind	To satiety	-	-	-
Carrots, raw	To satiety	-	16	X- LOW
Carrots, boiled	To satiety	-	41	LOW
Cassava (yucca), boiled	⅓ cup (1½ oz.)	1 carb	94	HIGH
Corn, kernels	½ cup (3 oz.)	1 carb	37 to 46	LOW
Corn on the cob	1 small	1 carb	48	LOW
Cucumber	To satiety	-	-	-
Eggplant	To satiety	-	-	-
Fennel	To satiety	-	-	-
Garlic	To satiety	-	-	-
Green beans, any kind	To satiety	-	-	-
Greenss (collards, kale)	To satiety	-	-	-
Legumes, dried, cooked	⅓ cup	1 prot	22 to 42	X-LOW- LOW
including black, cannellini, garbanzo, kidney, navy, pinto, soy, and white lima beans, lentils and split peas				
Legumes, chana dal	⅓ cup	1 prot	8 to 11	X-LOW
Lettuce, any kind	To satiety	-	-	-
Mushrooms, any kind	To satiety	-	-	-
Onions, any kind	To satiety	-	-	-
Parsnips	To satiety	-	52	LOW
Plantain, boiled	⅓ cup (1¾ oz.)	1 carb	40	LOW
Peas	To satiety	-	45	LOW
Peppers, all kinds	To satiety	-	-	-
Potato, new red, boiled	4 1-inch (5 oz.)	1 carb	59	MED
Potato, Russet, baked,	1 small (4½ oz.)	1 carb	111	HIGH
Potato, Russet, boiled	1 small (4½ oz.)	1 carb	76	HIGH
Potato, sweet Jersey, baked	½ medium (2⅔ oz.)	1 carb	94	HIGH
Potato, sweet Jersey, boiled	½ medium (2⅔ oz.)	1 carb	44	LOW
Potato, sweet orange, boiled	½ medium (2⅔ oz.)	1 carb	66	MED
Pumpkin, canned	1 cup	1 carb	64	MED
Spinach	To satiety	-	-	-
Squash, any kind	To satiety	-	-	-
Swiss chard	To satiety	-	-	-
Taro root	¼ cup (2 oz.)	1 carb	56	MED
Tomatoes, raw, cooked, canned, paste, sauce, or puree	To satiety	-	-	-
Turnips	To satiety	-	-	-
Water chestnuts	To satiety	-	-	-
Yam, true (bitter)	½ cup (2½ oz.)	1 carb	74	HIGH

Food	Serving Size	Units	GI Score	GI Range	Grams of Fat/serving

Protein Foods
Dairy and Egg Products

Dairy products make delicious and convenient protein snacks for a healthy eating plan. This table gives approximate grams of fat per serving, but read the label from your cheese, milk, or yogurt to determine how much fat you are ingesting. The fat in dairy products from pasture-fed animals contains a healthy omega-3 to omega-6 ratio fatty acids so can be consumed liberally, but limit fat from conventionally-raised cattle.

Food	Serving Size	Units	GI Score	GI Range	Grams of Fat/serving
Buttermilk	1 cup	1 prot	-	-	2
Cheese, hard, fat-free	1 ounce	1 prot	-	-	0
Cheese, hard, low-fat	1 ounce	1 prot	-	-	2
Cheese, hard, regular	1 ounce	1 prot	-	-	9
Cheese, mozzarella, part skim	1 ounce	1 prot	-	-	4
Cottage cheese, 1% fat	¼ cup	1 prot	-	-	0.5
Cottage cheese, 2% fat	¼ cup	1 prot	-	-	1
Cottage cheese, creamed	¼ cup	1 prot	-	-	2
Cottage cheese, dry curd	⅓ cup	1 prot	-	-	0
Cottage cheese, nonfat	¼ cup	1 prot	-	-	0
Cream cheese, nonfat	3 tbsp.	1 prot	-	-	0.5
(See page 222 for regular or reduced fat cream cheese).					
Egg substitute	¼ cup	1 prot	-	-	2
Egg, whites	2	1 prot	-	-	0
Egg, whole (large)	1	1 prot	-	-	5
Ice cream, sweetened with corn sweeteners or sugar	½ cup	½ prot/1 carb	51	LOW	4 to 12
Ice cream, no sugar added	1 cup	1 prot	-	-	4 to 12
Milk, cow's, 1% fat	1 cup	1 prot	-	-	3
Milk, cow's, 2 % fat	1 cup	1 prot	-	-	5
Milk, cow's, nonfat	1 cup	1 prot	-	-	0
Milk, cow's, flavored and sweetened	1 cup	1 prot/2 carb	26 to 31	LOW	0 to 10
Milk, cow's, whole	1 cup	1 prot	-	-	8 to 10
Milk, goat's, whole	1 cup	1 prot	-	-	10
Milk shake	⅔ cup	½ prot/2 carb	GI data not available		5
Milk, soy, sweetened	1 cup	1 prot/1 carb	31	LOW	5 to 20
Milk, soy, unsweetened	1 cup	1 prot	-	-	5 to 20
Pudding, sugar free	1 cup	1 prot/1 carb	40	LOW	3 to 8
Pudding, sweetened with corn sweeteners or sugar	½ cup	½ prot/1½ carb	40 to 47	LOW	3 to 8
Ricotta cheese, part skim	¼ cup	1 prot	-	-	5

Food	Serving Size	Units	GI Score	GI Range	Grams of Fat/serving
Ricotta cheese, regular	¼ cup	1 prot	-	-	8
Romano cheese	⅓ cup (1 oz.)	1 prot	-	-	8
Yogurt, flavored, no sugar added	1 cup	1 prot	-	-	0 to 8
Yogurt, plain	1 cup	1 prot	-	-	0 to 8
Yogurt, sweetened with corn sweetener, sugar or honey	1 cup	1 prot/2 carb	14 to 54	LOW	0 to 8

Meat, Poultry and Fish

Since meat, poultry and fish contain no carbohydrate, they may be eaten in a quantity sufficient to satisfy. The amounts given below for "serving size" are usually one ounce or the amount that will yield one protein unit (7 grams of protein) for the purpose of balancing these protein foods with the carbohydrate foods on the previous pages. However, for a meal you will probably eat 3 or 4 ounces of meat; the amount must be equal to or greater than the number of carbohydrate units you eat at that meal, which is two units at the most. If you eat meat from pasture-fed animals, the fat they contain has a healthy omega-3 to omega-6 fatty acid ratio so can be consumed liberally.

Processed meats are usually high in unhealthy fat and may contain sugar or corn sweeteners so should not be eaten on a regular basis. Check the package label to determine one protein unit (7 grams of protein) and how much fat you will consume.

As long as the meat, poultry or fish you are eating is unprocessed and healthily raised, do not be overly concerned about the portion size, but rather listen to your body and eat until your hunger is satisfied. As you can see from the listing for chicken or turkey, removing the skin (as recommended by standard weight loss diets) saves you just one gram of fat per ounce of meat, so don't deprive yourself if you enjoy the skin. Fat in meat slows digestion and makes your meal satisfy you longer.

Food	Serving Size	Units	GI Score	GI Range	Grams of Fat/serving
Bacon, raw weight	1 strip (0.8 oz.)	¼ prot	-	-	3 to 13
Beef, broiled, or ground beef, broiled or pan-cooked and thoroughly drained					
90% lean ground beef	1 oz.	1 prot	-	-	2 to 3
80% lean ground beef	1 oz.	1 prot	-	-	4 to 5
73% lean "regular" gr. beef	1 oz.	1 prot	-	-	7 to 10
Prime rib roast, ¼" trim	1 oz.	1 prot	-	-	8
Round (rump) roast or steak, ¼" trim	1 oz.	1 prot	-	-	3
Sirloin, ¼" trim	1 oz.	1 prot	-	-	3
Well-marbled steak such as T-bone, ¼" trim	1 oz.	1 prot	-	-	6
Bison (buffalo)	1 oz.	1 prot	-	-	1
Bologna	3 pieces (2 oz.)	1 prot	-	-	16

Food	Serving Size	Units	GI Score	GI Range	Grams of Fat/serving
Chicken or turkey, roasted					
Breast meat, no skin	1 oz.	1 prot	-	-	1
Breast meat, with skin	1 oz.	1 prot	-	-	2
Dark meat, no skin	1 oz.	1 prot	-	-	3
Dark meat, with skin	1 oz.	1 prot	-	-	4
Clams (meat only)	1½ oz.	1 prot	-	-	3
Crab or lobster meat	1 oz.	1 prot	-	-	0.2
Duck	1 oz.	1 prot	-	-	3
Elk or venison	1 oz.	1 prot	-	-	1
Ham, baked	1 oz.	1 prot	-	-	1 to 4
Hot dog, all beef	1½ (2¼ oz.)	1 prot	-	-	13 to 16
Hot dog, all turkey	1 (1½ oz.)	1 prot	-	-	8
Lamb leg, ¼" trim	1 oz.	1 prot	-	-	3
Oysters (meat only)	2½ oz.	1 prot	-	-	2
Pork chop, braised, ¼" trim	1 oz.	1 prot	-	-	5 to 7
Salmon, broiled	1 oz.	1 prot	-	-	2
Shrimp (meat only)	1½ oz.	1 prot	-	-	0.5
Trout, baked	1 oz.	1 prot	-	-	1
Tuna, water packed	1 oz.	1 prot	-	-	0.2
Turkey, ground (8% fat)	1 oz.	1 prot	-	-	2
White fish, poached, baked or broiled (cod, flounder, sole, halibut, etc.)	1 oz.	1 prot	-	-	0.2

Nuts, Seeds, and Nut Butters

Nuts, seeds, and nut and seed butters are great carry-along protein snack foods because they require no refrigeration. Almonds have not gone rancid when kept in my car for months. If your goal is to control inflammation, nuts and seeds are good sources of omega-3 fatty acids, so include them in your diet liberally. Although I could not find a GI score for chia seeds, here is information that indicates they can be consumed on a low-GI diet: http://www.mendosa.com/blog/?p=233

Food	Serving Size	Units	GI Score	GI Range	Grams of Fat/serving
Almond butter, natural[20]	3 tbsp.	1 prot	-	-	28
Almonds	1½ oz.	1 prot	-	-	22
Cashew butter, natural[19]	2 tbsp.	1 prot	-	-	16
Cashews	1½ oz.	1 prot	-	-	22
Chestnuts	5 (2 oz.)	1 carb/¼ prot	54	LOW	1
Hemp seeds[21]	4 teaspoons	-	-	LOW	-

---

20 Natural nut butters are made from nuts and salt and contain no sweeteners.

21 An estimated GI range for hemp seeds is here: http://www.formulazone.com/Help.asp?TID=ILUP&IID=075021&food=Hemp%20Seeds

Food	Serving Size	Units	GI Score	GI Range	Grams of Fat/serving
Macadamia nuts	3 oz.	1 prot	-	-	65
Peanut butter, natural[19]	2 tbsp.	1 prot	-	-	16
Peanuts, shelled	1 oz.	1 prot	-	-	14
Pecans	3 oz.	1 prot	-	-	61
Pine nuts	1 oz.	1 prot	-	-	14
Pumpkin seeds	1¼ oz.	1 prot	-	-	7
Sunflower seeds, shelled	¼ cup	1 prot	-	-	16
Tahini (sesame seed butter)[19]	2 tbsp.	1 prot	-	-	16
Walnuts, black	2 oz.	1 prot	-	-	32
Walnuts, English	1½ oz.	1 prot	-	-	28

Other Foods

Fats

The foods listed in this section do not contain significant amounts of protein or carbohydrates so they are not listed in the carbohydrate or protein food sections of this table and the "units" column below is blank. The information here is to help you know the amount of fat you eat per day. Don't deprive yourself however; avocados, many oils and dairy products from pasture-raised animals are great sources of healthy fats and make meals satisfy longer.

Food	Serving Size	Units	GI Score	GI Range	Grams of Fat/serving
Avocado	1 medium (7 oz.)	-	-	-	31
Butter	1 pat (1 tsp.)	-	-	-	4
Cream cheese	2 tbsp.	-	-	-	10
Cream cheese, low fat (Neufchatel)	2 tbsp.	-	-	-	6
Cream – table or light	2 tbsp.	-	-	-	6
Cream – whipping	2 tbsp.	-	-	-	11
Oils, cooking such as olive, canola, safflower, grapeseed, and nut oils	2 tsp.	-	-	-	9
Salad dressing					
Blue cheese	1 tbsp.	-	-	-	5 to 8
French	1 tbsp.	-	-	-	6 to 10
Italian	1 tbsp.	-	-	-	3 to 13

Other types of dressing – Read the nutrition label to determine the fat content

Food	Serving Size	Carb Units	GI Score	GI Range	Grams of Fat/serving

Snack Foods

Highly processed snack foods should be avoided by cancer patients and should be rare treats eaten in moderate quantities for healthy people. Dr. Cheryle Hart recommends dark chocolate for frequent controlled splurges because of its high level of nutrients that stimulate the production of neurotransmitters. With the information in this section of the table you will be able determine what size serving of a snack food is within the two carbohydrate unit (30 gram) limit for a meal or snack and how much protein you need to balance it.

Food	Serving Size	Carb Units	GI Score	GI Range	Grams of Fat/serving
Chocolate, dark, plain	1 oz.	1 carb	41	LOW	9 to 11
Chocolate, milk, plain	1 oz.	1 carb	41	LOW	8 to 10
Corn chips	1 oz.	1 carb	42 to 74	LOW- HIGH	8
Jelly beans	6 (¾ oz.)	1 carb	78	HIGH	0
Mars™ fun-size bar	1 oz.	1¼ carb	51	LOW	19
Popcorn, popped with oil	2¾ cups (1.1 oz.)	1 carb	65	MED	8
Potato chips	1 oz.	1 carb	51 to 59	LOW-MED	8

Sweeteners and Spreads

Food	Serving Size	Carb Units	GI Score	GI Range	Grams of Fat/serving
Agave[22]	4 tsp. (¾ oz.)	1 carb	19	X-LOW	0
Corn syrup[23]	1 tbsp. (⅔ oz.)	1 carb	115	HIGH	0
Grape jelly	1 tbsp. (½ oz.)	1 carb	52	LOW	0
Honey, single source	3 tsp. (¾ oz.)	1 carb	35	LOW	0
Maple syrup, pure	3 tsp. (¾ oz.)	1 carb	54	LOW	0
Orange marmalade	1 tbsp. (½ oz.)	1 carb	48	LOW	0
Strawberry jam	1 tbsp. (½ oz.)	1 carb	46	LOW	0
Sugars, pure					
Fructose	1 tbsp. (½ oz.)	1 carb	19	X-LOW	0
Glucose	1 tbsp. (½ oz.)	1 carb	100	HIGH	0
Sucrose (table sugar)	4 tsp. (⅔ oz.)	1 carb	60 to 68	MED	0

---

[22] The GI score given for agave is an average of agave scores which vary between different sources. All are in the extremely low GI range, however

[23] This GI score came from www.montignac.com/en/ig_tableau.php .

Appendix C
Allergies, Inflammation and Weight

There is a relationship between food allergies, inflammation, and weight gain. This appendix gives a brief overview of the subject, which is covered in detail in *Food Allergy and Gluten-Free Weight Loss*[1] and on the website www.foodallergyandglutenfreeweight-loss.com. Visit one of these resources to learn how the correct eating plan for you will help you slim down without hunger or deprivation.

Food allergies, inflammation and weight problems are intimately related. Eating foods to which you are allergic causes inflammation which makes your adrenal glands secrete hormones which destabilize your insulin and blood sugar levels. The high level of insulin affects the activity of two enzymes which cause your body to retain and deposit fat rather than burning it for energy. (See the last paragraph on page 28 to page 29 for details). Thus, food allergies can lead to weight gain, and a high amount of body fat can promote inflammation and exacerbate problems with allergies.

Excess body fat contributes to inflammation, although we may not be aware that we are experiencing silent inflammation. As we gain weight, our bodies do not add more fat cells. Rather, the fat cells we already have become larger and filled with more fat. The cells leak as they are increasingly stretched. Then immune cells called macrophages migrate to the area to clean up the mess. The macrophages release inflammatory substances in the fatty tissues as they are cleaning up.[2] This inflammatory response may be the mechanism behind many of the negative effects of overweight on health.

When your body counteracts this inflammation by producing anti-inflammatory substances, some of them interfere with the function of the hormone leptin. In optimally healthy people, leptin is responsible for automatically maintaining weight at their best level.[3] Some people do not gain weight no matter what they eat. If they overeat, their well-functioning leptin control system boosts their metabolism and decreases their appetite to restore them to their best weight. When leptin is made ineffective by inflammation, the dysfunction is called leptin resistance, meaning that even though you have normal or high[4] levels of leptin, your leptin does not work to suppress appetite and speed metabolism, so it is a struggle to achieve or maintain a healthy weight.

This may sound like a depressing vicious cycle. Excess fat leads to inflammation and the substances that counteract inflammation (which are necessary to keep silent

1 Dumke, Nicolette. *Food Allergy and Gluten-Free Weight Loss*. (Allergy Adapt Inc., Louisville, CO, 2012).

2 Galland, Leo, MD, *The Fat Resistance Diet*, (New York: Broadway Books, 2005), 33.

3 Galland, *The Fat Resistance Diet*, 32-33.

4 Leptin levels are usually high among those who are overweight.

inflammation from causing symptoms) make it impossible for the body's weight-control hormone, leptin, to function properly. Don't despair though – there is a way to break this cycle. There is also good news: As you slim down, leptin resistance abates, so when you reach a healthy weight, you should not have to struggle to maintain your weight. Your newly-functional leptin system will control your appetite and weight. Weight loss is actually not about calories; it is about controlling hormones such as insulin, cortisol, and leptin and decreasing inflammation.

So how do we reduce inflammation? A very important way is to control the type of fat we consume. Prostaglandins are made from the fats we eat. Some prostaglandins promote inflammation and some reduce it. (These anti-inflammatory prostaglandins are not the anti-inflammatory substances responsible for leptin resistance). The essential omega-3 fatty acids eicosapentaenoic acid (EPA) and docosahexaenoic acid (DHA) tip the balance toward the production of anti-inflammatory prostaglandins. Although optimally healthy people can make EPA and DHA from other omega-3 fatty acids, those of us with allergies may lack this ability so we must get preformed EPA and DHA. The best dietary source of these fatty acids is fatty fish. Most people need more omega-3 fatty acids than they can consume easily by eating fish, so benefit from fish oil supplementation. If you do not tolerate fish oil or prefer a more tasty way of consuming essential fatty acids, see the seed milk smoothie recipes on pages 188 to 189. I personally find that having a smoothie every day keeps the skin on my fingertips crack-free, unlike fish oil.

Some foods also have anti-inflammatory properties for a variety of other reasons besides the nature of their fat. These foods contain powerful bioflavanoids, carotenoids, and other anti-inflammatory substances.[5] They include ginger, cherries, blueberries, other dark berries, pomegranates and some other fruits, vegetables, seasonings, and beverages. These foods should be added to your diet in generous amounts to help control inflammation. For a list of these foods, see page 227.

Another and probably the most essential way to reduce inflammation is to stabilize and reduce insulin levels. In *The Anti-Inflammatory Zone*, Barry Sears, PhD describes his work with members of the Stanford University swim team during one summer and how he improved their stamina and performance by giving them EPA and GLA (another essential fatty acid, gamma-linolenic acid) in individualized regimens. However, when the school year started in the fall, their performance deteriorated and they became fatigued easily. Dr. Sears began to suspect that the cause was that high-carbohydrate processed dormitory food was raising their insulin levels. Library research confirmed his suspicion when he found a study which demonstrated that high insulin activates an enzyme that increases the production of pro-inflammatory substances. He had the swimmers change their diets and their performance improved. His conclusion was that following an eating plan which controls blood sugar and insulin levels results in the

---

5 Galland, *The Fat Resistance Diet*, 92-94.

balance of prostaglandins being more anti-inflammatory, resulting in less silent inflammation.[6] Although the goal of the swimmers was not weight loss, his findings also apply to those who wish to lose weight because when inflammation decreases, leptin becomes more active, and we lose weight more easily.

Some individuals are aware of their inflammation problems; they have allergic reactions, asthma, arthritis, inflammatory bowel disease, etc. Following a healthy eating plan for blood sugar control, taking a daily dose of fish oil in individually-correct amounts or consuming one of the smoothies on pages 188 to 189, and adding anti-inflammatory foods to the diet will help decrease inflammation. Those with food allergies must also eliminate their food allergens to control inflammation. Dr. Leo Galland writes about putting patients on diets designed to reduce inflammation and says, "those who were overweight began losing weight without even trying" as they saw their allergies, asthma, arthritis, or other inflammatory conditions improve.[7]

Therefore, a healthy eating plan should include three tools to improve health through controlling inflammation: (1) eating in a way that eliminates blood sugar and insulin spikes and maintains insulin at a relatively constant low level by following a linked-and-balanced, glycemic index controlled diet as discussed on pages 27 to 30; (2) the inclusion of a generous amount of anti-inflammatory foods in meals and snacks, and (3) the elimination of food allergens. If you eat this way to lose weight, your inflammatory health problems may improve, and if you do it to control inflammation, your weight should normalize. An additional benefit will be the normalization of your level of cortisol, the inflammation-dampening adrenal hormone. This may also lead to better sleep because excess cortisol depletes brain chemicals such at the neurotransmitter serotonin.[8]

You have much to gain from an eating plan that controls blood sugar levels and inflammation: hunger-free weight loss, improvement in inflammatory health conditions, better sleep, reduced risk of cancer or a cancer relapse, improvement in diabetes control and more. You have nothing to lose but some excess pounds. Perhaps you might consider giving glycemic controlled eating a try.

---

6 Sears, Barry, PhD, *The Anti-Inflammation Zone*, (New York, Regan Books, 2005), 215-216.

7 Galland, *The Fat Resistance Diet*, 32.

8 Beale, Lucy and Joan Clark, RD, CDE, *The Complete Idiot's Guide to Glycemic Index Weight Loss*, (New York: Alpha, 2005), 23, 27.

Appendix D
Anti-Inflammatory Foods

The foods in this section contain a variety of nutrients that moderate inflammation. Nuts, seeds, and high-fat fish such as salmon contain omega-3 fatty acids that dampen inflammation. Yogurt promotes the establishment of friendly intestinal flora and helps normalize immunity. However, most of the foods listed here quiet inflammation because of the wide variety of phytonutrients (bioflavanoids and carotenoids) they contain. Luteolin (found in green bell peppers and possibly other bell peppers) has an anti-inflammatory effect because it blocks the production of interleukin-6, a powerful promoter of inflammation. Green tea has a very potent anti-inflammatory effect due to its high level of catechin polymers, especially epigallocatechin gallate (EGCG).[1] Citrus flavanoids are found in grapefruit and oranges. Darkly colored fruits are potently anti-inflammatory because they contain high levels of anthocyanidins, so eat plenty of blueberries, cherries, and pomegranates. Resveratrol is found in red grapes and red wine. The vitamin A precursor beta-carotene is found in large amounts in carrots, broccoli, and arugula. Celery and celery seed contain over 20 anti-inflammatory compounds including apigenin.[2] Although this is a secondary effect of foods that dampen inflammation, the catechins in blueberries and green tea stimulate fat-burning in abdominal fat cells which promotes weight loss especially in the mid-section of the body.[3]

Most of the foods on this list come from the "Top 40 Superfoods" list in *The Fat Resistance Diet* by Leo Galland, M.D. A * denotes that this food was recommended as an anti-inflammatory food by another expert, Michelle Cook, footnoted below.

Although there are only four types of nuts and seeds on the top 40 superfoods list, other types of nuts and seeds also contain healthy fats that dampen inflammation. Individuals with food allergies should consume a wide variety of nuts and seeds rather than limiting themselves to the types listed here to prevent developing allergies to the nuts and seeds on this list.

Include generous portions of the foods below in your diet every day.

Fruits (Best eaten fresh and raw)
Apples
Blueberries (Use blueberries frozen without sugar if out of season).

1 Galland, Leo, MD, *The Fat Resistance Diet,* (New York: Broadway Books, 2005), 98.
2 Cook, Michelle. "13 Foods that Fight Pain." http://www.care2.com/greenliving/13-foods-that-fight-pain.html
3 Cook, Michelle. "12 Surprising Reasons to Eat More Blueberries." http://www.care2.com/greenliving/12-surprising-reasons-to-eat-more-blueberries.html

Fruits, continued

Cherries (Use cherries frozen without sugar if out of season).
Grapefruit
Oranges
Pomegranates
Red grapes*

Vegetables
Arugula
Bell peppers
Broccoli
Cabbage
Carrots
Celery*
Leeks
Onions
Romaine lettuce
Scallions
Shitake mushrooms
Spinach
Tomatoes

Nuts and Seeds (Raw, not roasted)
Almonds
Flaxseeds
Sesame seeds
Walnuts

Animal Protein Foods
Egg whites
Flounder
Salmon
Sole
Tilapia
Yogurt, plain (Mix in fruit and a little stevia if desired).

Herbs and Spices
Basil
Black pepper
Cardamom
Chives
Cilantro
Cinnamon
Cloves
Garlic
Ginger
Parsley
Turmeric

Beverages
Blueberry juice
Cherry juice
Ginger tea
Green tea
Pomegranate juice
Vegetable juice (mixed or carrot juice)

Appendix E
Additional Advice for Cancer Patients

Cancer patients can do much to support their bodies in the fight against cancer and lessen the chances of a recurrence. Diet, exercise, meditative breathing, and avoidance of plastic storage for water and food are discussed in previous sections of this book. This appendix contains a few bits of additional advice about miscellaneous subjects such as cell phones and learning more about helping oneself.

Although there is not definitive proof of a link between cell phone use and cancer, the international INTERPHONE study found an increased risk of brain tumors on the side of the head where cell phones were used in long-term users.[4] Individuals concerned about cancer risk should consider following the recommendations of Dr. David Servan-Schreiber for reducing the amount and strength of exposure to electromagnetic radiation from cell phones. His advice includes:

1. Distance yourself from your phone during calls. Use the speaker, a headphone, or a Bluetooth headphone. Distance yourself from other people who are talking on cell phones in crowded places also, if possible.
2. Don't make your calls during rapid travel when the phone will be working overtime to follow weak signals. If you are on a bus, etc. you will be doing other passengers a favor as well as protecting yourself by refraining from cell phone use there. Try to sit away from people who are talking on their phones while traveling at high speed.
3. Distance yourself from the phone when you are not planning to use it. Do not keep it on your night stand or in your bed at night. If you must keep it close, use the airline or off-line mode, which stops emissions.
4. Use your phone only for short calls. If you are planning to make a long call, wait until you can use a land-line phone. At home, have a land-line phone rather than a cordless phone which broadcasts the signal using technology similar to cell phones.
5. When you make a call, wait for the other person to pick up the call before you put your phone to your ear. The electromagnetic field will be less strong then.
6. Use text messages when possible.
7. Do not let children under the age of twelve have or use cell phones.
8. Choose your phone wisely. Look for phones with the lowest specific absorption rate (SAR) when you buy a phone.[5]

---

4 Servan-Schreiber, David, MD, PhD. *AntiCancer: A New Way of Life.* (New York: Penguin Group, Inc., 2009), 92.

5 Servan-Schreiber, 93.

It is natural for cancer patients in the throes of the initial crisis often just "do what the doctor said" rather than learning all they can. Although the diagnosis itself is overwhelming, and treatments may make you too tired or ill to do anything else. If and when you're able, learn as much as you can and become involved in decision making and every aspect of your treatment. Knowledge is power.

When you are able to do so, get the book *Anti-Cancer: A New Way of Life* by Dr. David Servan-Schreiber. Read and apply the health information it contains. Warning – the book also contains interspersed sections about his personal feelings and life. They may be too intense for you at first. If so, skip them. I suspect that you, like a friend of mine who skipped many parts of the book, will eventually read them. Then you will feel as if you're a member of a support group of two, knowing that he has had some of the same feelings you do. This may help you process your emotions.

Release negative emotions and parts of your life that are no longer important. Dispel feelings of helplessness. (See pages 40 to 42 for how to do this). Mend bridges. Live intentionally. Don't put off telling people that you love them. You actually may find that the "new way of life" is better in many ways.

Appendix F
Mold Remediation

When a mold problem develops in your residence, two things must be accomplished: (1) detection and diagnosis of the problem and (2) eliminating the source of the mold. The source and its location may be very obvious, such as a plumbing leak that has black or green growth around it. If the source is not obvious, you might need to hire an expert to do testing to find the cause of the mold problem and tell you how to solve it. I recommend hiring a well qualified expert who does testing and diagnosis only. If you hire an all-purpose remediation person who does both testing and cleanup, he may specialize in cleanup and be dismal at diagnosis. These "experts" may test and find a problem that is not the real source but is something that has been contaminated by the real source. After the "problem" is cleaned up or otherwise addressed, the "expert" may consider his job done. However, you will have made no progress on solving health problems because the real mold source will still be present.

Many people I've talked to have had to determine both the cause of and solution to their own mold problem. Incorrect diagnosis of the cause of the problem is very common. Perhaps the mold-allergic person is better at diagnosis than the expert because the sufferer has an internal mold sensor that tells whether the problem is really solved. Therefore, believe your own sensor no matter what a test or expert says. Unfortunately, sometimes it is impossible to reach "zero" with mold, and individuals can become so extremely sensitive to mold they have been living with for an extended time that some treatment or desensitization may also be needed for the internal sensor to say, "All is well."

Beware of the negative mold test if your internal sensor does not agree with it. Some species of mold emit spores sporadically; if an air sample is taken at any other time, the mold will not be detected. If there are a very small number of spores present, test results can look normal (i.e. show what would be expected from outdoor air) but a person who is highly sensitive to mold can still be reacting.

Here is the experience of an allergic engineer. Dust testing on his house revealed a high mold count, but the source could not be found. At that time, Johns Hopkins University did dust testing on samples that patients collected themselves. He sent them seven samples from various areas of his house, including his attic, for testing. The basement had the lowest result, other parts were intermediate, and the attic result was the highest. He was sure there had to be water leaking into his attic, but three roofers could not find a leak. Finally, the fourth roofer looked at the top of the joists. A tiny leak was landing on the top of one joist and running along the joist. The volume of water was too small to drip down to where it could be easily detected. This engineer is a good example of how we may need to be persistent when we, the patients, can tell there is a problem because we are reacting to it, although the rest of the world says "nay."

Therefore, hire experienced, competent people to do mold testing and diagnosis. (My only advice for how to find such a person is by word-of-mouth from satisfied clients). When they collect samples for testing, they should sample all possible areas that could be problematic. The testers should interpret the results of the testing and offer advice for solutions to the problem.

Since mold remediation is challenging, it is helpful to have an attack plan. The first step in eradicating the mold problem is to eliminate what mold needs to grow: water and food.[6] This may involve calling a plumber, roofer, or other repair service. If there is condensation forming in your home, a HVAC (heating, ventilation and air conditioning) repairman may be needed. Your mold tester should be able to recommend a company that has experience with the type of problem you have. After water issues have been addressed and contaminated construction materials have been removed, the area should be allowed to dry for a few days and then thoroughly vacuumed with a HEPA (high efficiency particle air) vacuum.[7]

If the problem beyond the scope of services provided by such repairmen, your mold tester should be able to refer you to a service agency to do cleanup. However, if you or a non-allergic family member is going to do the cleanup, there are precautions you should take. The first step is to remove all moldy materials wearing an N-95[8] mask, disposable gloves, and possibly protective clothing. If you do not wear protective clothing, remove and wash all your clothes when finished.

Also read the online California Department of Public Health article "Mold or Moisture in My Home: What Do I Do?"[9] to learn which materials must be removed and

---

6 *Mold or Moisture in My Home: What Do I Do?* California Department of Public Health Environmental Health Laboratory, https://archive.cdph.ca.gov/programs/IAQ/Documents/MMIMH_English_201610.pdf

7 *Mold or Moisture in My Home.*

8 N-95 means that the mask removes 95% of particles that are 0.3 microns in size or larger. The most important factor in how well an N-95 mask works to remove particles is how well it fits one's face and creates a seal at the mask edges. For example, I was advised to use an N-95 mask for cleaning that might stir up dust containing mold spores. The one-size-fits-all N-95 made by 3M™ that was recommended did not seem to work for me and also had a strong glue smell. When the mask was several months old, the glue smell had abated, but the mask smelled like perfume. When later I learned that fit was all-important, I ordered a size medium Moldex™ medical mask because it was free of PVC and latex. I hoped that I would be able to tolerate it because the manufacturers were aware that some chemicals should not be in masks. The mask fit well and I got a good seal on my face, but the Moldex™ mask also smelled like perfume. I could wear it for about five minutes before the perfume caused as much of a reaction as the mold from which the mask was supposed to offer protection. However, this mask seals well on the face and is a good option if perfume sensitivity is not a problem. For information about where to order Moldex™ masks, see "Sources," page 270.

9 *Mold or Moisture in My Home.*

discarded and which might possibly be disinfected and saved. After you have finished disinfecting or removing contaminated materials, let the area dry for two to three days and then vacuum thoroughly with a HEPA vacuum.

A 20% solution of hydrogen peroxide with a little liquid dishwashing soap added can be helpful for detection of mold, and in mild cases may also work for cleanup. I have used it in the kitchen and bathrooms for general cleaning to detect any mold I am not seeing. The recipe for making it is found on the next page.

This hydrogen peroxide solution is not a problem for the respiratory system, but it is hard on skin, so always wear disposable gloves when working with it. Spray it on suspicious areas. (I use it in bathrooms and kitchens on non-porous surfaces that it will not damage). If foam appears in a minute or so after you spray it on, this indicates organic matter, possibly mold. I have found that if there is a serious mold problem, the foaming is immediate and very vigorous. A spatter of dried tomato sauce or normal bathroom soiling produces only a few bubbles. The first less-than-helpful remediation man we had said if you keep spraying and wiping it will eradicate the mold. My experience was that this has a chance of working long-term only if the problem is very mild. More often than not, and for serious problems, if you spray the area again in a few days, foaming will occur again. In any case, the peroxide solution is good to use to scrub the area impeccably clean before proceeding.

If you spray and wipe repeatedly and it keeps foaming, or if an area foams again after a few days, you will have to use "big guns" such as Clorox™. (Do this only if you are not sensitive to Clorox™ or can get someone else to do the work). Use it with all the windows open to minimize its irritating effect on the lungs. After thorough cleaning, dampen the problem area with Clorox™, let it dry, and leave it overnight or longer. After you wash it off, spray with the hydrogen peroxide solution again to test for foaming. More often than not, Clorox™ has been effective long-term for me. However, mold may return, even after this treatment, if the area often gets wet.

Areas constantly re-exposed to water, such as around sink fixtures, will likely have a relapse eventually. A neighbor told me that she and other volunteers use vinegar to clean at her 125 year old church. After hearing this, I decided to use vinegar every time I clean around the sink fixtures, and it has worked well. I keep a spray bottle of 6% vinegar near the kitchen sink and in the bathrooms for routine cleaning and only use the peroxide solution occasionally to check for relapses (which have been mild and infrequent).

Once the mold problem is eliminated, consider using filtration to make and keep the environment as pure as possible. Consider purchasing portable HEPA filters, especially for bedrooms. We replaced our 34½ year old furnace with a new Lennox™ furnace that has a filter to remove particles down to 0.1 microns, which is smaller than the smallest mold spores. In addition, the filtration unit contains an ultraviolet light to kill mold, bacteria and dust mites. The furnace also has a heat recovery ventilation unit (HRV). This brings n fresh outdoor air, filters it, transfers the heat from the same volume of stale air to the fresh air, sends the fresh air out through the vents to the house, and discharges the stale air outside. For more about this furnace and portable HEPA filters, see "Sources," pages 268 yo 269.

To read more details of our experience with mold, see pages 279 to 284.

Hydrogen Peroxide Solution for Mold Detection

One 16 oz spray bottle, preferably with volume marks.
8 ounces of water
8 ounces of 40-strength hydrogen peroxide for bleaching hair
¼ teaspoon dishwashing liquid for hand washing dishes

Fill the bottle to the 8 ounce line with water. Add 8 ounces of 40-strength hydrogen peroxide purchased at a beauty salon supply store. Add ¼ teaspoon dishwashing liquid. Invert the bottle a few times to mix.

Appendix G
How To Read Food Labels

Commercially prepared foods are great savers of kitchen time, but we must know what we are buying and whether it is compatible with our specific diet. To determine if the food is right for us, we turn to food labels which promote wise shopping. Food labels offer two components: the "Nutrition Facts," which are in a box, and the ingredient list. The ingredient list is required by law to list ingredients in order of the quantity used with the ingredient that makes up most of the food listed first.

At the top of the nutrition facts box is the serving size and number of calories per serving. Do not obsess about calories. If you need to lose weight, calories are not what really count; hormones are most important. To prevent a food from looking too caloric on the label, the manufacturer may reduce the serving size to lower the calorie count, thus rendering the serving size unrealistic and the calories per serving nearly meaningless.

The next section of the nutrition facts lists the amount of fat, carbohydrate and protein per serving. For cancer patients, the amount of trans fats should be zero. On food labels zero may not mean zero, however, because government guidelines call two grams of trans fat per day a safe amount to consume. Cancer patients especially should totally eliminate trans fats, but everyone should try to avoid unhealthy fats. Read ingredient lists and eschew any food that lists hydrogenated fats or partially hydrogenated fats. If possible, choose foods made with healthy oils such as olive and canola or other acceptable oils such as coconut oil.

Nutrition Facts	
Imlak'esh Organics, Sacha Inchi	
Serving Size 1/4 cup (1oz / 28g)	

Amount Per Serving	
Calories 170	Calories from Fat 120

	% Daily Values*
Total Fat 13g	20%
Saturated Fat 1.5g	6%
Trans Fat 0g	
Cholesterol 0mg	0%
Sodium 150mg	6%
Total Carbohydrate 5g	2%
Dietary Fiber 5g	18%
Sugars 0g	
Protein 8.5g	

Vitamin A 0%	•	Vitamin C 0%
Calcium 4%	•	Iron 8%

*Percent Daily Values (DV) are based on a 2,000 calorie diet.

The carbohydrate section of the nutrition facts lists total carbohydrates, dietary fiber and sugars. If following a glycemic control diet, what matters is "net" carbohydrate (the amount of absorbable carbohydrate). This is calculated by subtracting the grams of dietary fiber from the grams of total carbohydrate. Every 15 grams of net carbohydrate (one carbohydrate unit) should be balanced in the same meal or snack with at least 7 grams of protein (one protein unit). Consuming more than 7 grams of protein with each carbohydrate unit is beneficial for many individuals.

"Sugars" includes both healthy sugars like the lactose in milk and unhealthy sugars such as high fructose corn syrup. Read the ingredient list and look for sugar, cane juice, corn syrup, corn sweetener, high fructose corn syrup, sucrose, glucose and dextrose. Avoid foods that contain these ingredients, especially if you are a cancer patient.

On the subject of milk, food labels on milk may have an important additional statement about recombinant bovine growth hormone (rBGH). (See page 13 for more about why we should avoid rBGH). If the milk is organic, the label will say that the milk does not contain rBGH. However, some milk that is not certified as organic, including economical grocery store brands, is also free of rBGH.

The label on my Kroger-brand milk says, "Our farmers pledge not to treat their cows with rBGH." Bravo for the farmers! This makes me feel comfortable with my family eating Kroger-brand cottage cheese as well. However, the FDA requires that these labels also say, "The FDA has determined that there is no significant difference between milk from rBGH-treated cows and non-rBGH-treated cows." In my opinion, this statement should be ignored. If an economical brand of milk does not say that the farmers pledged not to use rBGH, purchase Kroger or Safeway brand milk or read labels at other stores.

Finally, nutrition labels contain a listing of how much protein and a few vitamins and minerals are in one serving. The protein amount is helpful for balancing protein with carbohydrates as described above. The vitamins and minerals are listed as the percentage of the recommended daily allowance (RDA) that they provide for the nutrient. Keep in mind that these percentages are based on recommended daily allowances of nutrients that may be too low for people with compromised health.

Individuals who are on diets for food allergies, gluten intolerance, candidiasis or are on the specific carbohydrate diet, GAPS diet or low FODMAPS diet should read the ingredient list and not consume any foods that contain ingredients forbidden on the diets they are following.

Label-reading is essential for those on allergy and gluten-free diets because commercially prepared foods may contain hidden allergens or sources of gluten. These are foods or food additives which appear on ingredient lists disguised by unfamiliar names. For instance, if the ingredient list contains maltodextrin, people who are allergic to corn should not eat that food. A list of derivatives of common allergenic foods which can appear as disguised or hidden allergenic ingredients is on the next four pages. **This list may not be exhaustive.** Unfortunately, new additives are developed and food names change so other ingredients might be derived from your problem foods and may not be listed on the following pages.

Prepared foods that contain a certain allergen in their usual form also are included in this list. For example, bread is on the list as a source of wheat. However, not all bread is made with wheat; there are a number of gluten-and wheat free breads on the market. You must regularly read the labels of all foods purchased to see if you can or cannot eat them. Manufacturers change ingredients, so we need to re-read labels occasionally. If you find an ingredient not listed here, look it up online and try to determine its source.

See "Sources," pages 251 to 257, for prepared foods you might consider, but be certain to read the labels or online ingredient lists before you purchase them. The ingredient list may have changed since I compiled the "Sources" section. Enjoy the safe foods that you find and the time you save on preparing them.

Hidden Allergens and Food Derivatives to Avoid in Commercially Prepared Foods

WHEAT:

Adhesive stamps and envelopes. Do not lick them; apply water with a sponge instead.

Alcoholic beverages made from grains such as beer, whiskey, gin, and some vodka

Bulgur

Candy – some. Wheat flour may be used for dusting during processing.

Cooking oil spray – some

Couscous

Dextrin – some

Flavorings or extracts – Some contain grain-source alcohol.

Flour, durum flour, graham flour, gluten flour, wheat flour, semolina flour

Gluten

Grain-based coffee substitutes such as Postum™

Hydrolyzed vegetable protein (HVP) or hydrolyzed plant protein (HPP – some

Imitation seafood or sirimi. Some contain wheat starch as a binder.

Medications, prescription or over-the-counter. Some use wheat starch as a filler.

Modified food starch or modified starch – some

Monosodium glutamate (MSG)

Pasta, including those such as Jerusalem artichoke pasta made with semolina flour.

Poultry, self-basting – some

Processed and canned meats – some

Wheat germ, bran, or berries, cracked wheat

Wheat products such as bread, crackers, etc.

White (grain) vinegar

GLUTEN:

All of the items listed above under "Wheat" plus:

Alcoholic spirits – some. Canadian celiac groups say that distillation prevents gluten from entering the final product; American groups are not sure. Ask your doctor.

Caramel coloring, if imported source

Coffee – some. Flavored coffees may contain gluten. Freeze-dried coffee is the safest. Consult the manufacturer.

Grains, some in addition to wheat such as rye, barley, spelt, kamut and triticale. Oats might or might not be allowed; ask your doctor.

Herbal teas – A few contain malt.

Malt, malt flavoring, malt vinegar

Rice syrup – some

Soy sauce – some

Vegetable gum, vegetable protein – some

Vinegar – some which are made from grain. Canadian celiac groups say that distillation prevents gluten from entering the final product; American groups are not sure. Ask your doctor.

MILK:

Casein, sodium caseinate, or caseinate

Curds

Hydrolyzed vegetable protein (HVP) or hydrolyzed plant protein (HPP) – some

Lactalbumin

Lactoglobulin

Lactose

Medications, prescription or over-the-counter. Some use lactose as a filler.

Milk products such as butter, cheese, cream, etc.

Powder asthma inhalers contain lactose which may contain traces of milk

Powdered, evaporated, or condensed milk

Processed and canned meats – some

Whey

EGGS:

Albumin

Egg pasta

Egg products such as powdered or dried egg, egg yolk, or egg white

Egg substitutes such as EggBeaters™

Globulin

Meringue

Ovomucoid

Ovomucin

Ovovitellin or vitellin

Sauces such as mayonnaise, hollandaise, or tartar sauce

Wine – Some wines may be clarified with egg white.

CORN:

Adhesive stamps and envelopes. Do not lick them; apply water with a sponge instead.

Alcoholic beverages – some, especially sweet wines

Asthma inhalers and nasal sprays containing the HFA propellant

Baking powder – most contain cornstarch

Caramel coloring – some

Citric acid (made by growing *Aspergillus niger* on hydrolyzed corn starch)

Corn flour, cornmeal, corn oil, corn syrup, corn sweetener

Cornstarch – often used as a filler in supplements and medications

Dextrose

Dextrin – some

Egg substitutes such as EggBeaters™ might contain maltodextrin, etc.

Flavorings such as vanilla may contain corn syrup

Food starch – some

Fructose, which is also called levulose – most

Glucose – most

Grits

Hominy

Hydrolyzed vegetable protein (HVP) or hydrolyzed plant protein (HPP) – some

Imitation seafood or sirimi. Some contain cornstarch as a binder.

Instant tea – some

Intravenous solution most commonly used contains dextrose (5DW)

Maltodextrin – most

Medications, prescription or over-the-counter. Some use cornstarch as a filler.

Modified food starch – some

Paper and plastic items – Some plastic wraps and plastic or paper cups and plates may be coated with corn oil.

Poultry, self-basting – some

Powdered sugar (contains cornstarch)

Salt – Some contain dextrose to prevent caking.

Sugar alcohols such as sorbitol, xylitol, maltitol, etc. are usually made from corn.

Vitamin C – most. Some brands labeled as "synthetic" are actually manufactured from corn. Ecological Formulas™ makes tapioca-source vitamin C. See "Sources," page 271 for ordering information.

Xanthan gum – Usually produced by growing bacteria on a corn-source base.

SOY:

Cooking oil spray – some
Hydrolyzed vegetable protein (HVP) or hydrolyzed plant protein (HPP) – some
Lecithin
Margarine – Most margarine contains soy oil or lecithin
Miso
Processed meats – some
Shortening – most[1]
Soy flour, soy oil, soy meal, soy milk
Tamari, soy sauce, worcestershire sauce
Tempeh
Textured vegetable protein (TVP)
Tofu

YEAST:

All alcoholic beverages
Asthma inhalers and nasal sprays containing the HFA propellant
Black (fermented) teas[2]
Cheese
Enriched grain products – Most are enriched with vitamins made from yeast.
Malted products
Soft drinks which may contain fermented products such as root beer and ginger ale
Soy sauce and condiments which contain soy sauce
Vinegar (all kinds) and condiments which contain vinegar, such as mustard, pickles, etc.
Vitamins and vitamin enriched processed foods – some. Hypoallergenic vitamins may be yeast-free.
Yeast breads. Sourdough is not yeast-free, but if made with a traditional starter contains "wild" yeasts which some yeast sensitive people can tolerate.
Other foods: If your doctor puts you on a yeast-free diet, he or she may also advise you to avoid leftovers, fruit juices, mushrooms, dried fruits and spices, all types of tea, sugar, and other foods which may aggravate candidiasis.

---

1 For soy-free non-hydrogenated shortening, try Spectrum Naturals™ palm oil shortening. Palm oil is a naturally saturated but healthy fat, the best source of palmitic acid needed for mitochodrial function.
2 Other types of tea, including herbal tea, may contain a small amount of yeast or mold as a contaminant.

Appendix H
Bread Machine Information

In the early 1990s, programmable bread machines brought a major breakthrough in baking for individuals on gluten-free and allergy diets by producing non-wheat bread with very little effort from the baker. Usually the ingredients were added to the machine, a button or two was pushed, and in a few hours a wonderful treat was ready to eat.

"Which bread machine should I buy?" is a commonly asked question. The answer varies from person to person and from year to year. Like automobile manufacturers, bread machine manufacturers change their products often. Furthermore, the needs of each home baker are different. Ask yourself what you need: Will you be away from home and want to come home to a freshly baked loaf of bread to go with your dinner? If so, get a machine with a delayed cycle timer. Food allergies or other dietary requirements are other considerations, as is the amount of bread you or your family will consume. How often do you want to bake? If you have a large family or do not want to bake often, get a larger capacity machine. Do you have frequent power outages in your area? How long do the outages last? How much do you expect to use your machine? How much money can you afford to spend? How much money will the machine save you?

For people who must eat special bread such as those on food allergy and gluten-free diets, the last question is crucial. If by making your own bread, you will eliminate the weekly necessity of buying small, pricey loaves of commercially made allergy or gluten-free bread, paying more for a bread machine may be justified.

Almost any bread machine on the market can be used to make yeast bread with wheat, spelt, kamut or white rye flour or rice flour plus eggs and stabilizers. For yeast bread made using buckwheat, whole rye, quinoa, amaranth, oat or barley flour or rice flour without eggs and stabilizers, a machine on which the baker can control the length of the last rising time and the baking time is needed.

There are two possibilities for controlling the length of the last rising time before the bread bakes. In terms of initial investment in a bread machine, the more economical choice is to buy a machine with a bake-only cycle and a dough cycle that includes rising time as well as mixing time. You can use the dough cycle followed by the bake-only cycle to make your special bread, but you have to be present to stop the dough cycle and start the bake cycle after the bread has risen for just the right amount of time. Machines with bake-only cycles are usually available (although their makers change from year to year) and some low-priced machines can be used to make special breads in this way.

The option for controlling the last rising time that is more expensive (in terms of initial investment, but it will save time and money on bread in the long run) is to buy a truly programmable machine. Some machines are called programmable because they can be programmed for a delayed start to have bread ready at a certain time. However, with a truly programmable machine, the baker can program the length of various parts of the cycle such as kneading time, rising times, and baking time. The correct last rise and baking time are crucial for many allergy and gluten-free breads. In addition, programmable bread machines can compensate for environmental conditions that affect yeast bread such as altitude.

As with all bread machines, programmable models change frequently. Zojirushi was the first to introduce a truly programmable machine in the early 1990s with their BBCCS15 model, and they have continued to make excellent programmable machines. In the late 1990s I got a Zojirushi Home Bakery model BBCCV20 which I used to make buns plus several loaves of bread every week for over seventeen years including the years when my sons were hungry teenagers. The Zojirushi BBCCX20 which I currently own has served well as my primary bread machine for over fifteen years and is still going strong.

In about 2010, Zojirushi offered a new model, the BBCEC20, which is very similar to the BBCCX20 and previous Zojirushi models which have two kneading bars. I purchased this machine about seven years ago. I used its three programmable cycles to develop sourdough bread recipes made entirely in the machine using the Fermapan™ wheat- and gluten-free freeze-dried sourdough starter. (See pages 164 to 172 for these recipes). Since the BBCEC20 machine is very similar to the BBCCV20 and X20, I expect it to be a reliable, long-lasting workhorse like the previous models.

The large Zojirushi machines currently sold have a horizontally rectangular pan with two kneading bars and make large (2-pound) normal-shaped loaves of bread. The two kneading bars produce a mixing motion that includes both ends of the pan, so for most types of bread, the cook does not have to make sure that all the flour in the corners of the pan has been incorporated into the loaf. These machines' standard cycles include basic, whole grain, dough, quick basic, quick whole grain, and quick dough cycles, a cake (non-yeast) cycle, a jam cycle, a signal to add raisins for raisin bread on most of the cycles, and "homemade menu" programmable cycles. The machines' memory can store three homemade menu cycles which you can program to the time you want for any part of the cycle, including the last rising time, which is critical for allergy and gluten-free bread baking. For sourdough, you can program a cycle that mixes the sponge ingredients and then keeps them warm for up to 24 hours on the BBCEC20 model. This is ideal for making true sourdough. However, the newer BBPAC20 "Virtuoso" machine allows programming of a rise time of only up to 12 hours and incubates the dough at a higher temperature, which is not ideal for sourdough bread. This higher temperature may also cause failure of wheat-free and gluten-free bread recipes.

The BBCEC20 and BBPAC20 models also include a sourdough starter cycle. This cycle is not for true sourdough made with *Lactobacillus* bacteria as well as yeast, but rather enables you to ferment flour and yeast for two hours and then use this as a starter for a loaf of bread. This "sourdough" does not provide the advantages for blood sugar control offered by bread acidified by a long *Lactobacillus* fermentation.

The BBPAC20 "Virtuoso" machine has a few unique new features which, in my opinion, are not necessarily improvements. One is the machine's gluten-free cycle, which works well with the rice-potato starch recipes included in the manual, but it is a set cycle. Although the breads developed by Zojirushi for this cycle are very tasty, they are made with 60% potato starch and 40% brown rice flour. Potato starch is a highly refined starch from a high glycemic index (GI) food; rice is also high GI. In my opinion, a diet containing breads made from these recipes would increase weight gain, a common consequence of gluten-free diets containing rice-based foods. In contrast to the gluten-free cycle, the homemade menu cycles of Zojirushi machines offer the baker the flexibility needed to make many different kinds of special diet breads using a wide variety of non-wheat, gluten-free, grain or non-grain flours by allowing variation in any and all parts of the cycle. The homemade menu cycles make it possible to use almost any gluten-free or allergy flour successfully (in the older machines with a normal incubation temperature) and to compensate for factors such as altitude, etc. The variety of breads that can be made enables avoidance of another common consequence of standard gluten-free diets, namely developing an allergy to rice. (This is the reason for the book *Gluten-Free Without Rice* which is described on the last pages of this book).

Another feature of the BBPAC20 is that the machine stops whenever the lid is opened making it more difficult to make some gluten-free breads. Although it is important to keep the lid closed most of the time, I like to assist the initial mixing with a spatula for stiff allergy breads, such as quinoa or amaranth bread, to insure adequate development of the the "structure" of the guar or xanthan gum.

When making wheat sourdough with the BBPAC20 and the Fermapan™ freeze-dried gluten-free starter mentioned above, I noticed that after the initial 18-hour fermentation, the flour-starter-water mixture was more bubbly in this machine and had liquefied. The dough in the next step of the process also rose much more rapidly. I took the temperature of the dough in this machine and the BBCEC20 (the two machines were running in tandem) with an instant-read thermometer, and the readings were 78°F in the BBCEC20 and 92°F in the BBPAC20. I suspect that the higher temperature allows the yeast to metabolize more rapidly and overwhelm the *Lactobacillus*, thus resulting in a less acidic, less sour, higher glycemic index bread being produced by the BBPAC20 machine. The final hand-shaped loaf made from dough produced by the BBPAC20 was dense and had a coarse texture although it was proofed in the same place for the same time as an excellent loaf made from dough which came from the BBCEC20 machine. Additionally, the loaf from the BBPAC20 machine did not taste as tangy as usual.

I had been unable to make good amaranth bread with the BBPAC20 machine. The discovery that it incubated bread dough at 92°F explained the problem. I suspect that the higher temperature promoted faster rising which caused the bubbles of gas produced in the bread by yeast to over-expand and then collapse, thus producing a short, dense loaf which was gummy inside.

The final unique feature of the BBPAC20 is a heating element in the lid. This produces wheat bread that is as beautifully browned on the top as on the bottom and sides. However, for the types of gluten-free and allergy breads that make short loaves, it produces pale loaf tops.

The Zojirushi machines mentioned have quick cycles which can save you time. I use the quick yeast bread (basic and whole wheat) cycles to make whole wheat or spelt bread in about two hours. The quick dough cycle only takes about 40 minutes. These machines are very mellow kneaders and produce excellent spelt bread as a result.

The cake cycle of the Zojirushi BBCEC20 and BBPAC20 machines can be used to make non-yeast bread for allergy and gluten-free diets if you use a major delay in adding the liquid ingredients to the cycle. (Machines with an initial six-minute mix are better for quick breads). If non-yeast bread is all you and others who you bake for can eat, I would not advise investing in a bread machine. Quick breads are easy to make by hand, and the mixing and baking can be customized to the type of bread, thus giving the best results.

If you already own a bread machine that is not programmable and does not have a bake-only cycle and a dough cycle which includes rising time, you can still use your machine for the hard part of the job of making yeast bread which is the initial mixing and kneading. Measure out your ingredients into the pan and start the dough cycle. At the end of the first rise, remove the dough from the machine, stir or knead it briefly to deflate it, and put it in an oiled and floured loaf pan. Allow it to rise in a warm place until it is just under doubled in volume. Then bake it at 375°F for 30 minutes to 80 minutes. Very dense loaves, such as rye, take longer to bake, than for example, egg-free rice bread. Your bread is done when it pulls away from the sides of the pans, is well browned and sounds hollow when thumped on the bottom of the loaf.

For recipes and more information on making yeast bread with or without a bread machine, see pages 153 to 173.

Appendix I
Buteyko Breathing Experiences

My experiences with the Buteyko breathing method should be taken with a grain of salt. It has worked well for many people who are willing to be disicplined for just a few months; my experiences are atypical.

I find this method helpful but have not been able to re-set my CO_2 trigger to a level high enough to improve my breathing long-term because I have not been able to follow one command Patrick MeKeown gives in the training DVD which is, "Avoid your triggers." The "bottom line" is that doing three sets of the "steps" exercise per day and taking one to two half-hour walks sometimes makes me feel better for an hour or two and helps me be functional so I continue to do the exercises daily.

I might have quit Buteyko breathing early on if I had not been so desperate. I never received much benefit from inhaled asthma medications, my problems felt life-threatening at times, and the Buteyko "many small breath holds" exercise may have saved my life several times. Therefore, although I discontinued the exercises a few times times, I always returned and made a change or tried another exercise to see if I would get better results.

Had I been able to consult a Buteyko practitioner, I wonder if he or she might have known some tricks for how to make the exercises work as they should (as in increase my control pause two points per week) or have suspected continuous exposure to a trigger. Perhaps the practitioner would have said, "Come back for help when your doctor gets you on some kind of medication that controls your symptoms," because asthma symptoms cause overbreathing which interferes with progress.[1] Since I have never been free of symptoms, 1½ hours of Buteyko exercises plus walk(s) every day are not enough to reset the CO_2 trigger. The effect of the exercises in increasing the CO_2 level is undone by the negative effect of the fast and/or erratic breathing I fall into during sleep at night and for parts of the rest of the day when I do not give major attention to my breathing. However, the exercise and walks do give temporary relief, which is much better help than medication that rarely if ever worked. Breathing exercises also cause no unpleasant side effects.

It seems to me that the Buteyko breathing method makes these assumptions that may not be true for individuals who do not make progress:

1. The patient routinely takes asthma medication such as an inhaled steroid that helps prevent major symptoms and has a rescue inhaler (bronchodilator) that will relieve symptoms for at least a few hours.

---

1 Asthma symptoms are listed as one of ten causes of hyperventilation on pages 242 to 243 of this source: McKeown, Patrick, MA, H Dip. *Asthma-Free Naturally*. (San Francisco, CA, Conari Press 2008), 242-243.

2. The patient is able to avoid triggers at least part of the time.

3. The patient has asthma attacks rather than continuous asthma symptoms.

4. The patient can feel the "first urge to breathe" when taking the control pause rather than having an urge to inhale most of the time.

5. The patient is able to experience a relaxed exhale, i.e. airways aren't so tight that chest muscles must be used to force air out of the lungs most or all of the time.

Two changes occurred just before I had my first "Ah-ha" moment with Buteyko breathing. They were (1) the first step towards solving the mold problem in our home was taken when 1½ cups of moldy smelling black slime were removed from the bottom of our dishwasher, and (2) I took an LDA shot with very little mold exposure. This was accomplished by living in a tent in our back yard and only being in the house for quick bathroom visits and infrequent 10 minute showers during the three weeks when the lymphocytes induced by LDA were maturing. About a month after my shot, while on a routine daily walk on the bike path. I was mentally telling myself, "Small abdominal breath in, relaxed breath out, delay the next breath a little," while walking. Half way through the walk, I suddenly found myself breathing comfortably without the monologue, looking at the trees and sky and listening to the birds sing, and I was experiencing my first truly relaxed exhales. I was breathing correctly without even trying. The first half of the walk seemed to have boosted my CO_2 level enough to dilate my airways so the air could leave my lungs without help from muscles. Ah-ha! This is how Buteyko breathing was meant to work!

However, the improved response to Buteyko breathing disappeared when we were plunged into a cold, snowy winter closed up in a house with "mold bombs" going off in the kitchen. In March we finally received real help from a competent mold tester who told us how to cure our dishwasher of mold. We used the detergent he recommended, Cascade™ with the Power of Clorox™, for ten days, in spite of the fragrance in it being a chemical problem for me. Finally, even my husband could not stand the perfume. We switched to a Safeway™ brand dishwasher gel that said "contains chlorine bleach" on the label. This was a good change but still kept me exposed to milder perfume daily.

About the same time we switched to the Safeway™ dishwasher detergent, I made a change in my Buteyko breathing routine. I began doing the steps exercise instead of the reduced breathing exercise. I figured if steps was what children who cannot master the control pause should use, maybe I should give it a try. After a month or so I had increased my steps from the low 30s to the 50s. However, when the pollen got high, my steps were back in the 30s, with an occasional evening set in the 40s and 50s. Then the air quality was reduced by smoke from wildfires. However, I continued to do the steps exercise three times a day because if I miss these exercises, I feel worse.

I hope to gain some desensitization to pollen and mold with my next LDA shot which is coming up. I also hope to succeed in resetting my CO_2 trigger with Buteyko breathing after pollen and smoke triggers are lower or absent during the winter and I hopefully will be less sensitive in general due to the LDA shot. When I finally have built up a little tolerance for inhaled allergens and can avoid triggers I expect to make rapid progress with Buteyko breathing considering all the practice I have had. At some point I hope to update this book, including this appendix, and/or put a "happy ending" to this story on the website www.healingbasics.life .

For stories of two asthmatics who are now very fit and no longer suffer from asthma because of Buteyko breathing, see *Asthma-Free Naturally,*[2] pages 108 to 112. To learn about controlled clinical trials of the Buteyko breathing method, see *Asthma-Free Naturally,* pages 255 to 262.[3]

---

2 McKeown. *Asthma-Free Naturally*, 108-112.

3 McKeown. *Asthma-Free Naturally*, 255-262.

Appendix J
Table of Measurements

For some of the recipes you will need to measure less-common amounts of ingredients such as ⅜ cup or ⅛ teaspoon. The easiest and most accurate way to do this is to have a liquid measuring cup with ⅛ cup markings, a set of dry measuring cups that contains a ⅛ cup measure, and a set of measuring spoons that has a ⅛ teaspoon. Such kitchen equipment is available from the King Arthur Flour Baker's Catalogue (See "Sources," page 260). While you are waiting for your measuring cups and spoons to arrive or if you need to halve, double, or triple recipes, use this table.

$^1/_{16}$ teaspoon	= ½ of your ⅛ teaspoon measure	
⅛ teaspoon	= ½ of your ¼ teaspoon measure	
⅜ teaspoon	= ¼ teaspoon + ⅛ teaspoon	
⅝ teaspoon	= ½ teaspoon + ⅛ teaspoon	
¾ teaspoon	= ½ teaspoon + ¼ teaspoon	
⅞ teaspoon	= ½ teaspoon + ¼ teaspoon + ⅛ teaspoon	
1 teaspoon	= ⅓ tablespoon	= ⅙ fluid ounce
1½ teaspoons	= ½ tablespoon	= ¼ fluid ounce
3 teaspoons	= 1 tablespoon	= ½ fluid ounce
½ tablespoon	= 1½ teaspoons	= ¼ fluid ounce
1 tablespoon	= 3 teaspoons	= ½ fluid ounce
2 tablespoons[1]	= ⅛ cup	= 1 fluid ounce
4 tablespoons	= ¼ cup	= 2 fluid ounces
5⅓ tablespoons	= ⅓ cup	= 2⅔ fluid ounces
8 tablespoons	= ½ cup	= 4 fluid ounces
16 tablespoons	= 1 cup	= 8 fluid ounces
⅛ cup	= 2 tablespoons[1]	= 1 fluid ounce
¼ cup	= 4 tablespoons	= 2 fluid ounces
⅜ cup	= ¼ cup + 2 tablespoons[1]	= 3 fluid ounces
⅝ cup	= ½ cup + 2 tablespoons[1]	= 5 fluid ounces
¾ cup	= ½ cup + ¼ cup	= 6 fluid ounces
⅞ cup	= ¾ cup + 2 tablespoons[1]	= 7 fluid ounces
	or ½ cup + ¼ cup + 2 tablespoons[1]	
1 cup	= ½ pint	= 8 fluid ounces
1 pint	= 2 cups	= 16 fluid ounces
1 quart	= 4 cups or 2 pints	= 32 fluid ounces
1 gallon	= 4 quarts	= 128 fluid ounces

---

1 In my experience, measuring tablespoons are all a little scanty of $^1/_{16}$ cup so 2 tablespoons is a little short of ⅛ cup. Therefore, if you need to measure, for example, ⅜ cup of liquid and do not have a measuring cup with ⅛ cup markings, it will probably be more accurate to eyeball an amount halfway between ¼ cup and ½ cup than to use ¼ cup plus two tablespoons.

References

Baker, Sidney M., MD. *The Circadian Prescription*. Berkley Publishing Group, a division of Penguin Putnam Inc., New York, NY, 2000.

Blaylock, Russell L., MD. *Natural Strategies for Cancer Patients*. Kensington Publishing Corp., New York, NY, 2003.

Bowthorpe, Janie A, M.Ed. *Stop the Thyroid Madness* and *Stop the Thyroid Madness II: How Thyroid Experts are Challenging Inferior Treatments and Improving the Lives of Patients*, Laughing Grape Publishing, Dolores, CO, 2014.

Campbell-McBride, Natasha, MMedSci. *Gut and Psychology Syndrome*. Medinform Publishing, Soham, Cambridge, UK, 2010.

Crook, William G., MD. *The Yeast Connection*, 2nd Ed. Professional Books, Jackson, TN, 1984.

Davis, William, MD. *Wheat Belly*. Rodale, Inc., New York, NY, 2011.

Fallon, Sally with Mary Enig, PhD. *Nourishing Traditions*. NewTrends Publishing, Brandywine, MD. 2001.

Galland, Leo, MD. *The Allergy Solution*. Hay House, Inc., Carlsbad, CA, 2016.

Gottschall, Elaine, BA, MSc. *Breaking the Vicious Cycle: Intestinal Health Through Diet*. The Kirkton Press, Baltimore, Ontario, 1994, 2000.

McKeown, Patrick, MA, H Dip. *Asthma-Free Naturally*. Conari Press, an imprint of Red Wheel/Weiser, LLC, San Francisco, CA, 2008.

McKeown, Patrick, MA, H Dip. *Close Your Mouth*. Buteyko Books, Loughwell, Moycullen, Co. Galway. 2004.

O'Brien, Robyn. *The Unhealthy Truth: How Our Food Is Making Us Sick and What We Can Do About It*. Broadway Books, Random House, New York, NY, 2009.

Quillin, Patrick, PhD, RD, CNS. *Beating Cancer with Nutrition*. Nutrition Times Press, Inc., Carlsbad, CA, 2005.

Roberts, Barbara H., MD. *The Truth About Statins*. Pocket Books, a division of Simon & Schuster, New York, NY, 2012.

Rosenthal, Elizabeth, MD. *An American Sickness: How Healthcare Became Big Business and How You Can Take It Back*. Penguin Press. New York, NY, 2017.

Servan-Schreiber, David, MD, PhD. *AntiCancer: A New Way of Life*. Penguin Group, Inc. New York, NY, 2009.

Sources of Special Foods, Products, and Information

PREPARED FOODS

This section of "Sources" contains a list of some commercially made foods that you might be able to use on your diet. **READ THE LABELS** on these items before you purchase them; manufacturers change ingredients often and may have changed them since the time of this writing. Health food stores carry many of the items listed. Contact information is given for each company to help your health food store find foods they do not carry. Some of the companies listed welcome individual orders. Many of these companies make products in addition to those listed below which you also may be able to use. Visit company websites for up-to-date information about all of their products.

This list contains only "clean" foods and focuses mostly on those that do not contain common allergens. Therefore it is not exhaustive, but it should give you a starting point with companies that often also produce foods for those who want health-promoting foods but do not need to avoid wheat, gluten, dairy or other common allergens.

Websites change frequently; if you find a link that does not work in this section, a Google search often locates the product. At the time of this writing, an e-book with a live-links "Sources" section is planned. Please see www.healingbasics.life/livesources for more information.

ONE-WEBSITE SHOPPING for bone broth, cultured vegetables, sprouted grain bread, and nut butters made from soaked nuts

Wise Choice Market
#58 18th Street
Rouyn-Noranda, Quebec, J9X 2L5
Canada
Phone: (514) 613-1165
Email: info@wisechoicemarket.com
http://www.wisechoicemarket.com

The prepared foods offered on this website are not inexpensive. Since I have only purchased cultures from them, I have no experience with their foods, but you may find yourself in a situation where you cannot cook and have no one to shop for you. Having the right food is essential for health: Depending on your personal circumstances, choosing to simplify shopping by using one source and spending what is needed for food for the best recovery may be a wise decision.

Wise Choice Market, continued

If you are a cancer patient with wealthy friends who want to help, Wise Choice Market sells gift certificates here: http://www.wisechoicemarket.com/giftcertificates.php

If you have a helper or are healthy enough to cook, the Wise Choice Market website offers **free downloadable e-books** on how to make bone broth, cultured vegetables, cultured dairy products and more.

BAKED GOODS

Breads, buns, English muffins, waffles, tortillas, cereal and more made from a wide variety of sprouted grains, including many wheat-free and gluten-free breads.

Food for Life Baking Company, Inc.
P.O. Box 1434
Corona, CA 92878
(800) 797-5090 or (951) 279-5090
www.foodforlife.com
http://www.foodforlife.com/products

Bread made from a variety of sprouted grains, including gluten-free bread

Wise Choice Market
#58 18th Street
Rouyn-Noranda, Quebec, J9X 2L5
Canada
Phone: (514) 613-1165
Email: info@wisechoicemarket.com
http://www.wisechoicemarket.com/manna-bread/

Spelt bread, whole wheat sourdough and gluten-free bread, buns, rolls, tortillas, English muffins, etc.

Rudi's Organic Bakery
3300 Walnut Street Unit C
Boulder, CO 80301
(877) 293-0876 or (303) 447-0495
www.rudisbakery.com
https://www.rudisbakery.com/gluten-free/products/

Tortillas and Crackers

Food for Life™ brown rice and black rice tortillas plus wheat and corn tortillas

Food for Life Baking Company, Inc.
P.O. Box 1434
Corona, CA 92878
(800) 797-5090 or (951) 279-5090
http://www.foodforlife.com/products/tortillas

Spelt, wheat and gluten-free tortillas

Rudi's organic spelt, wheat, and gluten-free tortillas

Rudi's Organic Bakery
3300 Walnut Street, Unit C
Boulder, CO 80301
(877) 293-0876 or (303) 447-0495
www.rudisbakery.com
https://www.rudisbakery.com/gluten-free/products/

Rye crackers

Wasa Original Crispbread including sourdough rye crispbread
(These crackers are often available in health food stores).

Wasa LLC
885 Sunset Ridge Drive
Northbrook, IL 60062
800-924-WASA (1-800-924-9272)
http://www.wasa-usa.com/products/crispbread/sourdough/

BEANS – cooked dried legumes packed in glass jars

Jovial Foods
41 Norwich-Westerly Road
North Stonington, CT 06359
(877) 642-0644
Email: info@jovialfoods.com
https://jovialfoods.com
https://jovialfoods.com/product-category/gluten-free/beans/

BONE BROTH

Bone broth, organic beef, chicken and turkey

Bonafide Provisions
National Services
Carlsbad, CA 92011
(760) 683-9146
http://bonafideprovisions.com/

Bonafide Provisions broth also sold by Wise Choice Market - beef, chicken and turkey

Wise Choice Market
#58 18th Street
Rouyn-Noranda, Quebec, J9X 2L5
Canada
Phone: (514) 613-1165
Email: info@wisechoicemarket.com
http://www.wisechoicemarket.com
https://www.wisechoicemarket.com/bone-broth/

Bone broth - salmon and halibut

Wise Choice Market
#58 18th Street
Rouyn-Noranda, Quebec, J9X 2L5
Canada
Phone: (514) 613-1165
Email: info@wisechoicemarket.com
http://www.wisechoicemarket.com
https://www.wisechoicemarket.com/bone-broth/

CEREALS, HOT

Hot cereals are comforting and so easy to prepare that they are included in this section with the purpose of helping cancer patients. Soak these cereals overnight before cooking for ease in digestion and to neutralize phytic acid and enzyme inhibitors. Single rolled grains such as oatmeal from the health food store bulk bins are also a good choice for making hot cereal. However, many packaged hot cereals contain mixed grains. The packaged hot cereals listed below contain a single grain for individuals on rotation diets.

Bob's Red Mill rice, buckwheat, spelt, oat (including gluten-free oat), millet, barley, and rye hot cereals

Bob's Red Mill Natural Foods Inc.

13521 SE Pheasant Court
Milwaukee, OR 97222
(800) 349-2173
http://www.bobsredmill.com/organic-brown-rice-farina.html
http://www.bobsredmill.com/organic-creamy-buckwheat.html
http://www.bobsredmill.com/shop/cereals/hot-cereal/rolled-spelt-flakes.html
http://www.bobsredmill.com/shop/cereals/hot-cereal/organic-thick-rolled-oats.html
http://www.bobsredmill.com/shop/cereals/hot-cereal/gluten-free-organic-thick-rolled-oats.html
http://www.bobsredmill.com/shop/cereals/hot-cereal/millet-grits-meal.html
http://www.bobsredmill.com/shop/cereals/hot-cereal/rolled-barley-flakes.html
http://www.bobsredmill.com/shop/cereals/hot-cereal/organic-cracked-rye.html
http://www.bobsredmill.com/shop/cereals/hot-cereal/creamy-rye-flakes.html

Arrowhead Mills Rice and Shine Cereal

Arrowhead Mills

110 S Lawton Avenue
Hereford, TX 79045
(800) 364-0730
http://www.arrowheadmills.com/cpt_products/organic-gluten-free-rice-and-shine-cereal/

Pocono Cream of Buckwheat: 100% Buckwheat

The Birkett Mills

PO Box 440
Penn Yan, NY 14527
(315) 536-3311
Email: contact@thebirkettmills.com.
http://thebirkettmills.com/

CULTURED DAIRY PRODUCTS

YOGURT

Sheep's Milk Yogurt

Hollow Road Farms
Old Chatham Sheepherding Company
271 Hollow Road
Stuyvesant, NY 12173
(888) SHEEP60 or (518) 758-1881
https://berkshirefoodandtravel.com/old-chatham-sheepherding-company/

This is the rich and creamy sheep yogurt our local health food stores carry. Although this website doesn't have ordering information (just photos of the finished products), stores obviously are able to order it. Ask your health food store about carrying it.

Bellwether Farms
9999 Valley Ford Road
Petaluma, CA 94952
(707) 763-0993
Email: info@bellwetherfarms.com
http://www.bellwetherfarms.com/

This sheep yogurt is tasty but not as rich and satisfying as the Hollow Road Farm yogurt.

Goat Milk Yogurt

Redwood Hill Farm
2064 Gravenstein Highway North
Building 1, Suite 130
Sebastopol, CA 95472
(707) 823-8250
www.redwoodhill.com

OTHER DAIRY PRODUCTS

Goat Cheese

Mt. Sterling Cheese Corporation
505 Diagonal Street
Mt. Sterling, WI 54645
(608) 734-3151
Email: mtsterlinglund@yahoo.com
https://buymtsterlinggoatcheese.com/

Camel Milk, raw, pasteurized, kefir (all available fresh or frozen) and dried

Desert Farms Camel Milk
2708 Wilshire Boulevard
Santa Monica, CA 90403
(800) 430-7426
https://desertfarms.com/collections/camelmilk

I used Desert Farms frozen and dried milk when our local camel dairy had supply issues. The kefir ingredients say "kefir culture" but do not state whether or not it contains yeast. Although this milk is pricey, it is a good choice if there are no camels nearby.

CULTURED VEGETABLES

Cultured vegetables including carrots, beets and sauerkraut

Farmhouse Culture
182 Lewis Road
Watsonville, CA 95076
831-466-0499
Email info@farmhouseculture.com
https://www.farmhouseculture.com/

Wise Choice Market
#58 18th Street
Rouyn-Noranda, Quebec, J9X 2L5
Canada
Phone: (514) 613-1165
Email: info@wisechoicemarket.com
http://www.wisechoicemarket.com
https://www.wisechoicemarket.com/organic-raw-fermented-vegetables/

SUPPLIES AND INGREDIENTS FOR COOKING

BAKING INGREDIENTS, miscellaneous

Baking powder, corn-free

Featherweight Baking Powder
The Hain Celestial Group, Inc.
4600 Sleepytime Drive
Boulder, CO 80301
(800) 434-4246
http://www.hainpurefoods.com/products/product.php?prod_id=1842

Flavors and extracts, organic, gluten-, corn- and alcohol-free

Frontier Natural Products Co-op
P.O. Box 299
3021 78th Street
Norway, IA 52318
(800) 669-3275
www.frontierherb.com
Vanilla flavor
https://www.frontiercoop.com/frontier-organic-vanilla-flavoring-4-fl-oz/
Other gluten-, corn- and alcohol-free flavors including anise, lemon,
peppermint and orange
https://www.frontiercoop.com/catalogsearch/result/?q=alcohol+free+flavoring

Boyojian Lemon Oil

King Arthur Flour Baker's Catalogue
P.O. Box 876
Norwich, Vermont 05055
(800) 827-6836
http://www.kingarthurflour.com/shop/items/lemon-oil-1-oz

Gum, guar and xanthan

Bob's Red Mill Natural Foods Inc.
13521 SE Pheasant Court
Milwaukee, OR 97222
(800) 349-2173
http://www.bobsredmill.com/shop/baking-aids/guar-gum.html
http://www.bobsredmill.com/shop/baking-aids/xanthan-gum.html

Oils and non-hydrogenated trans fat-free shortening

Spectrum Naturals™ Oils
Spectrum Naturals™ Organic All Vegetable Shortening - palm oil only (soy-free)

Spectrum Organic Products, Inc.
5341 Old Redwood Highway, Suite 400
Petaluma, CA 94954 - or for customer support -
The Hain Celestial Group, Inc.
4600 Sleepytime Drive
Boulder, CO 80301
(800) 434-4246
http://www.spectrumorganics.com/spectrum-naturals/
http://www.spectrumorganics.com/product/organic-all-vegetable-shortening/

Rye flavor powder (gluten-free)

Authentic Foods
1850 W. 168th Street, Suite B
Gardena, CA 90247
(800) 806-4737 or (310) 366-7612
http://www.authenticfoods.com/products/item/37/Rye-Flavor

Thickener - Signature Secrets™ Culinary Thickener

King Arthur Flour Baker's Catalogue
P.O. Box 876
Norwich, Vermont 05055
(800) 827-6836
www.kingarthurflour.com
http://www.kingarthurflour.com/shop/items/signature-secrets-culinary-thickener-8-oz

Unbuffered vitamin C powder, tapioca source, made by Ecological Formulas™ and used for baking, soaking grains and salads

The Vitamin Shoppe
Customer Care Department
2101 91st Street
North Bergen, NJ 07047
(866) 293-3367
https://www.vitaminshoppe.com/p/cardiovascular-research-vitamin-c-tapioca-2000-mg-150-g-powder/cv-1038

Yeast, active dry and quick-rise, gluten-, corn- and preservative-free

> **Red Star™ Yeast and SAF™ Red Yeast**
> Universal Foods Corporation
> Consumer Service Center
> 433 E. Michigan Street
> Milwaukee, WI 53202
> (414) 271-6755
> http://redstaryeast.com/products/red-star/red-star-active-dry-yeast/
> http://lesaffreyeast.com/product/saf-instant-red/

The Red Star™ Yeast company is a good information source but does not sell direct to consumers. To purchase Red Star™ or SAF™ Red yeast in 1 or 2-pound bags, contact:

> **King Arthur Flour Baker's Catalogue**
> P.O. Box 876
> Norwich, Vermont 05055
> (800) 827-6836
> http://www.kingarthurflour.com/shop/items/saf-red-instant-yeast-16-oz
> http://www.kingarthurflour.com/shop/items/red-star-active-dry-yeast-16-oz

BAKING SUPPLIES AND EQUIPMENT

Bread machines, ⅛ teaspoon or ⅛ cup measuring spoons and cups, lemon oil flavoring, many types of flour, including rye flour and pecan and hazelnut flour/meal, and other baking ingredients and supplies

> **King Arthur Flour Baker's Catalogue**
> P.O. Box 876
> Norwich, Vermont 05055
> (800) 827-6836
> www.kingarthurflour.com

CHERRIES, TART for pies, frozen

> **King Orchards**
> 4620 N. M-88
> Central Lake MI 49622
> (877) 937-5464
> http://www.mi-cherries.com/can.htm

CULTURES FOR FERMENTED FOODS

Vegetable Culture - Caldwell Starter Culture for Fresh Vegetables ™

Caldwell Biofermentation Canada Inc.
579 Chemin de la Riviere
St. Edwidge, Quebec, J0B 2R0
Canada
http://www.caldwellbiofermentation.com/starter-culture.html

Wise Choice Market
#58 18th Street
Rouyn-Noranda, Quebec, J9X 2L5
Canada
Phone: (514) 613-1165
Email: info@wisechoicemarket.com
http://www.wisechoicemarket.com
https://www.wisechoicemarket.com/caldwells-starter-culture-vegetables/

Cultures for Health
200 Innovation Avenue, Suite150
Morrisville NC 27560
(919) 695-9600
https://www.culturesforhealth.com/natural-fermentation/fermentation-ingredients.html

Cultures for Health sells Caldwell Starter plus other cultures for vegetables and offers a helpful free e-book on lactofermentation when the webpage above is opened.

Cultures for Fermented Milks

GI Pro Start™ Yogurt Starter, gluten- and dairy-free

GI ProHealth Inc.
Box D-2
Fairhaven MA 02719
(877) 219-3559
Email: info@giprohealth.com
http://www.giprohealth.com/yogurtstarter.aspx

Cultures for Yogurt, Crème Fraiche, Sour Crème, Buttermilk, Kefir, Cheese, etc.

Cultures for Health
200 Innovation Avenue, Suite150
Morrisville NC 27560
(919) 695-9600
https://www.culturesforhealth.com/starter-cultures.html

Cultures for Acidophilus milk

Klaire Laboratories Therbiotic™ Factor 1 and *L acidophilus* SCD Compliant™ Formula

Klaire Laboratories
795 Trademark Drive
Reno, NV 89521
(888) 488-2488
http://www.klaire.com/prod/proddetail.asp?id=V771-06
http://www.klaire.com/prod/proddetail.asp?id=K-LAC

Sourdough cultures

Gluten-free live starter (dough)

Cultures for Health
200 Innovation Avenue, Suite150
Morrisville NC 27560
(919) 695-9600
https://www.culturesforhealth.com/gluten-free-sourdough-starter.html

Fermapan™ French-Style Sourdough Starter, gluten-free (freeze-dried)

King Arthur Flour Baker's Catalogue
P.O. Box 876
Norwich, Vermont 05055
(800) 827-6836
http://www.kingarthurflour.com/shop/items/french-style-sourdough-starter-5g

FLOUR for allergy and gluten free diets; many varieties of flour and starches such as tapioca starch and arrowroot

Bob's Red Mill Natural Foods Inc.
13521 SE Pheasant Court
Milwaukee, OR 97222
(800) 349-2173
www.bobsredmill.com

FLOUR, EINKORN (non-modern wheat, may be tolerated by the wheat-sensitive)

Jovial Foods
41 Norwich-Westerly Road
North Stonington, CT 06359
(877) 642-0644
Email – info@jovialfoods.com
https://jovialfoods.com
https://jovialfoods.com/product-category/einkorn/flour/

This company was founded and is owned by a family dealing with their daughter's allergies. They sell a variety of products including einkorn, the wild parent of all wheat that their daughter tolerates. They also wrote and sell a wonderful einkorn cookbook.

FLOUR, SPROUTED

Wise Choice Market
#58 18th Street
Rouyn-Noranda, Quebec, J9X 2L5
Canada
Phone: (514) 613-1165
Email: info@wisechoicemarket.com
https://www.wisechoicemarket.com/organic-sprouted-wheat-flour-5-lb-bag/
https://www.wisechoicemarket.com/organic-sprouted-spelt-flour-5-lb/

Shiloh Farms (wide variety of sprouted flours including many gluten-free flours)
191 Commerce Drive
New Holland, PA 17557
(800) 362-6832 x103
info@shilohfarms.com
http://www.shilohfarms.com/flours/

LACTOFERMENTATION SUPPLIES

Kraut Kaps™ and Crock Rocks™

Zatoba Products (formerly Primal Kitchens)
1425 North Market Boulevard, Suite 5
Sacramento, CA 95834
(916) 245-6087
http://zatoba.com/kraut-kap-3-pack/
http://zatoba.com/original-crock-rocks-3-pack/

FermentEm™ Airlock Kits

Kits for four or eight mason jars are available online from FermentEm™ or Amazon.com.

https://www.fermentem.com/products/fermentem-4-piece-kit?variant=10356671815
https://www.fermentem.com/products/fermentem-8-piece-kit?variant=14561877959
https://www.amazon.com/FermentEm-8-Piece-Fermenting-Kit-Fermentation/dp/B00VSJUICM

Silicone Mason Jar Seals

Silicone jar seals are available online from Amazon.com or Mason Jar Lifestyle

https://masonjarlifestyle.com/product/leak-proof-silicone-sealing-rings-for-mason-jar-lids/

MEATS AND BONES FOR BONE BROTH

Buffalo (bison) bones and meat:

North American Bison Cooperative
TenderBison
1502 1st Ave North
Fargo, ND 58102
http://tenderbison.com/
Phone: To order call Jeremy Anderson, 888-545-2499, extension 1

Meat from North American Bison comes in case quantities of about 10 pounds. The buffalo knuckle bones are specially cut and I have ordered 15 pounds. You can specify how many pounds you want, but there may be a minimum order weight.

Alpaca bones and meat

Many Pastures Alpaca
26219 Fremont Drive
Zimmerman, MN 55398
(612) 385-2187
http://manypastures.com/

Antelope and venison bones and meat

Broken Arrow Ranch
3296 Junction Highway
Ingram, TX 78025
(800) 962-4263
http://www.brokenarrowranch.com/Shop/

Elk bones and meat

Elk USA
Grande Natural Meat
PO Box 10
Del Norte, Colorado 81132
(888) 338-4581
http://www.elkusa.com/elk_meat.html

Guinea hen and other uncommon fowl for meat and bones

Specialty Meats and Gourmet
1810 Webster Street, #8
Hudson, WI 54016
(715) 386-6628
http://www.smgfoods.com/

Bones of common animals such as beef and chicken

U.S. Wellness Meats
PO Box 249
Canton, MO 63435
(877) 383-0051
Email: eathealthy@grasslandbeef.com
https://grasslandbeef.com/

U.S. Wellness Meats also sells sugar-free sausages, sugar and additive-free smoked bacon and more products made from pasture-raised anmials.

NUTS and SEEDS

Macadamia nut pieces (perfect size for drying) and many other nuts

Nuts.com
125 Moen Street
Cranford, New Jersey 07016
(800) 558-6887
Email: care@nuts.com
https://nuts.com/
Macadamia pieces: **https://nuts.com/nuts/macadamianuts/pieces.html**

Sacha inchi seeds
Imlak'esh Organics
6336 Lindmar Drive
Goleta, CA 93117
(805) 689-2269
Email: connect@imlakeshorganics.com
https://imlakeshorganics.com/products/sacha-inchi/

NUT BUTTERS

Nut butters made from soaked or sprouted nuts

Wise Choice Market
#58 18th Street
Rouyn-Noranda, Quebec, J9X 2L5
Canada
Phone: (514) 613-1165
Email: info@wisechoicemarket.com
http://www.wisechoicemarket.com/soaked-nut-butters/

NUT FLOUR FOR BAKING

Almond flour, blanched and finely ground, good for baking

Honeyville Inc.
1040 West 600 North
Ogden, UT 84404
(385) 374-9400
(888) 810-3212

http://shop.honeyville.com/products/flours/blanched-almond-flour.html/

SWEETENERS

Fruit Sweet™

Wax Orchards, Inc.
314 E 26th St.
Tacoma, WA 98421
(800) 634-6132
http://www.waxorchards.com/fruitsweet.aspx

Agave and Coconut Sugar

Madhava Natural Sweeteners
14300 East I-25 Frontage Road
Longmont, CO 80540
(303) 823-9000
http://madhavasweeteners.com/product/agave-amber/
http://madhavasweeteners.com/product/agave-light/
http://madhavasweeteners.com/product/coconut-sugar-2/

Stevia, enzyme treated white powder, filler-free

Berlin Seeds
5335 County Highway 77
Millersburg, OH 44654
(330) 893-2091

Berlin Seeds' stevia is the most purely-sweet tasting enzyme-treated stevia and is much less expensive than most enzyme-treated stevia. You may order by phone or request a catalogue and order by mail.

Protocol for Life Balance™

This supplement manufacturer that does not sell directly to consumers. Their stevia may be purchased from Professional Supplement Center.

Professional Supplement Center
5441 Palmer Crossing Circle
Sarasota, FL 34237
(888) 245-5000
http://www.professionalsupplementcenter.com/Stevia-Extract-powder-by-Protocol-For-Life-Balance.htm

OTHER PRODUCTS AND SERVICES

Some of the products listed in this section are not sold directly to consumers. In that case, a source for purchasing the product is given with as much information as is available which in some cases is only a web address.

AIR PURIFICATION PRODUCTS

Portable HEPA air filters

Austin Air Systems, Ltd.
500 Elk Street
Buffalo, NY 14210
(800) 724-8403
http://austinair.com/

The Allergy Store
18459 Pines Boulevard, #237
Pembroke Pines, FL 33029
(800) 771-2246
http://www.allergystore.com/air-cleaners/austin-air-healthmate-air-cleaners.html

I purchased an Austin Air™ HealthMate Junior (room-size) from the Allergy Store. The previous bedroom filter had died overnight, and when they heard my story, the sent the new filter the same day I ordered it even though I had submitted my online order with free shipping. It came by UPS ground, but there was no delay for order processing by the Allergy Store. After using it for about six weeks and finding that it made me feel much better than my previous filter, I purchased an Austin Air™ filter for areas up to 1500 square feet for our kitchen and main floor. These filters are made in the USA from metal rather than plastic so did not require out-gassing.

HVAC systems for Allergies

Lennox Heating and Cooling
2100 Lake Park Blvd.
Richardson, TX 75080
http://www.lennox.com/residential

At the time of this writing, Lennox is American-owned and their products are manufactured in the USA. Our previous Lennox furnace lasted 34½ years and was still working when we replaced it with a system that would provide state-of-the-art filtration.

Installer of Lennox systems in Colorado

> **Steele Brothers Heating, Inc**.
> 7147 Reynolds Drive
> Sedalia, CO 80135
> (303) 347-1958
> Contact: J.P. Richie. Please mention that you learned about Steele Brothers
>   in this book.

This company has very high review ratings and did a good installation job for us. The two air purification systems they installed were the Lennox **Healthy Climate Pure Air Filter System** and Lennox **HRV5-150 Heat Recovery Fresh Air Unit.**

CLEANING AND LIFESTYLE PRODUCTS

Chemically Safe Cleaning Products and Home Improvement Supplies

> **American Formulating and Manufacturing**
> 3251 Third Avenue
> San Diego, CA 92103
> (619) 239-0321
> https://www.afmsafecoat.com/
>
> **SafeChoice™ SuperClean™**
> https://www.afmsafecoat.com/products/cleaners-carpet-care/safechoice-super-clean
> https://www.needs.com/product/AFM_Super_Clean_Multi_Purpose_
> Cleaner_32/d_Cleaners_All_Purpose
>
> **Chemically-safe Sealants, Paint, Stain and Finishing Products**
> https://www.afmsafecoat.com/products

Microfiber cloths for cleaning

> **VibraWipe™**
> Email support@vibrawipe.com
> https://vibrawipe.com/
> https://vibrawipe.com/collections/microfiber-cloth
> https://www.amazon.com/VibraWipe-Microfiber-8-Pieces-ABSORBENT-
> STREAK-FREE/dp/B00CFALFXY

VibraWipe™ microfiber cloths contain 20% polyamide and pick up dust well even when used dry. This brand is a recent replacement for my former favorite cloths so I have not used them long enough to tell how well they last.

Gloves for cleaning, disposable

Allerderm™ disposable latex-free gloves, box of 100

> **Allergy One**
> 7375 N. Fresno Street, #101
> Fresno, CA 93720
> 800-989-0111
> http://www.allergyone.com/page/AO/PROD/aldrmDVEG

N-95 Masks for cleaning

Moldex™ disposable latex-free masks

> **Moldex™**
> 10111 W. Jefferson Blvd.
> Culver City, CA 90232
> (800) 421-0668
> http://www.moldex.com/respiratory-protection/disposable-respirators/healthcare-and-surgical/

Retail sales of Moldex™ masks

> **MacGill Discount School Nurse Supplies**
> 1000 N. Lombard Road
> Lombard, IL 60148
> (800)323-2841
> E-mail: macgill@macgill.com
> https://www.macgill.com/advancedsearch/result/?q=moldex+masks

Food storage products free of BPA, phthalates, and other carcinogens

Glasslock ™ glass storage containers

Sets of assorted containers, extra-large containers, etc.
http://glasslockusa.com/product-category/gift-box-sets/

Large and medium containers sold by The Container Store online or at local stores
https://www.containerstore.com/s/kitchen/food-storage/glass-ceramic/glasslock-rectangular-food-containers-with-lids/123d?productId=10032213
https://www.containerstore.com/s/kitchen/food-storage/glass-ceramic/glasslock-round-food-containers-with-lids/123d?productId=10032211

Cellophane bags and wrap

N.E.E.D.S. ((Nutritional Ecological Environmental Delivery System)
3160 Erie Boulevard East
DeWitt, NY 13214
(800) 634-1380
https://www.needs.com/prod_detail_list/s?keyword=cellophane

N.E.E.D.S. also sells supplements, personal care products and other supplies that are chemically pure and hypoallergenic

SUPPLEMENTS

Only a few supplements are listed here. All three companies sell many supplements; please search their websites to find others that are not listed.

N.E.E.D.S. ((Nutritional Ecological Environmental Delivery System)
3160 Erie Boulevard East
DeWitt, NY 13214
(800)-634-1380
https://www.needs.com/

N.E.E.D.S. sells supplements, personal care products, etc. that are chemically pure and hypoallergenic. See page 269 their URL for AFM SuperClean™.

Unbuffered vitamin C powder, tapioca source, made by Ecological Formulas

The Vitamin Shoppe
Customer Care Department
2101 91st Street
North Bergen, NJ 07047
(866) 293-3367
https://www.vitaminshoppe.com/p/cardiovascular-research-vitamin-c-tapioca-2000-mg-150-g-powder/cv-1038

Douglas Labs Bone CoFactors

Professional Supplement Center
5441 Palmer Crossing Circle
Sarasota, FL 34237
(888) 245-5000
http://www.professionalsupplementcenter.com/Bone-CoFactors-by-Douglas-Laboratories.htm

INFORMATION

Healthcare provider information

American Academy of Environmental Medicine (AAEM)
6505 E Central Avenue, #296
Wichita, KS 67206
(316) 684-5500
https://www.aaemonline.org/find.php

This website provides an online list of doctors who treat food allergies. Some AAEM doctors also treat thyroid problems with natural hormones (such as Armour™ Thyroid) or an individualized combination of T3 and T4. Call offices of doctors near you and ask if they have taken an AAEM thyroid course possibly taught by Dr. Alan McDaniel.

Armour™ Thyroid
http://www.armourthyroid.com/

In the past, the Armour website provided a list of physicians who treat patients with Armour™ Thyroid. Here is another website with a list which is searchable by location:

https://projects.propublica.org/checkup/drugs/1403?sort=state_id&utf8=%E2%9C%93

Information about asthma inhalers: reactions, prices, no generics, etc.

Soaring prices for asthma inhalers

http://article.images.consumerreports.org/prod/content/dam/cro/news_articles/health/PDFs/InhaledSteroidsFINAL.pdf , page 6

How the FDA and drug companies got free hand in price hikes

http://www.motherjones.com/kevin-drum/2013/10/heres-why-your-asthma-inhaler-costs-so-damn-much/

http://www.nytimes.com/2013/10/13/us/the-soaring-cost-of-a-simple-breath.html?pagewanted=all&_r=0

Potentially life-threatening reactions to the HFA inhaler propellant

http://www.consumeraffairs.com/health/hfa_inhalers.html?page=11

http://memec08.blogspot.com/2009/07/inhaler-propellant-and-corn-allergies.html

http://cornallergygirl.com/2013/10/16/corn-free-asthma-treatment/

Information about the Buteyko Breathing Method

An introduction to the Buteyko breathing method with video. Also explains how Buteyko Breathing can help with exercise and athletic pursuits.

http://articles.mercola.com/sites/articles/archive/2013/11/24/buteyko-breathing-method.aspx

Books and a DVD/CD resource for the Buteyko Breathing Method

McKeown, Patrick. *Asthma-Free Naturally*. San Francisco: Conari Press, 2008. This book is often found in libraries but should not be used alone for self-instruction without *Close Your Mouth* or the set below because it does not contain all the exercises and precautions.

McKeown, Patrick. *Close Your Mouth: Buteyko Clinic Handbook for Perfect Health*. Galway: Buteyko Books, 2004. This book contains all of the exercises and specifies physical conditions that determine whether each exercise is appropriate for you.

Buteyko Clinic Breathing Method 2 hour DVD of the training course, half-hour CD and Manual (*Close your Mouth*). The list price is $24.95 but at the time of this writing it costs $18.51 on Amazon.com. Purchase this set if you cannot take a course or visit a practitioner.

https://www.amazon.com/Buteyko-Complete-Instruction-Rhinitis-Permanently/dp/0954599691/ref=sr_1_1?ie=UTF8&qid=1505004309&sr=8-1&keywords=buteyko+breathing+method+dvd

Information about lactofermentation

Weston Price Foundation discussion of "why" as well as "how"

https://www.westonaprice.org/health-topics/food-features/lacto-fermentation/

Cultures for Health webpage with an offer for a free downloadable e-book called *Lactofermentation*

https://www.culturesforhealth.com/caldwell-starter-culture-for-fresh-vegetables.html

Caldwell's webpage which contains a how-to video for making cultured vegetables in the lower right corner of the page

http://www.caldwellbiofermentation.com/starter-culture.html
Lactofermentation information, continued

Segersten, Alissa. "How to Make Lactofermented Vegetables without Whey"

http://www.nourishingmeals.com/2012/02/how-to-make-lacto-fermented-vegetables.html

A Personal Postscript
Details of the Learning Experience

In the "Why You Must Help Yourself" chapter, I advised readers to read only about medical treatments that applied to them. The same principle applies to this section. My book *The Ultimate Food Allergy Cookbook and Survival Guide* also contains a personal postscript which my husband calls "fantast-yuck voyage." Amazingly, sometimes someone calls and says, "I have had the same experience with 'whatever' as you did and was glad to find out…" Therefore, I'm including the whole story here in case there is something someone might find helpful, but I also advise skimming it and skipping what doesn't apply to you. If you are battling mold, you may want to read pages 279 to 284 about our mold experiences, but avoid unnecessary yuck.

Three and one half years ago in spring, I got viral pneumonia. At that time, I had taken EPD or LDA (see pages 48 to 50) for over twenty years and my chemical sensitivities were mild to non-existent. A month or so after contracting the virus, I was in the grocery store and walked to the middle of the soap aisle to purchase some scent-free dishwashing liquid. As I reached for the bottle, my lungs tightened up to the point that I could barely breathe. I thought, "This isn't a virus, it's asthma." I had relatively mild asthma when I was young, but I had no trouble with it for over forty years before that day,

My allergy doctor put me on two inhalers, an inhaled steroid and Albuterol™, a fast-acting bronchodilator. I was told to use the Albuterol™ twice a day before using the inhaled steroid, or as often as every six hours if needed. The Albuterol™ was supposed to open my airways and help the steroid get to the deep recesses of my lungs. After the first week, I was to use Albuterol™ only "as needed." For a few days, things were looking up. After a week, I realized I needed the bronchodilator at least twice a day, often more, and was not going to be able to decrease its use it as the doctor had expected me to do after a week.

Along with inhalers I was given an important tool for gaining health at that first visit. My doctor's physician's assistant told me I should eat cultured vegetables to improve my intestinal flora which would help the asthma. She told me that asthma, and most chronic ill-health, can be helped by improving conditions in the gut.

Because I was not significantly improved at my next office visit, the doctor put me on a new inhaler containing a long-acting bronchodilator plus a much higher amount of inhaled steroid. He told me to continue using the Albuterol™ as a "rescue inhaler."

The doctor predicted that I would probably be feeling good in two weeks. I seemed slightly better for a few days, but then the side effects of the new inhaler, such as disrupted sleep, began to outweigh the benefits. The new inhaler also seemed to become less effective at controlling asthma symptoms the longer I used it.

In September, the doctor was finally pleased with the results of my pulmonary function test even though I didn't feel as if I had returned to anywhere near normal. I had read that asthma patients need to expect to live on inhalers for the rest of their lives. I didn't like that idea and really wanted to be able to go anywhere and breathe anything without consequences. All summer I had major problems with pollen to the point that I was trying to live inside most of the time.

Chemical sensitivities had also increased greatly. This became a problem because I had made a plane reservation to visit our younger son in the Washington DC area before I got pneumonia. I was uncertain about going. My husband said, "Go! Seeing John will be good for you." He was right.

About two days before my trip, a friend gave me another important tool for regaining my health. She told me about the Buteyko breathing method for asthma. I got *Asthma Free Naturally* from the library and took it with me on the trip.

In spite of having pre-treated with potent inhalers, I had difficulty breathing in the perfume-laden air of the plane. I practiced the Buteyko reduced breathing exercise for most of the four hour flight. Finally, my breathing began to ease. (Perhaps outside air was being brought into the plane as it descended). As the plane banked, I was able to see the ground, buildings and roads. A few minutes later, the pilot said we were approaching Dulles Airport and would land in about fifteen minutes.

Fortunately, the trip was good for me. There were no weeds anywhere nearby. All the ground was covered with asphalt, concrete, or well manicured landscapes. Other than grass, which had finished pollinating months earlier, most of the vegetation there was plants I had never seen before.[1] In addition, John had begun routinely walking around a nearby "lake." (It was a large pond surrounded by business buildings on three sides and manicured grass on the fourth). John made sure I accompanied him on his daily walks, and we even increased the pace over the week I was there.

I returned home more able to walk. Furthermore, the emotional boost of spending time with my son was good for my mental state. I began to feel more optimistic, in spite of an experience which showed that inhalers were really not an answer for me. One night while visiting John, I awakened unable to breathe. I used my Albuterol™ rescue inhaler. It took over forty five minutes to even begin to give me some relief, and then the slight improvement only lasted about fifteen minutes. During that brief interlude of improvement, I was able to begin using Buteyko exercises which helped and allowed me to relax and go back to sleep in an hour or so. I was out of the crisis in the morning.

In October, my older son, Joel, and I were scheduled to take our LDA injections. Because the patient instruction book says LDA is very effective for asthma, I expected it to greatly help my breathing problems. The shot-time protocol for asthma patients includes some time without inhalers, which are replaced with a "Prednisone™ burst"

---

1 Although I did not realize this at the time, not only was I away from problematic types of pollen, I also had a vacation from the types of mold in our house.

and an oral bronchodilator drug. The evening of my first day without inhalers, I felt as if a tremendous allergic burden had been lifted. I Googled "allergy to asthma inhalers" and – long story short – discovered that FDA had mandated that the propellant in all asthma inhalers be changed to hydrofluoroalkane (HFA) a few years earlier. This new propellant was made with corn-derived ethanol. I had been breathing small traces of corn and yeast to which I am allergic every time I used the inhalers for months.

Two days before our LDA shots, the mail brought an information set I had ordered containing the Buteyko breathing method training course DVD, CD, and copy of *Close Your Mouth*. (See "Sources," page 273 for where to get this set). Receiving this information made it possible, although not easy, for me to survive for the month after my shot. I knew that I could not go back to using the inhalers after the shot-time restrictions ended. If I had a night time crisis in breathing, the Buteyko exercise called "many small breath holds" helped somewhat, although it could take an hour or two to become effective enough for me to go back to sleep. Don't try this yourself!! The Buteyko books say to use the exercise for only *five* minutes, and then if it has not solved the problem, to use your rescue inhaler. Do what the Buteyko books say and follow your doctor's orders rather than living dangerously as I did. I made this risky decision because inhalers contained allergenic ingredients. I did not want to use them or to go to the ER and be treated with something that would destroy the potential benefits of my LDA shot.

When I saw my doctor after my LDA shot and told him what I had learned about inhalers, his eyes widened. He told me about trying, but finding it impossible, to get any information about the new propellant when the change occurred. The only information that the drug reps ostensibly had was that it was totally safe for his patients and much better for the ozone layer. He prescribed Budesonide ™, an inhaled steroid, and Albuterol™ administered by a nebulizer. Life felt less threatening than it had been without any inhaled asthma medication, but I still was not well and chemicals were still a real problem. I did notice that I could put my head on the floor to vacuum the hardwood floor under the bed with less distress, and the next spring I did better with pollen, so the LDA shot had done some good.

When I returned to the doctor in February, my pulmonary function test was worse than it had been at any time up to that point. He said, "We're going to have to look for things that are contributing to this asthma such seeing if you have a thyroid problem." Then he looked in my nose and said, "You have a sinus infection." He had seen pus draining from one of my sinuses. I had been doing saline nasal rinses routinely, and he had me add an antibiotic to them twice a day and said to call him in a week. I was quite reluctant to take oral antibiotics because killing normal intestinal flora is not what one wants to do with Crohn's disease. However, the antibiotic nasal rinses failed to clear up the sinus infection or help my breathing.

The next week the doctor put me on a two-week course of oral antibiotics. After ten days, I experienced a short time of some improvement in my breathing. The pulmonary function test I had after I finished the oral antibiotics showed good results, so I was cleared to take my LDA shot the following week.

Fortunately, the March LDA shot was a much less frightening experience than the fall shot. I was allowed to go back to using nebulized inhaled steroids the third day after my shot. However, a major factor in a brief time of feeling better was probably that part of the LDA protocol for me is to take a systemic anti-fungal drug the week before and five days after my shot. On the fifth day after my shot, I re-designed a cover for one of my books. My brain was in great shape if I could handle Adobe InDesign™ that well! Then things began to go downhill again. My breathing deteriorated. The diarrhea which had begun a few days after starting the oral antibiotic returned. After seven weeks of diarrhea with no improvement in spite of dietary intervention and tons of probiotics, I feared a Crohn's disease flare up so started the GAPs diet. (See page 37 for information about the GAPS diet).

When I returned to the doctor, my pulmonary function test was much worse than the previous "worst" test. Not only was air not getting out of my lungs well, it was not getting in. My pulse was 109 and my PO_2 (blood oxygen level taken with a finger-tip sensor) was low. The doctor talked about sending me to a pulmonologist, which I resisted because the local pulmonologists are part of a very conventional respiratory hospital where most allergy patients are treated with potent immunosuppressive drugs. Then he looked in my nose, throat, and mouth and said, "Yeast." He was so convinced that I had *Candida albicans*, and that he forgot about the pulmonologist and ordered immediate treatment with a systemic antifungal, Diflucan™. He also wanted a comprehensive stool test done, but it could not be done immediately due to my needing to avoid probiotics, etc. for three days before collecting it. Thus, I was to do the stool test while on Diflucan™. The doctor said, "We'll assume you have *Candida* and the test will show us the state of your digestion, what kind of bacteria are present, and if you have a resistant yeast."

He also began treating a not-very-obvious thyroid problem. My blood test showed a changed pattern from a test done five years previously. Although all the values were still in the normal range, the TSH and T3 were both at the lower limit of normal, and my TSH had been at the upper limit before. He suspected that my thyroid was getting worn out, which is very common among post-menopausal women.

The stool test results showed that I had impaired digestion, no *Lactobacillus*, no *E. coli*, a large amount of an opportunistic yeast that was resistant to all drugs, and a large amount of the opportunistic bacteria *Citrobacter freundii*. On the testing for "natural agents," both the yeast and *Citrobacter* were sensitive to uva ursi, which I began taking. I had taken tons of probiotics but was told by a nutritionist to take an all-*Lactobacillus* supplement at a different time of the day than the bifidus-containing mixed probiotic supplement I took. The GAPS diet had helped the diarrhea, but it took seven months to totally clear it up.

Because treating the sinus infection, my thyroid, and my intestinal flora had not helped the asthma, my allergy doctor ordered a dust test on our house. It took about three weeks to get the collector to take the sample and then over a month receive the results. I was impatient to fix anything that might be causing my problem. We had almost three months of steady rain that spring and summer and had experienced dark spots on the concrete in our basement, although the sump pump prevented water from coming in. So when our son John, who is an excellent cleaning helper, came home on a vacation, he and I did massive cleaning in the basement.

The dust test showed a high level of mold. I told my doctor about the cleaning we had done and he ordered another test to see if cleaning had solved the problem.

Then came a crisis. A small lump in my breast was diagnosed as Paget's disease, a rare form of breast cancer. Paget's disease cells migrate in the breast and out the nipple. The surgeon knew what I had as soon as he examined me because of the changes in my nipple made by the Paget's cells. The biopsy he took in his office at that first visit showed it was still all inside the duct in the sample taken, was grade two (medium aggressiveness) and was hormone receptor negative. I had a mastectomy. The rest of the tumor removed in the mastectomy was also in the duct only had not spread to any other parts of the breast or lymph nodes, making chemotherapy and/or radiation unnecessary, in the judgment of my oncologist who does not over-treat. Since the tumor was not receptive to hormone drugs, by the grace of God, I escaped all conventional treatments, which at that point I did not know to refuse.

I began reading books about natural and nutritional ways to prevent the recurrence of cancer. The diet I had been eating for many years for food allergies was in compliance with what I read in most ways. However, I did have some snacking habits that were less than ideal for keeping one's blood sugar stable. Therefore, I stopped eating fruits with a high glycemic index and snacked on easily-digested nuts most of the time. (See page 182 for the recipe for making nuts easy to digest).

When I read how cancer-promoting plastics are, I stopped drinking bottled water. I bought a water filter and glass food storage containers to keep from ingesting cancer-promoting chemicals from plastic ever again.

Our attention returned to the mold when the dust test results were high again. The cleaning we had done in the basement had not solved the problem. About three weeks after my surgery, a mold remediation man came to test our house. The air samples taken in the basement showed mold levels less than the amount usually found in outdoor air, but a random, just-to-compare sample taken in the living room was quite high.

When my husband heard that the main floor was the problem rather than the basement, he pointed out some dark stuff along the gasket in our dishwasher and told me to ask the remediation man about it on his second visit. I did, and the man said it was soap scum and to wipe it off. He did not do any testing on the dishwasher. He took a dust sample from the rug where he had set up his air sampling equipment before, which showed 38,000 viable *Alternaria* and *Aspergillus* spores per gram of dust. We got rid of the rugs immediately when we heard the results.

At this point in time, our son John was told that his company had lost its major government contract and that he was out of a job. In spite of a serious winter storm, he arrived home safely a week later, by the grace of God. I was very grateful for his presence and all of his cleaning help because I was not able to use the mastectomy-side arm normally yet. We did plenty of cleaning together during the seven months he spent finding a new job.

After the rugs were gone, more work awaited us. We did a major intensive whole house cleaning, followed by a dust test. The mold cout remained high. We then had our ducts cleaned, followed by another major intensive whole house cleaning and ventilation (since it was June by then). Shortly into the cleaning, after the living room had been cleaned, I noticed that my lungs became tight when I sat on the living room couch. The remediation man said to get it steam-cleaned, so we did, along with the chair that we had in the living room. Handling the family room drapes bothered me, so we took them to the cleaners. Because of their age and laminate backing material, they were washed with cold water and air dried. After this, I held them in my lap and hand sewed them with no problems.

We performed more dust tests. The basement and upstairs results finally were in the moderate range, but the main floor was still high at 34,000 viable spores per gram of dust. My doctor said to have the rest of our upholstered furniture cleaned, which fortunately was only the family room couch and dining room chair seats. Additionally, he said all the drapes should be cleaned. (They had all been run through the dryer several times already). The doctor also said to wash all the walls and seek out and clean every place I might have missed. This included the fire extinguisher in our kitchen, the inside of the piano, inside night lights, the smoke alarm, the back of a wall clock, etc. I'd already cleaned the back of everything else hanging on the walls and the unfinished back of our upright piano.

After this round of intensive cleaning and ventilation, I still was not breathing well, especially on the main floor of our house. I asked my husband to help me figure out what I had missed cleaning. After some thought, he suggested that I put Bioclean™ down the kitchen and dishwasher drains daily. (Bioclean™ is a bacteria-enzyme mixture that eats hair, grease, and other substances that clog drains). He had suspected a plumbing problem when he saw dark stuff in the dishwasher seven months earlier, and he was still suspicious about that area.

I started using the Bioclean™ on a Wednesday. At first it did not go down the dishwasher drain readily and had to be poured in six small portions. That weekend we left the house for about 48 hours. When we came home, the kitchen greeted us with a rotten egg odor. The dishwasher smelled the worst, but the odor was also coming from the sink.

I continued using the Bioclean™. Four days later, I could barely breathe in the kitchen, especially when the dishwasher was open. The next day I was able to pour the Bioclean™ treatment down the dishwasher drain all in one stream. I called the remediation man, and he said to get a product specifically for cleaning dishwashers. I got Glisten Dishwasher Magic™ Cleaner and Disinfectant, and the bad smell left. However, the "kitchen is killing me" feeling still remained. I continued using the dishwasher product at about eight times the recommended frequency. I also purchased the companion garbage disposal and drain cleaner and used it nearly daily.

As instructed by my doctor, I had sent in more mold tests three weeks after I finished the last round of cleaning. This waiting period included the week after the dishwasher drain was opened. When we received those test results, we learned that all three floors of the house showed mold spore counts ranging from 97,000 to 121,000 viable mold spores per gram of dust. Rather than getting the results by phone from the nurse, at my next office visit or in the mail as I had previously, my doctor called me on the phone with the results at about 6:30 pm the day he received the results.

The doctor asked, "What did you do? You really stirred up the pot!" After hearing what we had done, he said that we had finally found the *real problem* and to call the remediation man for advice about what to do to solve the problem with the dishwasher.

While I waited two days to talk to him, my son John did research on the Internet which recommended getting a plumber to snake our drains. My husband made an appointment for the plumber to snake the sink, dishwasher and sewer drains. When the plumbers arrived, they found they could not snake the dishwasher drain without breaking it. They snaked the kitchen sink and sewer drains and told my husband to get some ZEP™ drain cleaner and use it in the dishwasher drain.

My husband went to a family-owned hardware store for the ZEP™. The employee who told him how to use it also told him to clean the filter in the bottom well of the dishwasher that leads to the drain pipe. *What filter? What drain well? Why were we never told before that we should clean it?* When he opened the drain up, he found and removed 1½ cups of moldy-smelling black slime from the well of the drain. He also cleaned a large amount of black slime from a filter basket and a large-holed filter screen. We had finally rid our house of one source of growing mold, but it did not "cure" the kitchen completely. I did a three-week intensive housecleaning at this point and we lived with the windows open nearly full time in the, thankfully, unusually warm fall weather.

Since I was now seeking mold both in wet places and dusty places, I began cleaning the kitchen counter and the vanity tops in our bathrooms with the hydrogen peroxide solution on page 235. When I sprayed it around the kitchen sink faucet fixture, it instantly made a 1½ inch wide strip of very fine foam all the way around the faucet fixture. I cleaned and scrubbed it thoroughly and treated it with the hydrogen peroxide spray many times until the foaming stopped. Three days later, I sprayed around the fixture again, and the fine foam appeared again immediately. I asked for an early Christmas gift of a new kitchen faucet fixture.

When the plumber came and removed the old fixture, there was black crud underneath it. He quickly scraped the area to remove most of the crud and then went off to buy connectors to attach the new fixture to our old plumbing. While he was gone, I scrubbed the remaining black stuff off and treated the area with Clorox™. A second source of growing mold had been removed. This was again followed by intensive house cleaning and ventilation. After this, the kitchen no longer seemed as toxic to me, but when we closed up the house for the first snow, the whole house again seemed bad. The weather improved in about two weeks, so I could open windows to make cleaning more tolerable. I did major cleaning and ventilation, and began the three week countdown until we would do another dust test.

The first weekend in December, we harvested the last of the carrots and beets from our garden and I spent a lot of time at the kitchen sink. This included grinding skins from cooked beets down the garbage disposal. My breathing took a major turn for the worse that day, and continued to deteriorate. Two days later my husband discovered that our garbage disposal had a crack on the back side. He replaced it the next day during a major snow storm. We could not open the windows at the sub-zero temperature and being in the closed-up house after this third "mold bomb" went off was torture.

John's Hopkins had discontinued doing mold tests for which the client collected dust samples, and the local lab my allergy doctor was going to use did not allow people to collect their own samples. Therefore, I had made an appointment with a mold tester the lab recommended to collect samples at the three-week point after I finished cleaning. After the garbage disposal problem, I emailed the mold tester to cancel the appointment due to the house having become re-contaminated again by the garbage disposal aerosoling its moldy contents into the air. The tester recommended that we rent a HEPA air scrubber to eliminate the spores in the air, saying that it was more effective than opening windows. We were glad to hear there was an alternative to opening windows in the bitterly cold weather. We rented and ran an air scrubber and it seemed to help with the extreme rawness of my nose and airways, but its scent aggravated my asthma. The business that rented the air scrubber changed the filter between each rental. (This was a good idea because we didn't want to compound our problem by importing the previous customer's mold). Unfortunately, we suspected that the new filter was scented.

However, a seed had been planted in out minds. We now knew that filtration might be a way to treat the problem of winter living in a closed-up house with mold. In January we replaced our 34½ year old furnace with a Lennox™ furnace system that included a super-filter and indoor-outdoor air exchange unit. (See pages 268 to 269 for more about this system).

After the installation was complete, the severity of my asthma symptoms gradually decreased for about a month, but they never completely resolved. Then the kitchen started feeling much worse again. Exploration showed that dishwasher drain was again beginning to grow mold, in spite of my very aggressive use of the dishwasher disinfectant product.

I removed the dishwasher's filter basket and discovered it was covered with a white film that contained about a dozen tiny ($^1/_{16}$ inch or less) black spots. That minute amount of mold was enough to trigger major respiratory problems. I took all the removable parts from the bottom of the dishwasher, scrubbed them thoroughly, and soaked them in Clorox™ and water for a half hour before re-installing them.

In March, the mold tester recommended by the new lab came to collect air samples. He listened to the whole saga of the mold and asked me what dishwasher detergent we used. I said, "We used to use Seventh Generation™, but we switched to BioKleen™ a few months ago." He told me he had seen this kind of dishwasher problem with people who used Seventh Generation™ and they had successfully eradicated the problem. He said no matter what his test results were, we needed to begin using Cascade™ , not just any kind, the package had to say "Cascade™ with the power of Clorox™ and display the Clorox™ logo. That was what had worked for his clients with the same problem. I was concerned about being able to tolerate the scent that gives Cascade™ a bad reputation among allergic folks. He said that although an unscented stronger-for-cleaning detergent plus added Clorox™ would be a possible "plan B," I needed to give the Cascade™ a good try and open windows or do anything else to make it work. Because I could not find the recommended type of Cascade™ locally, that day I ordered some to be shipped to the nearest Target store.

My husband read online that Clorox™ was hard on the gaskets and plastic parts of dishwashers. I had already purchased CitriSolv™ dishwasher detergent for "plan B" that was not to be, so we used it for a few days. When checked in a couple of days, the filter basket in the bottom of the dishwasher was not oily as it always had been before.

We received the mold test results in a few days. All three floors of the house had reached the goal of being in the low range and the counts were much lower than the outdoor counts taken at the same time. However, we had a low number of *Aspergillus* spores remaining. The mold expert said that given the history of our mold problem, "treat no matter what" was the thing to do.

When the Cascade™ arrived, we began using it that evening. It was potently scented and made my lungs tighten up. I improved the situation somewhat by storing the "action-paks" in glass canning jars rather than the original non-sealing plastic container, which kept the cabinet beneath the sink from being as strongly perfumed and such a source of the scent. I left the kitchen, or preferably the house, while someone else unloaded the dishwasher. I only worked in the kitchen when I could have all the windows open. Rather than cleaning off and loading dishes into the dishwasher one at a time, I cleaned and saved dishes to put in the dishwasher all at once while holding my breath. The kitchen remained a hostile environment for me.

We used the Cascade™ for ten days. By that time, even my husband could not stand the scent. He said, "We have to find something that cuts grease well and contains bleach with less potent perfume." We found and switched to Safeway's Signature Home™ dishwasher gel that says "Contains chlorine bleach" on the back of the bottle. It was better, but still scented, and I had to be absent when the dishwasher was unloaded. I was grateful when the weather warmed up in mid-May which made having the windows open many hours per day possible.

In late June, the competent mold expert thought we could cease using chlorine bleach and perfume-containing dishwasher detergent. We switched to CitraSolv™ which is very good at cutting grease and food residue. The mold expert said, "See what happens and let me know," because his previous clients with dishwasher mold problems had switched to and then continued using Cascade™ permanently.

I have disassembled the bottom of the dishwasher and cleaned the filters every two weeks or more frequently since then and have found no sign of mold. The CitraSolv™ has kept our dishes and glassware sparkling clean and clear as new, so we are assuming that the dishwasher drain pipe is equally clean and contains no food residue to support mold growth.

Although still continually tight and congested, I have not had much major asthma except when our air was full of wildfire smoke. I am functional, able to work hard and am finishing this book. However, I have yet to reach "normal" because I seem to have lost most of the desensitization to inhaled substances provided by years of EPD and LDA.

Two weeks ago I took LDA. The final results of a treatment cannot be judged before three weeks because that is how long the lymphocytes take to mature. I also have not done things to test the shot such as liberalizing my diet or breathing in highly perfumed parts of the "real world." However, I'm noticing some signs that are very encouraging such as two incidents of about an hour of breathing freely and relaxed, more normally than in 3½ years. It was wonderful! I'm optimistic about getting to near-normal after this treatment takes full effect. However, the deadline to submit this book has come, so the final shot results will have to wait for an update of this book.

Take hope from this story and persevere.

Index

Recipes appear in *italics*. Informational sections appear in standard type.

A

Acidophilus Milk 122
Air filtration 234-235
 Recommended equipment 268-269
Allergy baking 84
Allergy shots
 Conventional 48
 LDA and EPD 48-49
Almond flour 90
Almond Pie Crust^{GF} 199 [1]
Alpaca Bone Broth 138
Antelope Bone Broth 139
Anti-cancer diet 25-27
Anti-candida diet 35
Anti-inflammatory foods 227-229
Apple Pie^{GFO} 205 [2]
Arnica, homeopathic 53-54
Asthma 13, 15-16, 20, 46-48
Asthma inhalers
 HFA propellant problem 46, 272
 Skyrocketing prices 46-47, 272
Autism
 Diet for 37-38

B

Baked Apples or Pears 106
Baked Potatoes or Squash, Oven 104
Basil Roughy 102
Bean soup recipes 178-180
Beans, Oven 103
Beef Bone Broth 137

Black Bean Soup 178
Blood sugar
 Dietary control of 25-26
Blueberry Pie^{GFO} 206
Bone broth 66-67, 128
 Chicken soup for colds study 128
 Health benefits of 67, 128
 Natural glutamate allergy 67, 128
Bone broth recipes 127-139
 Alpaca Bone Broth 138
 Antelope Bone Broth 139
 Beef Bone Broth 137
 Buffalo (Bison) Bone Broth 136
 Chicken Bone Broth 131
 Elk Bone Broth 134
 Duck Bone Broth 131
 Guinea Hen Bone Broth 130
 Turkey Bone Broth 128
 Venison Bone Broth 135
Bone "building" drugs 50-51
 Increase risk of fractures 50
 Incidence of esophageal cancer 50
 Incidence of osteosarcoma 50
 Side effect - osteonecrosis of jaw 50
Bread, glycemic index values of 215-216
 Lower GI score if sourdough bread 215
 or if made with stone ground flour, seeds, etc. 215
 Recommendations for type of bread 215
Bread Machine 100% Stoneground Whole Wheat Bread 158
Bread machine information 242-245

NOTES on ^{GF} and ^{GFO}

1 Gluten-free recipes are marked ^{GF}. This marking is used only with grain-containing or baked good recipes. All other types of recipes in this book are gluten-free: Unlike in restaurants or "normal" cookbooks, there is no flour added to thicken soup, etc.
2 Recipes which contain multiple ingredient list options, both gluten-free and gluten containing, are marked^{GFO} for "gluten-free options." The cook can choose a gluten-free ingredient list if needed. This marking is used only with grain-containing or baked good recipes.

Bread making instructions for
    Sourdough bread 160-163
    Yeast bread 153-154
Breathing 70-74
    Buteyko breathing, also see below 71-73
    Diaphragmatic best 70
    Meditative breathing for cancer 73-74
*Brownies, Nourishing Nut*GF 193
*Buckwheat "Rye" Bread*GF 157
*Buckwheat Sourdough Bread*GF 170
Buffalo (Bison) Bone Broth 136
Buteyko breathing 71-73, 246-248, 274
    Benefits of adequate CO_2 level in blood,
        lungs 71-72
    Natural treatment for asthma 71-73

C

Cabbage, Oven 104
Cancer and cell phones 230
Cancer prevention and recurrence prevention 10
    Avoidance of plastics 27
    Blood sugar level control 25-26
    Diet for 25-27
    Fruits and vegetables 26
    Recurrence lessened by taking charge 40-41
Cancer promoted by
    Bisphenol-A (BPA) 15
    Dairy products from cows treated with rBGH 13
    Feelings of helplessness 40-41
    High glycemic index foods 12
    Inorganic phosphates added to processed food 13
    Insulin-like growth factor (IGF) 26
Cancer rates
    Reduced by exercise 16
    Rising since 1940s 11
Cancer treatment, conventional 40-46
    Chemotherapy 43-45, also see below
    Little progress in 30 years 43
    Hormone drugs for breast cancer 45-46
Cancer treatment, nutritional
    May mitigate side effects of chemotherapy 44, 45
Candidiasis 30-31
    Diet for 35-36
    Caused by chemotherapy, some radiotherapy 45
    Connection to thyroid problems 36
*Carrot Cake*GF 196
Carrots, Oven 103

Cashews, not raw nuts 66
Celiac disease 33-35
    Gluten-free diet for 33-35
    Possible cause of 34-35
    Specific Carbohydrate Diet for 37
Celtic sea salt 67-69
    Do not use for cultured vegetables 69
Chemicals
    Carcinogenic 13, 15-16
    In personal care products and clothing 21
Chemotherapy 43-46
    Can cause food allergies, candidiasis 45
    Choose oncologist carefully 44
    Data manipulation 43-44
    Effective for some blood cancers 44
    Increases the risk of metastasis 44-45
    Rarely effective for solid tumor cancers 44
    Should be avoided without proof of spread 44-45
    Side effects 45
*Cherry Pie*GFO 206
Cherry soda 186
Chia seeds, good source of omega-3 fats 181
Chicken Bone Broth 131
*Chicken, Oven*GFO 99
Chicken Fricassee 98
Chocolate Cream Cheese Frosting 194
*Chocolate Layer Cake*GF, *Stevia-sweetened 194*
Cholesterol 55
    Decreased by Mediterranean diet 57
    Does not cause heart disease 55
    Essential for life in sufficient amounts 55
Circadian Rhythm Diet 30-31
Cleaning, non-toxic 20-21
*Coconut Pie Crust*GF 199
Combination diets 38-39
Cooking difficulties for cancer patients
    Ways to ease the burden 27, 81-83
    Prepared foods, sources 251-257
Corned Beef Dinner 96
Cranberry Soda 186
Cranberry Tea 192
Crispy Oven Sweet or White Potatoes 105
Crockpot Baked Beans 177
Crockpot Cooked Legumes 176
Crockpot recipes
    Meals and main dishes 95-98
    Bean Soups 178-180
Crockpot Roast Dinner 95

Crockpot Stew 97
Crohn's disease, diet for 36-37
Cultured dairy products 62-64, 120-122
  Cultures for 64, 261-262
  Factors for success in making 62
  Cleanliness in preparation 122
  Health benefits 120-121
  Homemade incubator for 62-63
  Milk used 63-64, 121
  Use of raw milk 122
Cultured Asparagus 118
Cultured Beans 115
Cultured Beets 111
Cultured Broccoli or Cauliflower 116
Cultured Carrots 110
Cultured dairy product recipes 122-125
Cultured Dill Pickles 112
Cultured Summer Squash 117
Cultured vegetable recipes 111-119
Cultured vegetables 60-61
  Airlocks for 108-109
  Best ingredients 61
  Cleanliness in preparation 61, 108
  Health benefits of 61, 108
  How to add to diet 108
  Glass weights for 109
  Use refined sea salt for 109
Cultures
  For cultured vegetables 60-61, 85
  For dairy products 85
  For sourdough bread 87-86
  Sources of 261-262

D

DEET mosquito repellent 21, 42-43
Dessert recipes 106-107, 193-207
Diabetes 11
  Diet for 27-30
  Statins increase risk of vascular disease 56
Dill Pickles 112
Dr. Baker's Rhythmic Shake 190
Duck Bone Broth 131

E

Easy dinners 94-107
Easy Fruit Crumble, No-Grain GF *198*

Einkorn 34, 263
Elk Bone Broth 134
Energy
  Improved by diet 30-31
  Correct thyroid treatment for 54-55
Enzyme inhibitors 64-66
Enzyme Potentiated Desensitization (EPD) 48-50
Exercise, moderate 22-23
  Beginning an exercise program 23
  For asthma 22
  For weight loss 22, 29
  Helps prevent cancer recurrence 23-23

F

Fat from animals
  Omega-3 to omega-6 fat ratio 12-13
  Healthy omega-3 to omega-6 fat ratio improves
    food taste 52
Fats, healthy choices 26
Fish in Papillote 100
Flour and Oil Pie Crust GFO *200*
Flour, types of 87-90
  Almond 90
  Gluten containing 88-89
  Non-gluten containing 89-90
  Non-grain flours 90
Food allergies
  And cancer 27
  Connection to overweight 224
  Desensitization 48-50
  Dietary control of 31-33
  Increased by chemotherapy, radiotherapy 45
  Increased by proton pump inhibitor drugs 51
Food allergy diets 31-33
  Elimination diet 31-32
  Rotation diet 32-33
Food labels, how to read 236-241
Food production, profit motives 12-14
Foods with anti-cancer activity 26-27
Fragrances, chemical
  Problems caused by 30
  How to eliminate 20
Fresh Fruit Tapioca 107
Frosting recipes 194-195
Fruit, anti-cancer properties 26-27
Fruit Sodas 186

G

Game meat 93
GAPS (Gut and Psychology Syndrome) diet 37-38
  Autistic children recover on 37
  For intestinal healing 37
GERD (gastro-esophageal reflux disorder) 52
  Natural treatment for 52
Ginger Ale 187
Ginger Concentrate 191
Ginger Tea by the Cup 191
Ginger Tea, Quick 192
Gluten-free diet 33-35
Glycemic control diet
  Principles of 28-29
  Steps to implement 29-30
Glycemic index (GI) values
  Definition 208
  How measured 208-209
  Using for weight loss 208-210
Glycemic Index Values for Foods, Table of 211-223
GMO foods, list of 32
GMOs (genetically modified organisms) 12, 13-14
  Food allergies due to 14, 31-32
Grains 64-65
  Enzyme inhibitors and phytic acid 65-141
  Nutrients provided by 141
  Sprouted grain flour 65
Grains, cooked 142-149
  Stovetop Cooked Grains^{GFO} *142-145*
  Oven Grains^{GFO} *146-149*
Guar gum 93
Guinea Hen Bone Broth 130

H

Health deterioration 11-14
  Causes 11-14
  Profit motives in food production 12-14
Health Dressing 126
Heartburn 52
  Drugs for and side effects 51
  Natural treatment 52
Heart disease
  Diet for 27-30
Helplessness 40-42
  Cancer outcomes 40-42
Herbed Yogurt Dressing 126

Hidden sources of gluten and food allergens 237-241
Home environment
  Cleaning 20-21
  Removing chemicals from 20
Home health care 82-83
Hormone drugs for reproductive cancers 45
Hunger
  Avoid for weight loss 28-29
  Indicates low blood sugar or high insulin 28
  Weight loss without hunger 27-30, 208-209
Hydrogenated fats
  Cancer patients must avoid 26
Hydrogen peroxide solution for mold 235

I

Ingredients, less common 84-93
Inflammation 224-225
  Relationship to overweight 224
  How to treat naturally 225
Inflammatory bowel disease (IBD)
  Specific Carbohydrate Diet for 36-37
Insulin level
  Cancer stimulation 26
  Determines whether fat burned or stored 28-29
  Relationship to weight 27-30
Intestinal bacteria, diets to control 36-38
Intestinal dysbiosis 41-42
Irritable Bowel Syndrome (IBS)
  Low FODMAP diet for 38
  Specific Carbohydrate Diet for 36-37

L

Leavening ingredients 91-93
  Acidic 91-92
  Baking powder 91
  Baking soda 91
Legumes 66, 174
  Enzyme inhibitors and phytic acid, how to
    neutralize 66
  "Gas" helped by preparation 174
  Nutrients provided by 174
Lemonade 185
Lemon Chiffon Pie^{GFO} *204*
Lemon Chiffon Pudding^{GFO} *205*
Lentil Soup 179
Leptin 224

Light Rye Sourdough Bread 169
Lima Bean Soup 178
Lipid hypothesis of heart disease 55-56
Low Dose Immunotherapy (LDA) 48-50

M

Meat, healthy choices 26
Medical decisions
  Know options and decide for self 9, 40, 42
  Personal circumstances and 44
Medical tests
  Take results with grain of salt 42
  May be misleading 50, 55
Mold remediation 232-235
  Air filtration 234-235, 268-269
  Cleanup 233-235
  Diagnosis of problem 232
  Precautions for cleaning 233
  Testing for mold 232-233
Mosquito repellents 42-43
  Vitamin B1 a non-toxic repellent 43
Multi-Bean Soup 179
Muffins, Nourishing GFO *149-151*

N

Natural killer (NK) cells 17, 23, 41
  And feelings of helplessness 41
Navy Bean Soup 178
No-Grain Easy Fruit Crumble GF 198
Nourishing Muffins GFO *149-151*
Nourishing Nut Brownies GF *193*
Nourishing Nut Pesto 183
Nourishing Nuts 182
Nourishing Seeds 182
Nut and seed recipes 182-184
Nut Milk 187
Nut or Seed Milk Smoothie 189
Nutrients in food
  Contribute to satisfaction 59
  Make food taste good 59
Nuts 66, 181
  Health benefits of
  How to neutralize enzyme inhibitors 66, 181
  Nutrients provided by 181
Nuts, Nourishing 182

O

Oil and Vinegar Salad Dressing 127
Osteopenia 50-51
Osteoporosis 50-51
Oven Baked 100% Stoneground Whole Wheat
  Bread 159
Oven Baked Potatoes or Squash 104
Oven Chicken GFO *99*
Oven Cabbage 104
Oven Carrots 103
Oven dessert recipes 106-107
Oven Grains GFO *146-149*
Oven main dish recipes 98-100
Oven Onions 104
Oven Peas or Beans 103
Oven Squash, Special 105
Oven Stew 98-99
Oven Sweet Potatoes or White Potatoes, Crispy 105

P

Pain medications
  Can cause liver damage 53
  Can increase intestinal permeability 53
  Can worsen food allergies 53
Pain, natural remedies for 53-54
Peanut anaphylaxis 21, 31
Peas, Oven 103
Pesto, Nourishing Nut 183
Pepper Steak 102
Personal care products and clothing 21
PET scan based on sugar uptake 12
Phytic acid problems 64-66
  Mitigated by raw milk 121-122
  Mitigated by good nutrition 141
Pie crust recipes GFO *199-202*
Poultry, Roasted 132
Poultry Stuffing, Quinoa GF *141*
Profit motives with
  Asthma inhalers 46-47, 272
  Bone "building" drugs that increase fractures 10
  Buteyko breathing ignorance 48
  Epi-Pen™ 46
  Food production 11-14
  Medical system 40-42
  Statins, no decrease in mortality 55-57
  Thyroid treatment 54-55

Proton pump inhibitor (PPI) drugs 51-52
   Dementia, kidney disease, fractures side effects 51
   Natural treatment 52
Pumpkin Pie^{GFO} 203
Pumpkin Pudding 203

Q

Quick and Easy Fruit Tapioca 106
Quinoa, rinse before cooking 141
Quinoa Pilaf or Poultry Stuffing^{GF} 141
Quinoa Raisin Bread^{GF} 154
Quinoa Sourdough Bread^{GF} 172

R

Radiotherapy 45
   Side effects 45
Recombinant bovine growth hormone
   (rBGH) 13, 237
Rhubarb Concentrate 190
Rhubarb Tea 190
Rice allergy 35
Rice Sourdough Bread^{GF} 171
Roast Beef, Bison, Lamb or Pork 101
Rotation diet for food allergies 32-33
   Required by cancer patients with multiple food
      allergies 27
RoundUp™ (glyphosate) 14
   Pre-harvest use on wheat leaves high residue 88

S

Salad dressing recipes 125-127
Salt
   Essential for nut preparation 181
   Whole salt good for health 67-69
"San Francisco" Sourdough Bread 164
Sauerbraten^{GFO} 96
Sauerkraut 113
Sea salt, whole unrefined 67-79
Seeds 66, 181
   Health benefits of 181
   How to neutralize enzyme inhibitors 66
   Nutrients provided by 181
Seed Milk 188
Seeds, Nourishing 182
Smoothie recipes 124, 189-190
Smoothie, Yogurt or Acidophilus Milk 124

Smoothie, Nut or Seed 189
Soda recipes 185-187
Sodas 12, 185
   Contain inorganic phosphates 13, 185
   Propaganda for 12
Sodium 68
   Amount in diet 68
   Balance with other minerals 68
   Ratio to potassium important 68
Soups, Legume 178-180
Sourdough bread instructions 160-163
Sourdough bread recipes 164-172
Sourdough Pancakes^{GFO} 151
Specific Carbohydrate Diet (SCD) 36-37
Spelt Bread 155
Spelt Bread, White 167
Spelt Bread, Whole 166
Split Pea Soup 179
Squash, oven recipes 104-105
Stevia 90-91
   Cooking properties 91
   Enzyme treated has neutral taste 91
   Import alert in the 1990s 49-50
   Improved glycemic index of foods prepared
      with 209
   Worldwide safe use for centuries 90
Stovetop Cooked Legumes 175
Stovetop Grains^{GFO} 142-145
Sugar consumption
   Rise in last century 12
   Propaganda from soda producers 12
   Stimulates cancer 12
Sweet Yogurt Dressing 126
Sweeteners 90-91
   List of allowed for cancer patients 25
   Nutritive, low GI 90
   Stevia 90-91

T

Tea recipes 190-192
Thyroid treatment 54-55
   Correct treatment 55
   Often mismanaged 54
Traditional diets 18
Trans (partially hydrogenated) fats 13
   Asthma resulting from 13
Transition to healthy diet and cooking 19-20
Turkey Bone Broth 128

U

Ulcerative colitis, diet for 36-37

V

Vanilla Cream Cheese Frosting 195
Vegetables, anti-cancer properties 26-27
Venison Bone Broth 135
Vitamin D 17
   Allergies, cancer, heart disease, etc. 17
   Osteoporosis 50-51
   Supplementation 17
Volkorn 100% Rye Bread 168

W

Water, bottled
   Carcinogenic chemicals from plastic 27
Water, distilled
   Do not use in yeast bread 92
   Leaches minerals if consumed routinely 92
Weight loss
   Balance protein and carbohydrate 29, 209
   Diet for 27-29
   No hunger 27-28
   No need for willpower 28
Whipped Cream 197
White Bean and Escarole Soup 178
Wheat flour 89
   High pesticide residue from pre-harvest spraying 89
Whole Wheat Bread 158-160
Whole Wheat Sourdough Bread 158-160

X

Xanthan gum 93

Y

Yeast bread
   Bread machine use for allergy and gluten-free
     bread 242-254
Yeast bread instructions 153-154
Yogurt 123
Yogurt or Acidophilus Milk Smoothie 124
Yogurt "Sour Cream" or Yo-Cheese 125

Helpful Books

In ***Healing Basics*** you will discover how to ***Prevent Cancer or its Recurrence, Achieve Ideal Weight without Hunger,*** and ***Build the Foundation of True Health.*** This book explores why Americans' health has deteriorated drastically and takes us back to basics of diet and lifestyle to prevent further decline and improve current problems. It also presents well documented information to help you decide on medical treatment wisely and explore natural strategies to use along with conventional treatment or alone. It contains 157 recipes, 95% of which can be eaten by those who must avoid gluten or food allergens, but which will be enjoyed by everyone. Also included is information on how to deal with food preparation when strength and time are in short supply and an extensive 24-page "Sources" section which will help you find prepared foods that fit your diet and also includes sources of special foods, products, services and information.

ISBN 978-1-887624-22-0. . . . . $29.95

Food Allergy and Gluten-Free Weight Loss gives definitive answers to the question, "Why is it so hard to lose weight?" It is because we have missed or ignored the most important pieces in the puzzle of how our bodies determine whether to store or burn fat. Those puzzle pieces are hormones such as insulin, cortisol, leptin, and others. Individuals with food allergies or gluten intolerance face additional weight-loss challenges such as inflammation due to allergies or a diet too high in rice. This book explains how to put your body chemistry to work for you rather than against you, reduce inflammation which inhibits the action of your master weight control hormone, leptin, and flip your fat switch from "store" to "burn." It includes 175 recipes and a flexible healthy eating plan that eliminates hunger, promotes the burning of fat, and reduces inflammation.

ISBN 978-1-887624-19-0. . . . . $29.95

The Ultimate Food Allergy Cookbook and Survival Guide: How to Cook with Ease for Food Allergies and Recover Good Health gives you everything you need to survive and recover from food allergies. It contains medical information about the diagnosis of food allergies, health problems that can be caused by food allergies, and your options for treatment. The book includes a rotation diet that is free from common food allergens such as wheat, milk, eggs, corn, soy, yeast, beef, legumes, citrus fruits, potatoes, tomatoes, and more. Instructions are given on how to personalize the standard rotation diet to meet your individual needs and fit your food preferences. It contains 500 recipes that can be used with (or independently of) the diet. Extensive reference sections include a listing of commercially prepared foods for allergy diets and sources for special foods, services, and products.

ISBN 978-1-887624-08-4. . . . . $29.95

Gluten-Free Without Rice introduces you to gluten-free grains and grain alternatives other than rice such as teff, millet, sorghum, amaranth, quinoa, buckwheat, tapioca, arrowroot, potato starch, and more. It gives you over 75 delicious recipes for muffins, crackers, bread, pancakes, waffles, granola, main and side dishes, cookies, and desserts. (Even ice cream cones!) With this book you can cook easily for a gluten-free diet without relying on rice. Whether you have celiac disease or food allergies, this book will make it easier and more enjoyable to stay on your diet and improve your health.

ISBN 978-1-887624-15-2. . . . . $13.95

Allergy Cooking With Ease, Revised Edition. This classic all-purpose allergy cookbook includes all the old favorite recipes of the first edition plus many new recipes and new foods. It contains over 300 recipes for baked goods, main and side dishes (including comfort foods), soups, vegetables, salads, ethnic dishes, and desserts including lots of cookies. There are "kid" recipes ranging from teething biscuits to no-grain cookies that could pass for Oreos™. Although there are several grain or grain alternatives given among the recipes for each type of baked food (muffins, crackers, etc.), this book has more "fun" recipes and does not cater to the rotation diet to the degree that *The Ultimate Food Allergy Cookbook and Survival Guide* does. If you are want to make your allergy diet a little more light-hearted, this is the book for you! It also contains an extensive sources section.

ISBN 978-1-887624-10-7. . . . . $24.95

Easy Breadmaking for Special Diets contains over 200 recipes for allergy, heart healthy, low fat, low sodium, yeast-free, controlled carbohydrate, diabetic, celiac, and low calorie diets. It includes recipes for breads of all kinds, tortillas, bread and tortilla based main dishes, and desserts. Use your bread machine, food processor, mixer, or electric tortilla maker to make the bread YOU need quickly and easily.

Third Edition – ISBN 978-1-887624-20-6. . . . . $24.95

Original Edition Bargain Book – ISBN 1-887624-02-3. . . . . $9.95

> With the bargain book we will include an insert of pages from the third edition about current bread machines, preparation of sourdough, and sourdough bread recipes.

Allergy and Celiac Diets With Ease: Money and Time Saving Solutions for Food Allergy and Gluten-Free Diets provides solutions to both the economic and time challenges you face. It shows how to shop economically, cook without spending all day in the kitchen, stock your kitchen for efficiency and good health, make the best use of your appliances, have good times with friends and family without breaking the bank, get organized, and be able to do this in limited time. This book contains over 160 money-saving, quick and easy recipes for allergy and celiac diets that those on "normal" diets will also enjoy. Over 140 of them are gluten-free. It includes extensive reference sections including "Sources" and "Special Diet Resources" sections to help you find the foods you need.

ISBN 978-1-887624-17-6. . . . .
$24.95

Do you need more fun in your life? *I Love Dessert but NOT Sugar, Wheat, Milk, Gluten, Corn, Soy, Unhealthy Fat...* can help you rediscover the enjoyment of simple pleasures. If you are on a restricted diet due to food allergies or gluten intolerance, you don't have to miss out on your favorite desserts any more. The book contains more than 300 easily-made recipes for almost any dessert you might want, all free of sugar, wheat, corn, soy, and unhealthy fats. Many of them are gluten-free. A very few of the desserts contain dairy products or eggs, but there are egg and milk-free alternatives for the same desserts. Many recipes are made with healthy new sweeteners such as agave and next-generation stevia (which is without the aftertaste that many dislike). When friends or family are having a treat, now those on special diets can join in.

ISBN 978-1-887624-18-3 . . . . $22.95

The Low Dose Immunotherapy Handbook: Recipes and Lifestyle Tips for Patients on LDA and EPD Treatment gives 80 recipes for patients on low dose immunotherapy treatment for their food allergies. It also includes organizational information to help you get ready for your shots.

ISBN: 978-1-887624-07-7. . . . . $12.95

BONUS ITEMS

Receive one bonus item **FREE with the purchase of two books** on these pages.

Healing Basics e-book with live links so all internet resources can be clicked on to take you to an information source or the seller of a product in the "Sources" section.

$11.99 or **FREE** with the order of **two** books on these pages

How to Cope With Food Allergies When You're Short on Time is a booklet of time saving tips and recipes to help you stick to your allergy or gluten-free diet with the least amount of time and effort. **Chose a paper copy** which will be shipped with your paper book(s) **or an e-book** which will be emailed to you as soon as your order is received.

$4.95 or **FREE** with the order of **two** other books on these pages

E-books

For information about e-books of all of the books on these pages, see <u>www.healing-basics.life</u> .

There is no shipping charge for e-books.

Order these books online by going to

<u>www.healingbasics.life</u>

or <u>www.food-allergy.org</u> ,

by mail using the order form on the next page

or from your favorite online bookseller.

Mail orders - Use the order form on the next page.

Shipping for mail-in orders:

Orders up to $9.99 – Add $4.00
Orders up to $34.99 – Add $6.00
FREE SHIPPING on any order over $35

Mail your order form and check to:
Allergy Adapt, Inc.
1877 Polk Avenue
Louisville, CO 80027

Questions about these books? or about international or **expedited shipping**? Call **303-666-8253** or email **foodalle@food-allergy.org**.

Thank you for your order!

Order Form

Send books to:

Name: _____

Street address: _____

City, State, ZIP code: _____

Email or phone number (for questions about order): _____

Item	Quantity	Price	Total
Healing Basics		$29.95	
Food Allergy and Gluten-Free Weight Loss		$29.95	
The Ultimate Food Allergy Cookbook and Survival Guide		$29.95	
Gluten-Free Without Rice		$13.95	
Allergy Cooking With Ease		$24.95	
Easy Breadmaking for Special Diets – Original Edition Bargain Book Third Edition		$9.95 $24.95	
Allergy and Celiac Diets with Ease		$24.95	
List other book(s) from previous pages here:			
Circle the bonus item of your choice: *Healing Basics e-book with live links* *How to Cope with Food Allergies e-book* *How to Cope with Food Allergies paper book*		**1 FREE with 2 book purchase**	
Order any **TWO** books and get *How to Cope* or the ***Healing Basics e-Book* FREE!**	Subtotal		
	Shipping – See chart on the previous page		
	Colorado residents add 4.1% sales tax		
	Total		

An extra order form is on the next page.

Order Form

Send books to:

Name: _____

Street address: _____

City, State, ZIP code: _____

Email or phone number (for questions about order): _____

Item	Quantity	Price	Total
Healing Basics		$29.95	
Food Allergy and Gluten-Free Weight Loss		$29.95	
The Ultimate Food Allergy Cookbook and Survival Guide		$29.95	
Gluten-Free Without Rice		$13.95	
Allergy Cooking With Ease		$24.95	
Easy Breadmaking for Special Diets – Original Edition Bargain Book Third Edition		$9.95 $24.95	
Allergy and Celiac Diets with Ease		$24.95	
List other book(s) from previous pages here:			
Circle the bonus item of your choice: *Healing Basics e-book with live links* *How to Cope with Food Allergies e-book* *How to Cope with Food Allergies paper book*		**1 FREE with 2 book purchase**	
Order any **TWO** books and get ***How to Cope*** or the ***Healing Basics e-Book* FREE!**	Subtotal		
	Shipping – See chart on page 295		
	Colorado residents add 4.1% sales tax		
	Total		

www.ingramcontent.com/pod-product-compliance
Lightning Source LLC
Chambersburg PA
CBHW082351270326
41935CB00013B/1587